Shame and Modern Wr

Shame and Modern Writing seeks to uncover the presence of shame in and across an array of modern writing modalities. This interdisciplinary volume includes essays from distinguished and emergent scholars in the Humanities and Social Sciences, and shorter practice-based reflections from poets and clinical writers. It serves as a timely reflection of shame as presented in modern writing, giving added attention to engagements on race, gender, and the question of new media representation.

Barry Sheils is Assistant Professor in twentieth and twenty-first century literature at Durham University, where he is also an associate director of the Centre for Cultural Ecologies. He is the author of *W.B. Yeats and World Literature: The Subject of Poetry* (Routledge), and co-editor of *Narcissism, Melancholia and the Subject of Community* (Palgrave).

Julie Walsh is Lecturer in Psychosocial and Psychoanalytic Studies at the University of Essex, and a psychoanalyst in private practice. She is the author of *Narcissism and Its Discontents* (Palgrave), and co-editor of *Narcissism, Melancholia and the Subject of Community* (Palgrave). She is also a member of The Site for Contemporary Psychoanalysis.

Routledge Interdisciplinary Perspectives on Literature

For a full list of titles in this series, please visit www.routledge.com.

Shame and Modern Writing

Edited by
Barry Sheils and Julie Walsh

Routledge
Taylor & Francis Group
New York London

First published 2018 by Routledge
52 Vanderbilt Avenue, New York, NY 10017
2 Park Square, Milton Park, Abingdon, Oxon OX14 4RN

First issued in paperback 2020

Routledge is an imprint of the Taylor & Francis Group, an informa business

© 2018 Taylor & Francis

Library of Congress Cataloging-in-Publication Data
CIP data has been applied for.

ISBN 13: 978-0-367-66701-6 (pbk)
ISBN 13: 978-1-138-06727-1 (hbk)

Typeset in Sabon
by codeMantra

Contents

Acknowledgments

Chapter 2, "Montaigne's Writing: 'Honteux Insolent'?" by Elizabeth Guild was first published in *Montaigne Studies*, XXVII, 1–2 (2015), 99–112, and is republished with the kind permission of the editor. Chapter 12, 'On Writing-Up: Shame and Clinical Writing' by Julie Walsh with Oliver Sacks was first published in *Exchanges: the Warwick Research Journal*, 1 (2013), and is republished with permission of the author.

A symposium on 'Shame and the Act of Writing' in 2014 funded by the Institute of Advanced Study and the Humanities Research Centre at Warwick University gave this work its initial impetus; we are grateful to all those who participated. We would also like to thank Marc Botha, Geoff Gilbert, and Arthur Rose for their contributions, witting or not, to the evolution of this volume, and Rick de Villiers at Durham University whose sharp and timely editorial work was truly helpful.

Notes on Contributors

J. Brooks Bouson is Professor of English at Loyola University Chicago in the United States. In her scholarship and teaching, she has focused on twentieth and twenty-first century women's literature and she has a long-standing interest in the empathic dynamics of the reader/text transaction, which grows out of her application of Heinz Kohut's psychoanalytic theory to the study of literature in her book *The Empathic Reader: A Study of the Narcissistic Character and the Drama of the Self*. More recently, she has turned to the study of emotions in literature, shame in literature, and trauma and narrative. In addition to her book *The Empathic Reader*, she has published scholarly books on contemporary women writers, including *Brutal Choreographies: Oppositional Strategies and Narrative Design in the Novels of Margaret Atwood*; *Quiet As It's Kept: Shame, Trauma, and Race in the Novels of Toni Morrison*; *Jamaica Kincaid: Writing Memory, Writing Back to the Mother*; *Embodied Shame: Uncovering Female Shame in Contemporary Women's Writings*; and *Shame and the Aging Woman: Confronting and Resisting Ageism in Contemporary Women's Writings*. She also is the editor of four recent critical collections: *Critical Insights: Margaret Atwood*; *Margaret Atwood: The Robber Bride, The Blind Assassin, and Oryx and Crake*; *Critical Insights: Emily Dickinson*; and *Critical Insights: Margaret Atwood's The Handmaid's Tale*.

James Brown is Associate Research Fellow in the Politics Department at Birkbeck College, University of London, having previously been a lecturer at Middlesex University. He is the convenor of the Guilt working group in the Birkbeck Centre for Social Research. He publishes at the intersection of cultural theory and political philosophy on topics such as liberal democracy, violence and romantic feeling.

Thomas Docherty is Professor of English and Comparative Literary Studies at Warwick University. He specializes in the philosophy of literary criticism, in critical theory, and in cultural history in relation primarily to European philosophy and literatures. Recent work has been done on matters of cultural policy related to international higher education. He has published over ten books, including: *Confessions: The Philosophy* *of Transparency* (Bloomsbury, 2012); *For the University* (Bloomsbury, 2011); *Aesthetic Democracy* (Stanford UP, 2006); *Criticism and Modernity* (Oxford UP, 1999); *After Theory* (Routledge, 1990); and *Postmodernism* (Harvester/Columbia UP, 1993).

Martin Paul Eve is Professor of Literature, Technology and Publishing at Birkbeck, University of London. He is the author of four books: *Pynchon and Philosophy: Wittgenstein, Foucault and Adorno* (Palgrave, 2014), *Open Access and the Humanities: Contexts, Controversies and the Future* (Cambridge University Press, 2014), *Password [a cultural history]* (Bloomsbury, 2016), and *Literature Against Criticism: University English and Contemporary Fiction in Conflict* (Open Book Publishers, 2016), as well as many journal articles. In addition, Martin is the director of the Birkbeck Centre for Technology and Publishing, is a founder and director of the Andrew W. Mellon Foundation-funded Open Library of Humanities platform, was a member of the HEFCE Expert Reference Panel for open-access monographs, and is a member of the Jisc National Scholarly Communications Advisory Group.

Zlatan Filipovic is Research Fellow in English Literatures at the University of Gothenburg and a Senior Lecture at the University of Jönköping, Sweden. He has a PhD in English & Comparative Literature from Goldsmiths, University of London, focusing on Paul de Man and the ethics of writing, currently revised for publication. His published work has focused primarily on the ethical implications of poststructuralism in theory and modern literature. He is currently also working on a monograph considering the ethics of shame in Levinas's writing and the way it informs our understanding of diasporic identities in modern fiction.

Sheldon George is Associate Professor of English at Simmons College in Boston, Massachusetts. He directs the English Graduate Program and teaches courses on American and African American literature, along with courses on cultural and literary theory. His scholarship focuses primarily upon African American literature and culture, and on Lacanian psychoanalytic theory. His most recent publications include a Lacanian reading of Toni Morrison's *Beloved* that appeared in *African American Review* and a co-edited special issue of the journal *Psychoanalysis, Culture and Society* on "African Americans and Inequality." His new book *Trauma and Race: A Lacanian Study of African American Racial Identity* was published by Baylor University Press.

John Goodby is Professor of English Literature at Swansea University and a specialist in modern poetry. He is the author of *Irish poetry since 1950: from stillness into history* (2000) and, as an international authority on Dylan Thomas, author of *The Poetry of Dylan Thomas:*

Under the Spelling Wall (2013) and *Discovering Dylan Thomas: A Companion to the Collected Poems and Notebook Poems* (2017). His annotated edition of Thomas's *Collected Poems* appeared in 2014. He has also published translations of Heine, Soleïman Adel Guèmar (with Tom Cheesman), Reverdy and Pasolini, and his own recent poetry includes *The No Breath* (Red Ceilings, 2017). Between 2009 and 2012 he was co-organizer of the Hay Poetry Jamboree with Lyndon Davies, and in 2011 he founded the Boiled String series of poetry chapbooks. He is currently editing the 'lost' fifth notebook of Dylan Thomas (with Adrian Osbourne), and an anthology, *The Edge of Necessary: Welsh innovative poetry 1966–2016*.

Elizabeth Guild lectures in French at the University of Cambridge; recent publications focus mainly on Montaigne, for instance, *Unsettling Montaigne: Poetics, Ethics and Affect in the Essais and Other Writings* (D.S. Brewer, 2014). She is also a psychoanalytic psychotherapist and is one of the founders of The Site for Contemporary Psychoanalysis.

Kaye Mitchell is Senior Lecturer in Contemporary Literature and Co-Director of the Centre for New Writing at the University of Manchester, UK. She is the author of two books – *A.L. Kennedy* (Palgrave, 2007), and *Intention and Text* (Continuum, 2008) – and editor of a collection of essays on Sarah Waters (Bloomsbury, 2013) and of a special issue of *Contemporary Women's Writing* on experimental women's writing (2015). She is Co-Editor of the OUP journal, *Contemporary Women's Writing*. Her work-in-progress includes a monograph on the politics and poetics of shame in contemporary literature (for which she received a Humboldt Foundation Research Fellowship for Experienced Researchers in 2014–15), an edited *Companion to Women's Experimental Literature, 1900-Present* and a co-edited collection on British avant-garde writing of the 1960s.

Christopher John Müller is Associate Fellow at the Centre for Critical and Cultural Theory, Cardiff University and a Senior Associate Teacher at the Department of English, University of Bristol. He is the author of *Prometheansim: Technology, Digital Culture and Human Obsolescence* (Rowman & Littlefield, 2016), which includes a translation of 'On Promethean Shame' (by Günther Anders). Further publications and translations include: 'The Obsolescence of Privacy (by Günther Anders)', *CounterText: A Journal for the Study of the Post-Literary* (2017), 3 (1): 20–46 and 'Desert Ethics: Technology and the Question of Evil in Günther Anders and Jacques Derrida', *Parallax* (2015), 21 (1): 42–57. His main research focus lies on the completion of *Shame: Artifice and The Exposure of Life* (working title), a monograph that presents shame as an affect shaped by the generative relationship between humanity and technology.

Thomas Osborne is Professor of Social and Political Theory at the University of Bristol. His current research interests are in the direction of political theory and political ethics, focusing on topics to do with trust, representation, liberalism, political fear and populism. He currently holds a Leverhulme Major Research Fellowship covering these areas.

Denise Riley's books are *War in the Nursery: Theories of the Child and Mother* (1983), *'Am I That Name?' Feminism and the Category of 'Women' in History* (1988), *The Words of Selves: Identification, Solidarity, Irony* (2000), *The Force of Language* (with Jean- Jacques Lecercle; 2004), *Impersonal Passion: Language as Affect* (2005) and *Time Lived, Without Its Flow* (2012). Her poetry collections include *Marxism for Infants* (1977), *Dry Air* (1985), *Mop Mop Georgette* (1993), *Penguin Modern Poets* series 2, vol 10 (with Douglas Oliver and Iain Sinclair; 1996), *Selected Poems* (2000), *Say Something Back* (2016) and *Penguin Modern Poets* series 3, vol 6 (with Maggie Nelson and Claudia Rankine; 2017).

Oliver Sacks was a renowned neurologist and author. Dr Sacks was born in London. He earned his medical degree at the University of Oxford (Queen's College) and the Middlesex Hospital (now UCL), followed by residencies and fellowships at Mt. Zion Hospital in San Francisco and at University of California Los Angeles (UCLA). As well as authoring best-selling books such as *Awakenings* and *The Man Who Mistook His Wife for a Hat*, he was clinical professor of neurology at NYU Langone Medical Center in New York. Dr Sacks completed a five-year residency at Columbia University in New York, where he was professor of neurology and psychiatry. He also held the title of Columbia University Artist, in recognition of his contributions to the arts as well as to medicine. He was a fellow of the Royal College of Physicians and the Association of British Neurologists, the American Academy of Arts and Sciences, and the American Academy of Arts and Letters, and was a fellow of the New York Institute for the Humanities at NYU for more than 25 years. In 2008, he was appointed CBE.

Barry Sheils is Assistant Professor in English Literature at Durham University, where he is also an Associate Director of the Centre for Cultural Ecologies. He is the author of *W.B. Yeats and World Literature: The Subject of Poetry* (Routledge), and co-editor of *Narcissism, Melancholia and the Subject of Community* (Palgrave).

Charles Turner is Associate Professor of Sociology at Warwick University, UK. His publications include *Modernity and Politics in the Work of Max Weber* (Routledge, 1992) and *Investigating Sociological Theory* (Sage, 2010). He has edited *Social Theory After the Holocaust* (Liverpool University Press, 2000), *The Shape of The New*

Europe (Cambridge, 2006) and *The Sociology of Wilhelm Baldamus: paradox and inference* (Ashgate, 2010).

Julie Walsh is Lecturer in Psychosocial and Psychoanalytic Studies at the University of Essex, and a psychoanalyst in private practice. She is the author of *Narcissism and Its Discontents* (Palgrave), and co-editor of *Narcissism, Melancholia and the Subject of Community* (Palgrave). She is also a member of *The Site for Contemporary Psychoanalysis*.

1 Introduction

Shame and Modern Writing

Barry Sheils and Julie Walsh

It is not uncommon for the opening statement of a new academic work to impress upon the reader a self-consciousness concerning the legitimacy of its very existence; to call into question the terms of its own offering as if to outwit the shame of redundancy – of not being wanted, read or enjoyed. "Given the state of the field, who now needs a further book on X, Y or Z?" If such a sentiment is familiar, so too will be the conviction with which the book in question then answers itself: "it is precisely because of the present configuration of cultural, political or economic exigencies that the need for a book on X, Y or Z is most pressing." With a prudent deployment of the chiasmus, the author has let us know that she is (already) all-knowing with respect to the prospect of her own exposure, a little like being both the emperor in his birthday suit and the bystander who calls him out on it. Might it be that such a play of modest self-effacement and barefaced self-advertisement has a special resonance for the production of writing from within the Academy? As the editors of this volume, we answer "yes." Two of shame's constituent components – knowing and seeing – are symptomatically heightened in a modern university system in which the operations of knowledge production and the directives of visibility – being seen to know – collide. But might it also be that, irrespective of institutional setting, the very act of writing – be it the private diary entry, the functional to-do list, or the crafted and much redrafted excerpt of literary prose – will inevitably leave on the page a residue or trace of shame? Again, our response would be affirmative. And to justify this double "yes" we must address with care the terms of our engagement, defending the contention that there is no such thing as a writing devoid of shame, but also allowing that shameful writing has different modes through which its histories and affective intensities interact.

This introduction provides an opportunity to argue for the intrinsic relation between shame and writing, while also reflecting on the pronounced tendency in the contemporary moment towards nominating "shame" as a phenomenon worthy of analysis. In other words, there are two interleaving concerns. The first seeks to identify shame in existing writing practices by acknowledging an economy of affective transfer between writer, reader and text, operating in excess of representation. At one level, this economy is manifested through the anecdotes of writerly subjectivity: reflective inhibition, intense frustration, the abjection of the body encountering an impossible task, useless feelings (common to poet and bureaucrat) when confronted with the empty page and the command to write. There are also the humiliations of finding oneself to have been already written; as well as the errors, missteps and solecisms that slip from the pen, there is the essential reduction of being metricized and forever more "on the record." Yet, as we know from the years of "theory," such ordinary anecdotes persist as textual figures, or deconstructive aporias inside every work we deem legible. And, once acknowledged, they testify to more than subjectivity, but to the linguistic act itself and the force of expulsion required by even the most impersonally scientific prose. What Jean-Jacques Lecercle nominates the "constitutive remainder" of language, the endless contamination of word and world, and the means by which writing consistently fails to be an autonomous structure of meaning, suggests an important point of apposition here: namely, that "[b]efore it is a practice, language is a body – a body of sounds." Thus the violence of language, Lecercle emphasizes, "is to be taken at its most literal, as body penetrating body."[1] The sound of writing, then, beyond the tip tap of the keyboard or the scratch of the pen, is the sound of a body entering into relation with other bodies, where the risk of shame is ubiquitous.[2]

Our second concern is with the descriptive purchase of the word shame today when thinking about the fact and force of writing-as-exteriorization. There is little doubt that over the last three decades shame has been enjoying a period of discursive prominence, both within the institution of the university as the subject of academic writing, and in culture more broadly as a theme deserving of serious attention. It is not difficult to suggest several reasons why this might have become the case. (1) *The ongoing transformation of the public sphere and the rise of so-called identity politics, which have been cast in fresh light by the internet and new media forums.*[3] The public space and the people who occupy it have further fragmented, it seems, not simply into political, but also ontological segregations, with online persona granted a means of addressing themselves beyond any intended, or even recognizable, audience. Such an unprecedented circulation of opinion has undoubtedly made it more difficult within the "world" of Twitter, Facebook, WikiLeaks, etc. to define lines of trespass. Indeed, it can hardly be ignored that we are writing this book in the age of President Trump whose media presence relies on emotional hyperbole and *ad hominem* attacks and is at the same time surrealistically imprecise (e.g. "you are fake news"[4]). It is this imprecision, virtually obscuring an adjudicated object of interest, which induces in his opponents feelings of shortcoming before the task of formulating a proportional response – a response that will be adequately seen or heard – as well as the shameful temptation to shout-over or to simply disavow and close down all future attempts at engagement. In this way, our understanding of the historical moment converges with reflection upon the vicissitudes of our affective lives. (2) *Theorizing within the biopolitical paradigm, broadly conceived according to Michel Foucault's designation of a shift from the politics of territorial sovereignty to the government of populations.*[5] Though the modern globalizing university is itself an agent of 'governance,' there have been, within its frame, specifically through studies of sex, sexuality, race and colonialism, attempts to confront the shame of the institution. To frame biopolitical ordinances is to make conspicuous that shameful line between those bodies given the opportunities of formation and those rendered disposable through organized processes of representation. (3) *The emergence of the Environmental Humanities.* "Species shame" may yet be regarded skeptically as a specifically Western pathology, or even as a displaced Malthusian anxiety concerning overpopulation, but the hypothesized advent of a new geological epoch wherein the effects of human culture are said to have irremediably altered the planet's ecosystems marks an important paradox of university discourse. As an epoch commonly dated to the first Atomic bomb in 1945, itself a result of the Manhattan Project's hypertrophic research practices, what is now sometimes called the Anthropocene provides a good example of the university turning upon the shame of its own history. (4) *The turn to affect.* Though canonized in anthologies such as *The Affective Turn: Theorizing the Social* (2007) and *The Affect Theory Reader* (2010), affect remains a difficult term to delineate, sometimes associated with the materialism of modern brain science, and sometimes with the reputed demise of poststructuralism.[6] Affect is often distinguished from emotion,[7] and in the most general terms used to signal investments in prelinguistic embodiment, generative intensity and the inassimilable relations of *becoming* (see, for example, Patricia Clough, Brian Massumi, and, always standing in the background, the work of Gilles Deleuze).[8] In the most optimistic readings, affect offers us a radical contrast to theories of emotion that conservatively bind us to an already coded world of objects. For Silvan Tomkins, the mid-twentieth-century psychologist whose work, introduced by Adam Frank and Eve Kosofsky Sedgwick, has proven so influential in this field, shame/humiliation takes its place as one of nine basic affects.[9] Importantly, within this psychobiological paradigm, shame is not determined by particular scenes: although a certain scene might be "culturally scripted" to direct and contain our shame – say, a child being beaten by an adult – we cannot say of it that is it *necessarily* shameful.[10] This is because the intensity of an affect remains independent of (autonomous from) the object it attaches to.[11] As we shall see throughout this volume, shame has most often come to occupy a space between affect and discourse: on the one hand pointing towards the auto-affective capacities of embodiment, and on the other to the reflexive component of being ashamed (the shame of shame, or shame's impropriety), which involves the suspicion that we are feeling someone else's shame, or, indeed, that our felt shame disregards, *affectively* short-circuits, the attempt to understand its historical conditions.

If academic writing in the Humanities and Social Sciences has conventionally been granted a critical function, and more lately a melancholic cast of mind (consider the influence of Judith Butler's work), then perhaps, with the fourfold tendency towards shame just outlined, it has become, at last, a truly confessional mode. Certainly we can say of recent works (especially by those working within anti-colonial and queer paradigms) that there is an increased recognition of the embodied relations that stand at the heart of our knowledge economies, which has consequences for our understanding of academic writing conventions. Whether it is Jacques Derrida standing wet and naked before his cat, Elspeth Probyn receiving an email from an angry, humiliated colleague, or Sedgwick facing the empty space where the Twin Towers once stood, the shame idiom has come to involve the interpenetration of personal anecdote with theory.[12] Dodie Bellamy (whose life writing is discussed further by Kaye Mitchell in this volume) writes of how oppressive she finds the impersonality of academic essays: "how exciting – and important – [it is] to undermine the patriarchal hegemony that created the MLA Style Sheet." Or, as she puts it more succinctly a page later: "what the fuck I wanted to do was to shit on academic pretension."[13] Inevitably, such confessions are as narcissistic as they are honest: as invested in the affective capacities of being an embodied self as in the admission of particular historical transgressions. In this context, the noticeable move away from the term guilt towards shame in university writing (a longer-term trend discussed further below) stands alongside the ubiquity of J.M. Coetzee's *Disgrace* (1999), a novel whose protagonist David Lurie is a Communications Professor (erstwhile Comparative Literature Professor) transgressing the terms of his office by sexually accosting a student.[14] Lurie's adamant refusal to display his shame in the University's Committee of Inquiry, which he deems an improper and performative extrapolation from the rationalization of his admitted guilt, haunts the rest of the novel. Having initially dismissed as *unnecessary* his personal humiliation before others, by the end of the book, once associated to a series of violent humiliations in the South African countryside, including the rape of his daughter by local men (or boys) and the hopeless labor of euthanizing unwanted dogs, Lurie comes to embody the very *necessity* of shame. *Disgrace* is a novel in which the university discourse can be no more separated from the decolonizing politics of South Africa than the exchangeable abstractions of the law can be separated from the shameful entanglements of non-exchangeable bodies contesting space.

With this chastening coordinate in mind, we introduce the essays in this volume – all originated from the American and European university systems. While it is clear that this work, like any other, can be read for what it omits, we aim to draw together two facets of shame through the question of literary and academic writing. First, the general shame produced by all writing: that of being superfluous, of exposing more than it seems necessary to expose. And second, the historical situations which force us to read shame's general auto-affective character in more specifically political ways. After giving further thought to the general dynamics of shame – its pathology, tense, and questionable, though mythopoeic, universality – we shall consider three particularizing histories which underlie, we suggest, the constituency of modern writing: the shame of the anthropological gaze, the shame of bearing witness to historical catastrophes, specifically the Holocaust, and the shame of acknowledging the structural violence of colonization.

Shame, Writing, Action

We can begin, then, by considering the grammar of shame. The first and quite obvious observation to note is that shame can be deployed as a noun and as a verb.[15] And yet it is rare that we encounter the abstract noun "shame" without at least the implication of action, and of movement. If I am paralyzed by shame, trapped *within* the confines of my own self, it is probably because I have been caught *out*. While it is me who feels exposed, trapped in my body, it is also always my body entered into a relation with other bodies – I am ashamed when I find myself delineated or differentiated by being out of place. As Liz Constable reminds us, there is a sense in which shame cannot be said to 'belong' to anybody, despite being very much about the problem of belonging.[16] Another way of putting this, in keeping with the most famous depiction of shame in the canon of European art, Masaccio's *The Expulsion from the Garden of Eden* (1425), is to say that shame is scenographic rather than, strictly speaking, psychological: it is a felt condition which also has to be *seen* to be felt, and which therefore always elucidates something of the space in which it occurs. It is an internal feeling which actively founds the external background against which it can be witnessed. Related to this scenic visualization of my own shame, is the phenomenology of vicarious shame, a common and yet somehow extraordinary experience of shame's mobility, in which the witness, ostensibly standing outside the scene, suddenly becomes the object within. More spectacular than a voluntary identification with others, understood as sympathy or compassion, say, vicarious shame potentially rips through the contours of the subject, throwing into disarray the formal distinctions between inside and outside, background and foreground.

The best known of several attempts in mid-twentieth-century French philosophy to capture the interscopic and vicarious predicament of shame is Jean Paul Sartre's discussion of the look [le regard], specifically the interaction between the transcendent subject perceiving others [les autres] in the world and the same subject finding himself being looked at by the Other [l'Autrui]. For Sartre it is the enigma of the Other's unperceivable eyes (those which are looking at me!) which allows me to apprehend my own vulnerability: "that I have a body which can be hurt, that I occupy a place and that I can not in any case escape from the space in which I am without defense."[17] The snooping man outside the door, leaning over the keyhole, feels footsteps behind him: he is *seen* looking, and thereby given a situation, revealed to himself as fallen *into* the world. "It is shame or pride which reveals to me the Other's look and myself at the end of that look. It is the shame or pride which makes me *live*, not *know* the situation of being looked at," writes Sartre; and later, that pride or shame is "the feeling of being finally what I am but elsewhere, over there for the Other."[18] In Sartre's account, there is something inherently shameful about ego formation, about the fact that "I have my foundation outside myself."[19] It is the Other who confers upon me a boundary, and who spatializes and temporalizes myself beyond (in excess of) the terms of a transcendent subjective consciousness. In the grand tradition of Hegelian phenomenology, what is most shameful is that I depend upon the freedom of the Other's look in order to recognize myself.

Emmanuel Lévinas, writing before Sartre in 1935 on the theme of escape, and more precisely on the *inescapably* of being oneself, recalls us to a very ordinary instance of the self's spilling over itself: "The sick person in isolation, who 'was taken ill' and who has no choice but to vomit, is still scandalized by himself."[20] Here shame arises with the confusion between bodily isolation and exposure before the Other, and is manifest through an act of physical expulsion which is at once an illness and a catharsis, a depletion and a surplus of being. The scene poses a question, not unrelated to the question posed by the scene of writing: *is this vomit me?*

If shame threatens to disrupt our boundaries in this way, leaving us stripped of the confidence to be proprietorial (*am I merely an object in someone else's world?*), we might also expect it to disturb our language. Indeed, the prefix "dis," suggesting division or dual motion (a two-way-ness), gives us a ready clue to the work that shame does: in the work of dislocation, displacement and dispossession, shame enacts an undoing or a becoming undone – *I am shattered, and out of place.* And yet, equally, in its proximity to disgust, and what Silvan Tomkins has called "dissmell," shame enacts a recall to the finitude of the body – *I am sequestered here, smelling my own death.* This duality, of being at once displaced and inescapably oneself, is the ontological enactment of shame as a private feeling which always elaborates a public world. The subject who feels ashamed is never quite alone; and contrariwise, the subject who calls down shame upon another, availing of the *dis* of disgust or disrespect, never quite belongs to the public world in the way he imagines. If I have put you in your place in the name of some public law or morality, then the chances are that in the process I have displaced myself. This is what the sick man in isolation and the offended man in the street demonstrate, together: that shame is a relational and double-dealing sentiment, and that the shame of shame invariably rebounds.

Tomkins's work is especially rich when describing the rebounding dynamism of the shame affect. His most pithy definition of shame as "the incomplete reduction of interest or joy" draws our attention to those social attachments that obdurately remain after the self-protective work of inhibition or closure has taken place.[21] Here, the scene underlying all such attachments is psychoanalytic in character, performing the disruption of the infant-mother gestalt: the infant's turning away, determinative of the ego, remains nonetheless dependent upon the nourishments of the maternal world. This withdrawal or contraction of self, combined with persistent interest in the Other, sets the terms for all subsequent scenes of social shame. Such scenes are, of course, empirically diverse, as well as being paradoxical, and they place a writerly demand upon those who would seek to describe them. Indeed, Tomkins's writing on this topic is "astonishingly heterogeneous" according to Sedgwick and Frank; it "nurtures, pacifies, replenishes, then sets the idea in motion again."[22] Certainly it delights in qualifications and indeterminate catalogues, to an extent that Sedgwick and Frank deem almost Proustian, and its speculative accounts of subjective experience bring the scientific ambition of his project (to map the basic affects) and the idiosyncratic nature of his expression into perilously close agreement. Here is an example we have picked out in which it is clear that Tomkins has a writing *style*:

> Let us consider next the varieties of sources of shame which arise from love, friendship, and close interpersonal relationships. If I wish to touch you but do not wish to be touched, I may feel ashamed. If I wish to look at you but you do not wish me to, I may feel ashamed. If I wish you to look at me but you do not, I may feel ashamed. If I wish to look at you and at the same time wish that you look at me, I can be shamed. If I wish to be close to you but you move away, I am ashamed. If I wish to suck or bite your body and you are reluctant, I can become ashamed. If I wish to hug you or you hug me or we hug each other and you do not reciprocate my wishes, I feel ashamed. If I wish to have sexual intercourse with you but you do not, I am ashamed.[23]

With all these "ifs" we are assured that these are imaginative, rather than strictly clinical, vignettes, pointing out shame's mimetic character, and relating it to the reflexivity of the look – the looking and being looked at of Sartre's regard. However, the phenomenology of the look is not the whole point in Tomkins's text; the point is also the too-muchness of the writing. Tomkins sets out to catalogue examples of shame, but since there is no totality of circumstances which would make this open-ended list scientifically comprehensive, we are drawn to its rhetorical wantonness ("If I wish to suck or bite your body and you are reluctant..."). Sedgwick and Frank's fascination with this style can be restated as the realization that shame is not simply what Tomkins writes *about*; it is *in* his writing. The pleasures of reading and writing shame – pleasures forever adjoined to reluctance, repetition, frustration and block – are not merely incidental to the theme.

We can elucidate this point by considering a literary example from George Eliot's 1876 novel *Daniel Deronda* in which the phenomenology of a blush (that attributed to Gwendolen Harlath, one of the novel's two major characters) collides with the demands of narrative sense.[24] Gwendolen is vexed to have been seen blushing, and so performs the self-protective gymnastic of wheeling away from company:

> If any had noticed her blush as significant, they had certainly not interpreted it by the secret windings and recesses of her feelings. A blush is no language: only a dubious flag-signal which may mean either of two contradictories. Deronda alone had a faint guess at some part of her feeling; but while he was observing her he was himself under observation.[25]

Gwendolen laments the fact that the blush has entered her into an interscopic social relation before, or outside of, linguistic representation. This is a lament which poses a formative question to the narrative order, the blush being at once prelinguistic ("no language") and productive of excessive linguistic signification ("If any had noticed her blush as significant, they had certainly not interpreted it by the secret ... of her feelings"). In one view, we can conclude, in Brian Massumi's phrase, that "skin is faster than the word," which is to say that it registers an order of temporality capable of interrupting narrated time: Gwendolen's blush provides a trace of affective intensity which reveals the narrative order of the novel to be a form of cover-up, sense disguising nonsense.[26] And yet, the very same blush is also readable as the iteration of narrative convention, specifically within the romantic-political arena of the Victorian novel, the conventional prolepsis of a character's red face anticipating an idealized sexual and social union: that Gwendolen blushes and Deronda sees her blush establishes the decorous terms of erotic estrangement which we expect to be overcome over the course of the narrative. Ultimately, however, the narrator's reflections on the contradictoriness of *any* blush gesture beyond Gwendolen's specifically psychological reasons for wanting to deny her blush a meaning, and move us to the novel's striking failure to fulfill a romantic union between Gwendolen and Deronda: the narrative expectations established by the conventions of reading skin are disappointed. Accordingly, the meaninglessness of the blush, its apparent absurdity, points us beyond character to plot; and then, through the false expectation of plot, to the act of writing itself (before any narrative order has been imposed) to the biographical figure George Eliot, or Mary Anne Evans, sitting at her desk, negotiating between the impulse to write and the cover-up of having written.

Most mythic accounts of shame recount this cover-up in the past-historic tense, thus performing the fall from Paradise into language which is also their explicit theme. Sigmund Freud, for example, in *Civilization and Its Discontents* invites us to consider how shame is intimately associated with the anthropomorphic act of genital exposure that occurred when mankind assumed an "upright gait." Shame was first provoked in man when, moving from four legs to two, his genitals became "visible and in need of protection" (*Scham* in the German, also connoting the male genitals).[27] To say that there must have been such an exposure covered-over in the past, at least in an imagined past, is to suggest that the feeling of shame is temporally as well as spatially arranged. This accords with Giorgio Agamben's treatment of the biblical Fall in his essay "Nudity."[28] Agamben stresses that the mythic fall into Original Sin marks the passage from nakedness to nudity, where the former was a mythic state without shame and the latter an event *in time*: Adam and Eve suffer not because of the present fact of their bodily nakedness before God, but rather through God's inference of their nudity beneath the fig leaf.[29] Nudity *happens*; it is something to be *activated*: we can at any moment be denuded of our clothes, conventions, the labors of our civilization, including of language. Which is to say, like Adam and Eve, we exist in anticipation of a return to our original disgrace – our denuded bodies which can never be naked again. Sharing affinities with the critical questioning of the philosopher and the obscene demand of the sadist to "make flesh appear," the shameful consciousness operates through narrative as the possibility of its unraveling. It is when we *know* that language covers us that we feel historically vulnerable to being exposed.[30]

What is most remarkable about the previously quoted passage from *Daniel Deronda*, then, is that its discursive intervention comes so close to denuding its own narrative elaboration ("no language"), thereby exposing the scandal of writing itself. It comes close to confessing, in other words, the contingent (not already meaningfully coded) interaction between a body and the text. Whilst in anthropological or psychobiological terms the blush is taken for a conventional manifestation of shame, once figured in literature it also potentially reflects a doubleness inherent to the narrative act: writing as sublimation up and away from the body into measured linguistic exchange; and writing as desublimation, a writing against, which returns always to an unexchangeable body's relation to itself. Helen Merell Lynd has written suggestively of how certain modern-period texts give exceptional focus to specific body parts – Dimitri Karamazov's hideous big toes, for example, or Phillip's clubfoot in W. Somerset Maugham's *Of Human Bondage*.[31] In such cases, acknowledged shame is indexed to a single body's relation to itself; the characters in these novels suffer not primarily because of exposure before others, but rather due to the necessity of bearing unrelenting witness to themselves. Shame, offers Jacqueline Rose, is "the only affect which works internally, passing from one to another part of the self."[32] The blush illustrates such an understanding: transferential in nature, it also presents a kind of proof of the shameful body as auto-poetic; it is the beacon for a subjectivity generating its own content in significant separation from a larger, more objective history.[33] Such dissociation of character from plot is a familiar modernist trope, of course, as is the sense of affective disproportion which accompanies it. Lynd establishes this out-of-jointness through the character of Joseph K. in Kafka's *The Trial* who translates the impersonal circumstances of his abduction by the Law into the pain of personal failure: he felt "the shame of being delivered into the hands of these people by *his* sudden weakness" (emphasis ours).[34] The loss of a comprehensible position within a broad network of symbolic meanings at once reduces and intensifies K.'s experience of selfhood: the ashamed self becomes an excessive burden.

It remains unclear, however, whether shame is the cause or the effect of such a characteristic falling short of a storyline, since the formal disconnect produced by K.'s removal from the assurances of plot (a plot in which we might eventually find out who has been spreading lies about Joseph K.) also ensures that the author-function is contaminated by the affective life of the protagonist. To say, for instance, that K. is Kafkaesque, though stopping just short of saying he is indeed "Kafka," nonetheless sustains the suspicion that through the impersonality of the written form moves the personality of the artistic self. Likewise, Henry James's prefaces or Virginia Woolf's essays offer more than secondary explanations to those works they are often seen to accompany; rather, they supplement and interpenetrate, even potentially undermine the formal cohesion of the authors' named fictions. For Sedgwick, in her essay "Shame, Theatricality, and Queer Performativity: Henry James's *The Art of the Novel*," James's prefaces are "a strategy for dramatizing and integrating shame, in the sense of rendering this potentially paralyzing affect narratively, emotionally, and performatively productive."[35] The writer emerges, shy and exhibitionist, as the reader of his own work.

Of course, this view goes against a certain orthodoxy concerning modernism: if everybody knows that Leopold Bloom in his spit is a *Joycean* artist of the everyday, it still seems a temerity befitting a writer like Wyndham Lewis to suggest that J. Alfred Prufrock and T.S. Eliot share key personality traits. And yet attempts to join the phenomenological and autobiographical to the textual, to place the figure of the writer struggling with the demand to write within a textual frame, are also, in part, readings against the institutionalization of high literary accomplishment. What is now commonly called life writing, as well as blurring the line between fiction and autobiography, often returns us to the figure of the writer: not the institutional author, the proper name who has always already written, but the precarious bodily self, who is actively entering into contingent relations with itself and other selves.

This kind of writing often invokes its own heritage, including, importantly, classical modes of plain speech, which have been traced genealogically by Foucault as the tradition of parrhēsia. Eschewing the techniques of rhetoric and persuasion, and drawing attention to the vulnerability of the speaker, who was often speaking against the received opinions of those in power, Foucault tells us that classical plain speaking (risky or fearless speech) fulfilled the double function of political and personal critique: from the Cynics to Socrates "there [was] a relation between the rational discourse, the logos, you are able to use, and the way that you live."[36] However, Foucault is also careful to distinguish the classical act of speaking plainly through the wisdom of personal experience (ethos) from more modern, Christianized conceptions of confession where the emphasis is upon a sinful and sexualized body. The Greek Cynic Diogenes masturbating in public (a physical manifestation of his many indecorous barbs at those in power), though situated at the very edge of the "parrhēsiastic contract," was yet imbued with the dignity of critique: his was a shameless act designed to call out social contradictions as well as advertise his own ethos. In modern, specifically Christianized terms, however, any such understanding is bound to be further overdetermined according to a reading of spiritual or psychopathological symptoms.[37] Similarly, though the essential value of risky speech in Ancient Greece was that of speaking truth to power, the tendency of modern confession is rather towards identification with the Law;[38] modern autobiography, instead of exemplifying a critical-philosophical position taken up against the sophistry of the state, is more usually concerned with an aberrant life, which has to somehow be written or spoken *out* of existence.

This fate of philosophical "truth" imprisoned within the neuroses of the modern subject is detectable within life writing where the declarative determination to be honest and artless is accompanied by the taint of self-aggrandizing vanity; most famously perhaps is the case of Rousseau's autobiographical writings – his *Confessions* and solitary promenades – in which the political object of his unusually honest scrutiny becomes difficult to distinguish from the range of his persecutory identifications. Recently, Karl Ove Knausgaard's series of memoirs *My Struggle* has enjoyed considerable success by describing in shame-filled terms the author's attempt to escape his shame through writing about it.[39] The separation of this work from classical risky speech is manifest: sick with the conceit of literary fiction, Knausgaard doesn't write to reveal his life as exemplary or even "interesting," but rather to declare it an unusually wounded one. Several times throughout the volumes he abruptly interrupts the flow of his conventional memoiristic accounts of the past to take us to the present-tense scene of authorship: the writer sitting at his desk engaged in writing what we are reading:

> It is now a few minutes past eight o'clock in the morning. It is the fourth of March, 2008. I am sitting in my office, surrounded by books from floor to ceiling, listening to the Swedish band Dungen and thinking about what I have written and where it is leading.[40]

In other words, the narrative fabric unravels, denuding the author of narrative certainty while sticking to the necessity of his subject matter. What is thematically necessary for Knausgaard, the self to which he returns, is also necessarily a deformation of plot. As he puts it most programmatically towards the end of Volume 2:

> Over recent years I had increasingly lost faith in literature. I read and thought this is something someone has made up. ... Living like this, with the certainty that everything could equally well have been different, drove you to despair. I couldn't write like this, it wouldn't work, every single sentence was met with the thought: but you're just making this up. It has no value. ... The only genres I saw value in, which still conferred meaning, were diaries and essays, the types of literature that did not deal with narrative, that were not about anything, but just consisted of a voice, the voice of your own personality, a life, a face, a gaze you could meet. What is a work of art if not the gaze of another person? Not directed above us, nor beneath us, but at the same height as our own gaze. Art cannot be experienced collectively, nothing can, art is something you are alone with. You meet its gaze alone.[41]

Here we can see how the author's stipulation against fiction, and his narcissistic itemizing of his own life, though not inviting emulation on ethical grounds, may yet be deemed exemplary as a mode of singularizing the self. Famously, Deleuze expressed a similar ambition in his essay "Literature and Life": "The shame of being a man – is there any better reason to write?" For Deleuze, true writing must accept the challenge of *becoming* other than man: "in writing, one becomes-woman, becomes-animal or-vegetable, becomes-molecule."[42] Contemporary strategies of shamelessness, distantly related to the Cynicism of Diogenes, though less objectively critical, exist in order to corrupt preexistent or generic cultural narratives, which are seen as the representative forms of manhood (standing in for the phallus, symbolic power, and so on). Accordingly, the value of a confession such as Knausgaard's, which aspires through shame to shamelessness, is that it permits, in Deleuze's terms, for life to be "singularized out of a population rather than determined in a form" – it attempts, in other words, to escape "its own formalization."[43]

This view is an affirmative one, and characteristically modernist in its commitment to the non-preexistent. However, while we may want to celebrate any such means of confronting "the shame of being a man," especially if it promises a reconfiguration of the body through language, therefore disrupting the reproduction of symbolic power, we must also concede that we are, initially at least (as is obvious from the record of Deleuze's examples, including Witold Gombrowicz, J.M.G. Le Clézio, André Dhôtel, D.H. Lawrence and Kafka) writing only of men. There is indeed a long line of "honest men," from Augustine through Montaigne to Rousseau and Knausgaard, who have been granted the license to deconstruct the edifice of their cultural authority as men. Consequently, their detailed abjections have been more easily transformed into spiritual virtues. Just as the humility of reading many books (an academic modesty borrowed from the poets) can translate into the institutional fame of being "well read," so the humiliations of failure, specifically the failure to write, can transform into canonicity (see the remarkable case of Samuel Beckett). A woman writer, by contrast, seldom granted the same historical prestige, is also often denied the terms of a heroic contest with authority. As feminist scholars continue to remind us, not only has much female memoir been precipitously understood as "hysterical," and in this way denied a priori the dignity of "truth," but female writing – as reflected on by Woolf and Hélène Cixous, among others – is less acquainted, whether by circumstance or design, with the prospect of escape.

Shame*less*ness, or the ridding of oneself of neurosis, Freud once suggested, is something more often met with among men – a statement replete with implications for female authorship: if women are thought incapable of working through their shame, then what they write of themselves can only be treated as evidence of a pathological condition (indeed the Freudian association of shame with "genital deficiency" is hard to separate from its characterization as "a feminine characteristic *par excellence*").[44] It is worth pondering the force of such a preconception once more as we reanimate our argument that shame attends every act of writing, as a necessity, but also a strategy. We might further infer that shame is an historical device which entraps a woman just as soon as it exposes a man in the foolhardy presumption of transgression or escape.[45] If it's true that shame adheres to all bodies that write, then even a cursory look at the record of *what* gets published and *how* tells us that shame does not adhere to all writing bodies in the same way.

Historicizing Shame

For Liz Constable shame presents a "vicissitudinous ethics" of community; for Christopher Lebron it poses a realignment of method when thinking about political justice; Jennifer Biddle conceives of shame as the problem of anthropological looking, whilst it remains "an arm of the law" for Martha Nussbaum, and an old tool for Jennifer Jacquet, though with potentially new uses.[46] According to David Halperin and Valerie Traub, shame is "the otherwise" of gay pride; for Francis Broucek (quoted approvingly by Sedgwick and Frank) it is "the keystone affect" in self-psychology and for the sociologist Thomas Scheff it is "the master-emotion of everyday life."[47] Timothy Bewes reads colonial shame as the cultural form that helps us think the absence of forms; whilst for Giorgio Agamben shame marks a bearing witness to our own passivity when confronted with the inhuman reductions of biopolitical regimes.[48]

We have already suggested some reasons why shame might have risen to such prominence in recent years, but equally significant is the comparative retreat of the term guilt. The old complaint that psychoanalysis, for example, treats of guilt but not of shame – in other words that it neglects the body – might now be reversed: where is guilt in the face of so many shame publications? This deserves some further thought; because if focusing on shame indicates a progressive acknowledgment that sovereign laws, their means of adjudication, depend upon prior mechanisms of inclusion and exclusion, as well as processes of identification and interpellation, and that the "human" scale of their operation belies the inhuman determinations of material history (capitalism), then it also suggests a return, a backsliding we might say, from the law-abiding citizen to the question of personal character. In this sense, shame attaches to characters more than to citizens. By way of illustration we might introduce two character-types met with in the contemporary sociopolitical landscape, both of whom call forth the question of shame in a way that seems to take precedence from the question of guilt or innocence: the stateless migrant, and the whistle-blower. Both these characters are familiar figures of excess: the former as the constitutive outsider of settled convention who bears the burden of selfhood in excess of any measured distribution of social affect (to be without papers *sans-papiers* is to be all body); the latter because she reveals the inconsistency of the system to which she belongs. Both are also figures of shame, shamed and shaming, who, we'd suggest, are complementary in so far as they reveal together how the ordinary function of institutional or state power purveys shame whilst remaining shameless in itself. For our present purposes, it is also worth noting that whistle-blowing is most often an act of writing or rewriting, carrying the insider language of institutions across an established border. However contested the legacies of Edward Snowden, Julian Assange or Chelsea Manning remain, each character, though in very different ways, has borne the burden of their actions as whistle-blowers, embodying a tragic statelessness in stark contrast to the bodiless language of the state institutions they opposed. Such an exorcism of institutional bad faith, by no means identical to the migrant experience of being involuntarily outcast or destitute, does at least adjoin that experience; it brings shame to shame and enters into a relation with the Other who is outside and not allowed in, the Other who has to bear the burden of the self without any guarantee of legal representation.

Rob Halpern's recent poetry collection *Common Place* (2015) exercises the dangerous prerogative of the whistle-blower.[49] Throughout the collection the poet performatively transcribes the autopsy of Al Hanashi Muhammad Ahmad, a detainee of the Guantánamo Bay holding facility who died with a ligature around his neck in 2009. Halpern copies the institutional language which incarcerated, taxonomized and ultimately mortified Al Hanashi's body ('*Autopsy No (b) (6). ID No. (b) (6).*'), contaminating this language with his own supplementary reflections, and, inevitably in the process, carrying it over and out of its 'proper' context.[50] The work reads as an attempt to *feel* impersonal language personally, an effect mostly achieved through the sexualization of the institutional register. An example:

> Ligature: The ligature is collected as evidence by the NCIS at the scene and examined by the prospector and the observing civilian medical examiner prior to autopsy. The ligature is almost identical to the elastic band of a white brief, medium size 34-36, issued to the detainees at the detention facility. The ligature consists of two segments, with a combined aggregate length of approximately 23½″ and width of approximately 1″. The smaller of the two segment measures 6½″ in length. The ligature fibers are elongated and distorted at the junction of the two cut edges c/w the history of cutting the ligature at the twisted part. There are no bloodstains on the ligature. Boredom distracts and numbness disorients, but arriving at that period I become acutely aware of my body as I write. The word "ligature" excites me and my left hand begins caressing my thigh.[51]

The immeasurability of Halpern's desire, its proper to improper border crossing here, addresses in Al Hanashi someone doubly removed from the possibility of communication: a figure of migration detained outside the law, and a man who is dead. Nonetheless he also conjures an awkward physical intimacy: "It makes no sense for my hard-on to shame me, opposing the stiffness of his body."[52] Halpern's language, ethically perilous as a conscious admission of complicity in the exploitation of the silenced Other, and vulnerable to censure on the grounds that it expresses narcissistic pathology rather than political or philosophical truth, exhibits a short-circuited relation which can only raise the "senseless" prospect of shame: a repeated interest which repeatedly falls short of meeting with its object.

> This is not a wet dream, it's a poem, and I want to believe it needs to be written, not simply that it can be. But the degree to which my

writing sublimes in private yearning is the degree to which it yields to civic embarrassment.[53]

The shameful necessity of Al Hanashi's fate, its literal inescapability, shames the gratuitousness of Halpern's voluntary act of transcription: they relate according to a conspicuous, unbridgeable difference. No matter how the poet wishes for the necessity of a muse, the impersonality of the work to provide the formal alibi for his writerly ambition, he is recalled to the embarrassing inadequacy of his identifications.

Halpern's project as a writer is also of course a readerly one, reading into and implicitly against the institutional languages which organize Al Hanashi's body. If the institution shames its object by reproducing it as a knowable, quantifiable entity, the critical and poetic response is to ask how the institution can be made to feel or recognize its own shame, beyond merely delegating it to a scapegoat. Halpern's historical coordinates include the recent American wars and other illicit involvements in Iraq, Afghanistan and elsewhere; but his indictment of institutional impersonality – fixing the body biometrically, and constricting its narrative possibilities to the zero point where an autopsy becomes its most apt expression – is general. There is a point of apposition here between the dilemmas of the poetic "I," and the figure of the blush as a sign of excessive subjectivity falling short of plot or historical narrative. We might say of Halpern's "lyric" mode that it performs the experience of too-much-face when confronting the involuntary and faceless deformations of the world.

Famously Charles Darwin characterized the blush as "the most peculiar and the most human of all expressions": an issue of subjectivity, in other words. Yet he also went on to explain it in objective terms as "the relaxation of the muscular coats of the small arteries, by which the capillaries become filled with blood; and this depends on the proper vaso-motor centre being affected."[54] The blush, then, is biographical *and* biometric. But what Darwin doesn't fully investigate is how the material triggers he describes are related to particular psychical and historical representations: to what extent do fantasy and imaginative identification *overdetermine* the manifest phenomenon of a red face? How can a blush be *known* if its causes are endlessly confused with its effects? This confusion is most evident when the process of identifying the blush as a material bodily phenomenon is shown to produce the humiliation it claims to study, as in the following quotation:

> [Dr. J. Crichton Browne] gives me the case of a married woman, aged twenty-seven, who suffered from epilepsy. On the morning after her arrival in the Asylum, Dr. Browne, together with his assistants, visited her whilst she was in bed. The moment that he approached, she blushed deeply over her cheeks and temples; and the blush spread quickly to her ears. She was much agitated and

tremulous. He unfastened the collar of her chemise in order to examine the state of her lungs; and then a brilliant blush rushed over her chest, in an arched line over the upper third of each breast, and extended downwards between the breasts nearly to the ensiform cartilage of the sternum.[55]

Sally Munt has noted the soft pornographic imaginary which underwrites this passage ("agitated and tremulous") and which Darwin's scientific literalism is not in a position to reflect upon.[56] However, it is important to appreciate that the objectifying regard of Darwin and the Doctor in this scene does not straightforwardly negate the female patient's subjectivity, but rather determines its institutional conditions. The married woman's blush remains a blazon of self-enclosure and mute retreat, a subjectivity communicating itself through institutional space in oblique and painful ways.

In his essay "Shame, or On the Subject," Giorgio Agamben transfers a similar thought to the institution of the Nazi death camps. We have considered the blush of the writing subject who falls short of plot (Gwendolen's "no language"), and the blush of the objectified patient, possibly bearing witness to her own objectification (Darwin's "married woman"). For Agamben, these two positions together infiltrate the dilemmas of Holocaust testimony. His paradigmatic example comes from Robert Antelme's *L'Espèce humaine* (1947), in particular from his written account of a young Italian student who "turned pink" after being interpellated by a member of the SS: "*Du komme hier!*"[57] In this unforgettable scene Agamben finds the "I" "overcome by its own passivity": the student has entered into a fundamental relation with his own physiological or "bare" life.[58] "In shame, the subject ... has no other content than its own desubjectivisation; it becomes witness to its own disorder, its own oblivion as a subject. This double movement which is both subjectivisation and desubjectivisation is shame."[59] Agamben generalizes this moment – the bearing witness to the material deformation of oneself – so that not only is it paradigmatic for all Holocaust testimony, but it captures in an especially vicious historical circumstance the fundamental task undertaken by the lyric subject of poetry. The lyric "I" offers testimony as the only remainder of the human when the subject's humanity has been deformed or destroyed.

We might wonder, in this regard, whether the unbearable particularity of the Italian student's case – his autopoiesis standing in excess of the historical circumstance of mass extermination – really connects to the long tradition of poetic testimony where, according to Agamben, the language of shame stands in the place of a "missing articulation"?[60] Are we really to imagine poetic experiment on the page as continuous with the Italian student's experience when confronted with his own death? The Italian student doesn't get to write his own poetry (neither did Al Hanashi);[61] rather, he has to be witnessed witnessing himself by

Antelme, and therefore, might be said to mark less the exemplary moment of poetic self-testimony, than its crushing defeat. This is a point of consternation for Ruth Leys in her 2007 study *From Guilt to Shame: Auschwitz and After.*[62] Leys suggests that Agamben, as well as potentially dehistoricizing the specificity of what happened at Auschwitz, specifically misreads Antelme. For Antelme the "pink face" is not simply the phenomenological mark of shame – a subject facing desubjectivisation – but a textual sign transposed to other figures including at one point to a German baby, signaling "aliveness or vitality."[63] In other words, for Leys it is significant that Antelme's writerly strategies refuse the institutional reduction which equates the pink face to humiliation: "Attention to Antelme's own thematisation of pink in the text suggests a different meaning, one that emphasized not the issue of desubjectivisation and shame but of human relatedness and responsibility."[64]

This is part of Leys's larger argument against shame as it replaces guilt in the discourse on Holocaust testimony. Shame, for Leys, indicates a turn away from complex questions of complicity, intentionality, fantasy and transference – all terms of linguistic inquiry which allow us to connect bearing witness to "survivor guilt" – towards what she calls a kind of biopolitical literalism: bearing witness to oneself as pure materiality to be manipulated. Agamben's reading of Antelme is a recent example of this turn according to Leys, inspired by the (re)turn to affect and the new literalism of the (anti-psychoanalytic) materialism of neuroscience.[65] Writing is deprived of fantasy in this register, enacting in the same breath a return to Darwin and an omission of Freud.

Leys's argument is invaluable to us for two reasons: first, it demonstrates, by the scope of its genealogy of writing about the Holocaust, the reality of the discursive shift from guilt to shame. Beginning with a discussion of the concept of "survivor guilt" linked to "identification with the aggressor" (suggested by Bruno Bettleheim in 1943, framed by William G. Niederland in the early 1960s, and articulated also in Primo Levi's writings), Leys goes onto note that from 1979 on writers who were concerned to challenge the Freudian underpinnings to survivor guilt (especially the problematic implications of the victim's identification with the aggressor) turned to shame as an embodied, materialist alternative to the complexities of transference and fantasy. "There is a marked tendency in recent trauma theory to treat the traumatic event as something that leaves a 'reality imprint' in the brain," she writes "an imprint that in its insistent literality testifies to the existence of a timeless historical truth unaffected by suggestive-mimetic factors or unconscious-symbolic elaboration."[66] She nominates Terence Des Pres, Lawrence Langer, as well as Agamben, as writers whose work has extended this interpretation.

The second value of Leys's argument is how her account of guilt as both "suggestive-mimetic" and "unconscious-symbolic" usefully complicates the guilt-shame distinction. She is not content to reproduce the commonplace opposition between shame as a bodily, ontological concern with our being, and guilt as a mental and moral concern with our deeds. Rather Leys defends guilt as an *emotional* descriptor underpinned by psychoanalytic theory: a theoretical framework which insists that guilt can come before the act, and that *feeling* guilty can be revealed as a cause as much as a consequence of particular deeds. Indeed, following the work of Herbert Fingarette, Leys defends a psychoanalytic conception of guilt against existentialist philosopher Martin Buber who considered the question of "real" guilt to be beyond the province of psychoanalytic enquiry: "there exists real guilt," Buber avers, "fundamentally different from all the anxiety-induced bug bears that are generated in the cavern of the unconscious."[67] For Buber, the moral destiny of man depends upon his standing in an *objective* relation to others. The gendering of this heroic transparency before the Other is probably not insignificant: the active as opposed to the neurotic mind, a legal reality as opposed to an unconscious motive, a man standing objectively in the world as opposed to a not-man entangled, dependent, or embattled by the extent of their identifications with and through others. By defending guilt on the basis of its emotional complexity rather than its objective facticity, Leys espouses a distinctively modern position. As James Brown points out in this volume, it was only in 1901– coincident with the rise of psychoanalysis – that guilt was first defined in the OED as a subjective *feeling*. Consequently, although Leys's intention seems to be to separate guilt from shame along an historical axis, and make the case for the moral complexity of guilt feelings as against the material literalism of shame, she is also contributing to a broader modern discourse in which it has become more and more difficult to distinguish the ostensible facticity of the former (guilty or not) from the affective intensity of latter. After all, the discursive turn to shame, and the affect theory that underlies it, is not the wholesale rejection of psychoanalysis which Leys depicts it as being; rather, as noted above, Tomkins's mid-century theory of the affects drew on traditions of post-Freudian psychoanalytic writing which emphasized the preoedipal mother-infant relation in particular. It may be, then, that instead of only literalizing the body and fixing the wound temporally and spatially in morally unsophisticated ways, shame also points us towards even more complex and disordered identifications unregulated by the traditional fable of oedipal contest between the law of the father and the son.

It is not only in the discourse of Holocaust testimony that the terms of guilt and shame have been disputed and conflated. In anthropology, too, shame and guilt have been said to define particular cultural formations. Writing in the 1930s, Margaret Mead found only two of what she called "guilt cultures" out of a selection of thirteen distinct "primitive peoples": two cultures, that is, whose ethos was competitive and/or individualistic (rather than cooperative) and therefore closer to the Western

European form.[68] The remaining eleven more cooperative cultures were more likely to be controlled by shame. A "shame culture," for Mead, is one in which "the individual is controlled by fear of being shamed, he is safe if no one knows of his misdeed." In guilt cultures, on the other hand, the individual must atone for his taboo deed in order to "reestablish the internal balance of the personality." Mead is careful to allow that shame cultures do not rely exclusively on external or group sanction: shame too, she writes, "can be internalized within the individual mind."[69] But the distinction remains categorical nonetheless, between a culture that believes in atonement – the ability to exchange one deed for another – and a culture that believes in the humiliation of character. The most famous amplification of Mead's distinction is Ruth Benedict's work of 1946, *The Chrysanthemum and the Sword*, a text which, even as it was produced on a war footing, tasked with accounting for the psyche of America's enemy, the Japanese, is careful not to attribute to its general distinction between shame and guilt cultures the status of incompatibility. Both Mead and Benedict, it must be said, though determining a contrast and even a contest in Benedict's case between shame and guilt, also rely on the modern convergence between the two terms: to speak of a guilt culture, after all, allows that guilt is felt and expressed rather than simply adjudicated. Perhaps it should not surprise us that a conceptual opposition belies some deeper ideological historical confusion, but it remains noteworthy nonetheless. For example, Benedict's historically incentivized research question *why do the Japanese not surrender?* is answered according to the dictates of shame: to surrender for a Japanese soldier would be to wear an ineradicable stain on one's character. The American soldier feels less shame at being captured. The implication is that the American soldier can forgive himself his capture because he knows a future deed is able to atone for it. Underlying this interpretation, however, is the additional premise that the American soldier is able to treat his own captivity *impersonally*, because he has, according to the structure of a guilt culture, abstracted himself from his own experience. By implication at least, he understands himself to be a unit of capital for exchange in an economy of indebtedness, and therefore bears less personal responsibility for his fate. We can discern in this example an unstated convergence between Benedict's understanding of guilt culture and Nietzschean and Weberian analyses of modern capitalism's structural alliance with Christianity. Considering the political asymmetry which underlies Benedict's guilt-shame opposition (remember American guilt culture has just emerged victorious from war), and the soft imperialism never far from the surface of her project, it is not difficult to read beneath her characterization of guilt culture, as favored for its dynamic means of atoning for past sins, a handbook for the expansion of global markets. Benedict professes admiration for the discipline and self-care of the average Japanese, but equally she praises the cunning of

General McArthur for how he has managed to flatter traditional Japanese attitudes the better to succeed with a modern political occupation. In other words, instead of being a conceptual distinction, the shame-guilt contest is fundamentally ideological, with the former term standing in for noncapitalist or "primitive" cultures, posing the problem of assimilation, and the latter for a dynamic and expressive modernity.

Read in this light, the title of our volume will seem oxymoronic: the more pertinent pairing would be *guilt and modern writing*. Certainly, this is how E.R. Dodds extrapolated from the Mead-Benedict tradition in his 1951 study of the Ancient Greeks.[70] What separates us Moderns from the culture of Sophocles and Euripides, contends Dodds in *The Greeks and The Irrational*, is the essential difference between our guilt and Greek shame. We might want to be careful about endorsing such an "us and them" formulation, however, because it has evolved by means of an alliance between anthropological scholarship and post-war *realpolitik*, and also because such categorical distinctions belie the contaminations of anthropological practice. Jennifer Biddle puts this second point well with reference to her work with the Warlpiri people:

> anthropologists intentionally put themselves in the out-of-place, in the wrong place, and thus, the place occupied by shame. Even if it is never taught in undergraduate courses, this is the first principle of the ethnographer's sensibility ... Field work, like shame, exalts self-difference.

Notwithstanding the fact that Benedict carried out no field work when writing *The Chrysanthemum and the Sword* – many of her major Japanese informants were acculturated Americans – Biddle's point is wholly pertinent to the shame culture discourse. If the anthropologist's major transgression is that of not looking away (a writerly transgression too we might surmise), then the discourse which formalizes and legitimizes the gaze is stimulating the shame it claims to uncover. In this context, Ukai Satoshi has written of the self-perpetuating identification of Japan as a "shame culture": Japan enters our globalized modernity with this reductive characteristic, known even to itself through such mediations from abroad.[71] But for Biddle there can be no atavistic retreat behind borders where one cannot be seen; it is not simply that anthropologists should be ashamed of themselves and desist with their practice, but rather that they should acknowledge shame as a way of addressing institutional impunity when it comes to knowledge production, and interrogate the always personal experience of shame's projective, mimetic and contagious characteristics.

Bernard Williams is another writer who has disputed the tidiness of the shame-guilt distinction. Though not an ideology critic, and in some sense offering a belated response to E.R. Dodds, the major point of Williams's argument in *Shame and Necessity*[72] is to challenge what he sees as the unhistorical privileging of guilt in the modern period.[73] Williams finds lodged within the Greek term aidôs (for Dodds the signifier of ancient shame) values which have become associated with guilt, including indignation, reparation and forgiveness.[74] If the ancients combined aspects of both guilt and shame, Williams surmises, then our modern guilt culture must also contain aspects of shame. Indeed, if we want to give the full picture of our ethical lives, we must make the effort to countenance shame. What is intriguing reading Williams's work today, which converges upon a dispute with a strict Kantian belief in the autonomy of the subject acting in accordance with a universalisable moral principle, is how the conclusion that shame and guilt cannot be kept decisively apart – either historically or psychologically – becomes itself a kind of ethical content. So, for example, considering the primacy of guilt as it turns us "towards victims" – enquiring about the harm done to others and the terms of reparation – Williams points out how such a guilt morality is only equipped to weigh voluntary or conscious actions. Only shame, he writes, can consider times when personal failings played a role in harming others where no harm was consciously intended. Only shame can square up to the involuntary or unconsciously motivated consequences of action, actions which seem more born of necessity than will. Thus, he writes, "shame can understand guilt, but guilt cannot understand itself."[75] Another way of putting this might be that shame is a necessary supplement to guilt. Of course, its concern with personal character, situated within a world of heteronomous attachments to others who bear witness to the self, conveying esteem and disappointment, can be read as narcissistic when pitched against the ideal of guilt culture's other-directed concern for the victim. Yet, as Williams concludes in the postscript to his book, once "guilt comes to be represented simply as the attitude of respect for an abstract law,"[76] removed in other words from consideration of personal anger or fear which produces actions and potentially victims, then its other-directed virtue is devoid of intimacy and sunk by its inflated estimation of the capacity of the rational autonomous mind to hold a moral purview of the world.[77] Put more bluntly than Williams puts it: a principle of justice once historically reified as a universal cultural value can be used to perpetuate rather than address the suffering of victims.

More recently in his work *The Color of Our Shame: Race and Justice in Our Time*, Christopher Lebron has shown how Williams's recuperation of shame's modernity might apply to the specific circumstance of race in America. Whilst we might easily imagine shame attaching itself to the racialized subject – the subject known according to her race – Lebron's study seeks to transfer this phenomenological or psychological fact into a kind of intellectual method: shame is a way to stipulate the difference between what is and what potentially might be the case within a given formal system of justice. In other words, instead of, as we might expect, appealing to the neutrality of the law (the idea that everyone is equal before the law) as a militation against the determination of character on racial grounds, Lebron suggests, following a Williams-like argument, that we use the question of character and shame in order to make sure the law functions. Like Williams, he offers critique of Kantian systems of morality, specifically John Rawls's distributive theory of justice which models fairness in strategic ignorance of historical conditions of subjectivity. The problem with Rawls's formal model is that although by its light it is unreasonable to defend slavery – and this, says Lebron, is in accordance with the contemporary practice and attitude of most law-abiding American citizens – it is not unreasonable to ignore the *effects* of slavery. This "reasonable ignorance," and the problem it infers, cannot be addressed according to a further appeal to the law – by a subscription to a rule of distribution however stringent – but only by returning us to the ethics of shame. Such an ethics "implicates us in coming up short on our own account, on account of principles and standards for which we have expressed a prior standing preference."[78] In other words, shame isolates the difference between the formality of the law to which we adhere and the fulfillment of social justice which the law might possibly permit. Instead of eradicating shame, then, Lebron wants to generalize it and put it to work: all Americans should be ashamed, which, in the specific case, is to say all Americans should be racialized insofar as they have not actualized the equality written into their law.

Those writing in a critical postcolonial perspective will find little to surprise them in Lebron's argument, except perhaps his philosopher's faith in the law's ultimate consistency. For Timothy Bewes in his 2011 study *The Event of Postcolonial Shame*, the historical play of identity and difference is the organizing principle of both shame and colonialism, extending to all scholarly ethnographies and underlying too the production and persistence of race, which interrupts the purely formal value of the law.[79] Whereas for Lebron shame is a goad working within the terms of the law, as a means of realizing its formal promise of equality, for Bewes shame can only produce the rupture of form and content.[80] Through shame – in the "event" of shame – all formal strategies of representation are rendered inadequate. It is telling that for Bewes, "shame is an event of writing."[81] Pointing both to Holocaust testimony and to contemporary postcolonial literature, he says that we don't simply write *about* shameful scenes that once happened, or happened over there, giving them a frame and a salutary meaning which can be represented here and now; rather, we encounter shame by and through writing as the inadequacy of the frame and the collapse of meaning. It's not simply that the content of the experience being described exceeds the form of its description (those unspeakable horrors, etc.), but rather that through this excess shame is communicated.[82] Shame is an event which produces between the writer-subject and her object the thought of the absence of form.[83] This is an important shift, from content to form (lessness), because it reminds us, in the first place, that the shame of a destitute other must rebound upon her witness; and in the second place, because it reveals that at the heart of the conceit of formally objectifying experience – *doing justice* to things – lies an unredeemable subjectivity and a perspective founded on exclusion and ignorance.

Bewes's reading of shame as a formal concern, especially pertinent for the ethnographic quandaries of postcoloniality, returns us to the obscure terms of inclusion and exclusion which constitute the field of representation. Given this emphasis on the political margins of form, the point at which it breaks down, we might suggest that his study underplays the importance of sexuality, especially as questions concerning the communicability of lived experience and the instability of social relations across political boundaries often come to express their irresolution through the ambiguity of sex. Queer theory's formative engagement with shame comes through Sedgwick's essay "Shame, Theatricality and Queer Performativity" in which she characterizes its double movement, "painful individuation" and "uncontrollable relationality," as, for queer people, the first structuring fact of identity – identity however without the secure standing of an essence.[84] In broader social terms, queer shame has come to query the politics of gay pride (it is "pride's otherwise" in David M. Halperin and Valerie Traub's language) where pride is seen to appeal for legitimation to the political center, and to be tending, in this way, towards assimilation within normative power structures. Shame is productive, in Sedgwick's unapologetically literary sensibility, when there exists a recognition that accompanying its pain is the possibility opened up by non-assimilation and by the excitement of unsanctioned pleasures. This is no resting place, however, since, even allowing for shame's queer pleasure, the politics of shaming – the asymmetric power relations shame too often implies – persist.

The tension between queer and more conventional political readings of shame is well represented in the anthology *Gay Shame*, edited by Halperin and Traub.[85] This volume risks becoming exemplary for how it showcases its own shame as an institutionally sanctioned writing project. Not only does it advertise its own shortcomings and dismemberments (those writers who refused on political grounds to be included in the publication) but the terms of inclusion and exclusion become quite uncertain as particular contributors insist on expressing within the work their exception from it. As the editors explain in the Introduction, they had conceived the original academic conference "in such a way as to make the prospect of publishing the proceedings unlikely, if not impossible," for reasons of scope and inclusivity: the ambition to connect queer scholarship to broad social movements, and to encourage the involvement of different nonacademic groups including sex workers and local activists.[86] The feeling that we are indeed reading writing that should have been impossible, a form annulling itself in the event – in this case the event of the original conference – emerges most obviously through two pieces included in the volume which are *almost* not there. The first is entitled "An Open Letter to Douglas Crimp" (not an academic paper) by Lawrence La Fountain-Stokes, quoted in full in the editors' introduction. La Fountain-Stokes addresses Crimp's reading of Andy Warhol's "Screen Test #2" in which the drag queen Mario Montez is objectified and humiliated. For Crimp, Warhol's film is not simply voyeuristic but "shows a performer in the moment of being exposed"; in Mario's "irresistible, resplendent vulnerability" (73) we witness his shame, but "a shame that we accept as also ours, but curiously ours alone."[87] The erotics of this contagion are rebuked by La Fountain-Stokes for the way its abject heroism for shame entirely neglects, renders invisible, Mario Montez's race. Does it matter that it is a nonwhite body being shamed? And who are we to witness, and narcissistically appropriate, this shame for ourselves, in our strange isolation? Are we inevitably white – as white as Andy Warhol? As a corrective to such assumptions, La Fountain-Stokes invokes the racially alert and consciousness-raising shame writing of Frantz Fanon and Audre Lorde, among others, and stipulates the specificity of Munoz's identity (performative or not) as a queer Puerto Rican. The second nearly absent contribution is that of Leo Bersani who in his less-than-a-page contribution, as well as expressing his "disappointment" with the conference, takes the opposite view from La Fountain-Stokes. For Bersani, Crimp's paper was the only genuine attempt to consider shame in its "psychic dimensions." For too many, he writes, the politically correct interpretation offers itself: shame is imposed from without by "evil heterosexism" which it is in all our interests, and all our pleasures, to overcome.[88]

There is something unsettled about the conception of shame which emerges from this debate: marking on one side the productivity of non-assimilation in the lives of queer subjects and on the other the effect of political reduction and oppression along the lines of race. This conflict is further explored by Judith Halberstam, who attended the conference but refused publication of her paper within the volume. Halberstam professes "gay shame" an anachronistic idea, suspecting that "shame" prefers white male subjects abjecting themselves before history; it is, she suggests, the feeling of castration, a powerlessness akin to feeling feminized against their will which excites the authority of white gay shame.[89] For Halberstam, the specter of the shamed other (non-white, non-male) means that questions of race necessarily intersect with those of sex and gender.

This position resonates with Biddle's point, mentioned above, regarding anthropology and the taboo on looking – the transgression of crossing borders which, she remarks, is also always sexualized.[90] Biddle adds that when anthropology is shown up or shamed in this way, shown up to be less than objective, the fact that the "best known anthropological practitioner is a woman" is by no means adventitious: "infamous indeed is Margaret Mead, with all the sexual and sexist undertones implied; conjoined as she and her work have become where the travel, the exotic places, her various husbands and lovers and sex itself, metonymically all unite."[91] It is the ideological canard of "Woman" here who is at once shameless enough to dare to look, and crippled by shame, othered by her involvement in a foreign element. Shamed or shameless, Mead, in this view, is not given the license granted to gay white men of *experimenting* with the erotics of contagion. Halberstam argues that "shame for women, and shame for people of color plays out in different ways and creates different modes of abjection, marginalization, and self-abnegation; it also leads to very different political strategies": these, she concludes, are structural rather than ego-based.[92] The details of this politics are not spelt out, though it is clear that Halberstam is unhappy with the diversity and extent of the shame archive as it currently exists.

Jessica Berman has recently asked "Is the Trans in Transnational the Trans in Transgender?" concluding that the comparison is at least worth making if bodies crossing borders are also, necessarily, bodies reconfigured.[93] The further question, one which emerges through trans discourse, is *how* these bodies get reconfigured and whether they are readable in their complexity as such? If, in one story, the white man ventures abroad, encountering there the queer, painful excitement of castration, then, in another story, it is up to the not-(white)man to interrupt that journey and put an end to the perennial *Fort Da!* of a man playing with his penis. A woman is not a man, but, as Simone de Beauvoir once reminded us, neither is she a eunuch.[94] It is by re-addresing the archive of women's experiences, therefore – experiences of subjects who are neither phallically endowed, nor *fixed* by the logic of deficiency – that we can arrive seriously at the task of transition. If, in one story, ours is the age of shame, in another story, according to Halberstam and others, including contributors featured below, it might yet become the age of shame giving way to something else.

This book does not propose to formulate shame as a single idea or concept – hence the diversity of theoretical approaches to the topic – though it does contend, as the foregoing account of overlapping discourses suggests, that, for good or ill, shame has come to bear considerable cultural weight in the modern period. The essays that follow connect shame to the character of the writing self representing her own failure to write; to the blurring of the distinction between legal and psychological conceptions of guilt; and to various modern critical projects – postcolonial and feminist – which insist on the historical character of the law and the violent imperatives of looking and framing and reproducing knowledge. Organized in rough chronological order, the essays provide something of a genealogy of shame's modernity as it infiltrates the practice of writing, beginning with Montaigne and Shakespeare, moving through Rousseau and into the twentieth and twenty-first centuries. Because shame troubles the object of institutional knowledge, and because the writers writing here are working in some form within American or European institutions, we end with a series of reflections on the university, and academic writing as it is practiced today.

Notes

1 Jean-Jacques Lecercle, *The Violence of Language* (London: Routledge, 1990), 229.
2 "One does not speak [or write] *of* things or states of affairs, one speaks *in the midst* of states of affairs ('à même les états de choses')" (Ibid., 226).
3 Jon Ronson's popular book *So You've Been Publically Shamed* (Picador, 2015) makes explicit the role of the internet in the contemporary instrumentalization of shame as a moral tool, or as a failure of judicious impersonality in debate. In this volume, Martin Eve considers how the internet has shaped the publishing norms of academic writing.
4 Locatable as a symptom of so-called post-truth politics, one of Trump's signature declarations "you are fake news," brings to mind Brian Massumi's analysis of the "affective means" through which Ronald Reagan maintained his leadership:

> It wasn't that people didn't hear his verbal fumbling or recognize the incoherence of his thoughts. ... He was a communicative jerk. ... Reagan transmitted vitality, virtuality, tendency, in sickness and interruption. ... Reagan was many things to many people, but always within a general framework of affective jingoism. Confidence is the apotheosis of affective capture.
>
> Brian Massumi, Parables for the Virtual: Movement, Affect, Sensation (Duke University Press, 2001), 41–42

5 Michel Foucault, *Security, Territory, Population: Lectures at the Collège de France, 1977–1978*, ed. Michel Senellart and trans. G. Burchell (New York: Picador, 2007); *The Birth of Biopolitics: Lectures at the Collège de France, 1978–1979*, ed. Michel Senellart and trans. G. Burchell (London: Palgrave Macmillan, 2008).
6 Patricia Ticineto Clough and Jean Halley, eds., *The Affective Turn: Theorizing the Social* (Durham, NC and London: Duke University Press, 2007); Melissa Gregg and Gregory J. Seigworth, eds., *The Affect Theory Reader* (Durham, NC and London: Duke University Press, 2010).
7 Jonathan Flatley, for example, writes that whereas "*emotion* suggests something that happens inside and tends toward outward expression, *affect* indicates something relational and transformative." See Jonathan Flatley, *Affective Mapping: Melancholia and the Politics of Modernism* (Harvard University Press, 2008), 12. Sara Ahmed, however, has argued convincingly against positing a clean distinction between emotion and affect, not least because the "contrast between a mobile impersonal affect and a contained personal emotion suggests that the affect/emotion distinction can operate as a gendered distinction." See Sara Ahmed, *The Cultural Politics of Emotion*, 2nd ed. (Edinburgh University Press, 2014), 207.
8 Patricia Ticineto Clough, *Autoaffection: Unconscious Thought in the Age of Technology* (Minneapolis: Minnesota Press, 2000); Massumi, Op. cit.
9 Eve Kosofsky Sedgwick and Adam Frank, eds., *Shame and Its Sisters: A Silvan Tomkins Reader* (Durham, NC and London: Duke University Press, 1995).
10 Ahmed offers a necessary reminder *vis-à-vis* Tomkins: it is not enough to say that cultural scripts channel our biological affects in certain directions, we must also admit that cultural scripts – the script of the stranger, say – *generate* affects, including shame, by creating general receptacles for affect using historically particular images: is the black face more strange than the white face; and is it therefore more "natural" that I attach the affect

of fear there? "Sticky" is the term Ahmed uses to designate the emotional *and* affective dimensions which underlie all research. We are attached to our knowledge in various complicated and complicit ways.

11 Massumi, Op. cit., 35.
12 Jacques Derrida, *The Animal That Therefore I Am*, trans. David Wills (New York: Fordham University Press, 2009); Elspeth Probyn, *Blush: Faces of Shame* (Minneapolis: Minnesota University Press, 2005); Eve Kosofky Sedgwick, *Touching, Feeling: Affect, Pedagogy, Performativity* (Durham, NC and London: Duke University Press, 2003).
13 Dodie Bellamy, *When the Sick Rule the World* (South Pasadena, CA: Semiotext(e), 2015), 53, 55.
14 John M. Coetzee, *Disgrace* (London: Secker & Warburg, 1999).
15 Ranjana Khanna has spelt out some of the intricacies of shame's grammar in the following passage:

> Is it always in response to a regulative ideal? Is it constituted through that regulation? Or is it organic? Is it a state in itself, or is it a dynamic entity even if not always public in the most literal sense? Whether verb (to shame) or noun (shame) one has to consider whether some kind of action is involved in both. Is it transitive or intransitive? Reflexive or not? Does its action pass over to an object or not? Is it a response to an object, or a function of being-in-the-world?
>
> Ranjana Khanna, "Fabric, skin, *honte*-ologie," in *Shame and Sexuality: Psychoanalysis and Visual Culture*, eds. Claire Pajaczkowska and Ivan Ward (Hove: Routledge, 2008), 159–179

16 Constable argues that the experience of shame

> needs to be understood as both an *intrapsychic* and *intersubjective* lens through which a sense of belonging is magnified or shattered, an affect intensely linked to what it means to belong, to the processes of fitting in, as well as to those of becoming a misfit.
>
> E. L. Constable, "Introduction: States of Shame," *L'Esprit Créateur* 39, no. 4 (1999: 3–12), 6

17 Jean-Paul Sartre, *Being and Nothingness: An Essay on Phenomenological Ontology*, trans. Hazel E. Barnes (Oxon: Routledge Classics, 2003 [1943]), 282.
18 Ibid., 284–285, 291. We can note that Sartre seems to share with the poet William Blake the intuition that "Shame is Prides cloke." William Blake, "The Proverbs of Hell," in *The Complete Poetry and Prose of William Blake*, ed. David V. Erdman (Berkley: University of California Press, 2008), 36.
19 Sartre, Op. cit., 284.
20 Emmanuel Lévinas, *On Escape [De l'évasion]*, trans. Bettina Bergo (Stanford, CA: Stanford University Press, 2003 [1935]), 67.
21 Silvan Tomkins in Sedgwick and Frank, *Shame and Its Sisters*, 134.
22 Eve Kosofsky Sedgwick and Adam Frank, "Shame in the Cybernetic Fold," in *Shame and Its Sisters: A Silvan Tomkins Reader*, eds. Eve Kosofsky Sedgwick and Adam Frank (Durham, NC: Duke University Press, 1995; 1–28), 3.
23 Silvan Tomkins, "Shame-Humiliation and Contempt-Disgust," in *Shame and Its Sisters*, eds. Eve Kosofsky Sedgwick and Adam Frank (Durham, NC: Duke University Press, 1995: 133–178), 152.
24 See also W. Ray Crozier's, "The Blush: Literary and Psychological Perspectives," *The Theory of Social Behaviour* 46, no. 4 (2016: 502–516), 503.

25 George Eliot, *Daniel Deronda* (Oxford: Oxford University Press, 2014), 354.

26 Massumi, Op. cit., 25.

27 Sigmund Freud, *Civilization and Its Discontents* in The Standard Edition of the Complete Psychological Works of Sigmund Freud, vol. XXI (London: The Hogarth Press and the Institute of Psycho-analysis, 1961 [1930]), 99.

28 Giorgio Agamben, "Nudity," in *Nudities*, trans. David Kishik and Stefan Pedatella (Stanford, CA: Stanford University Press, 2010), 55–90.

29 Ibid., 68.

30 Ibid., 74.

31 Helen Merell Lynd, "The Nature of Shame," in *Guilt and Shame*, ed. Herbert Morris (Belmont, CA: Wadsworth Publishing Company, 1971: 159–202), 160.

32 Jacqueline Rose, *On Not Being Able to Sleep: Psychoanalysis and the Modern World* (London: Chatto and Windus, 2003), 4. Another way of framing this point is that metonymy, which Roman Jakobson famously considered the major device of realist fiction, nominating the synecdochic details used by Tolstoy as exemplary (Anna Karenina's handbag, the bare shoulders of a female character in *War and Peace*), breaks down as the physical part begins to confound the organizing intelligence of the narrator who wanted to put everything into symbolic relation (Roman Jakobson, *Fundamentals of Language*, 2nd ed. (Berlin and New York: Mouton de Gruyter, 2002 [1956]), 90–96).

33 Socially and narratively speaking (in terms of modest witness) the blush is both a defense against, but also an oblique invitation to the Other's desire. It is also synesthetic, where synesthesia originally, in physiological discourse, referred to a stimulation applied to one part of the body felt in another. The blush we might say is exemplarily synesthetic since it registers a feeling or sensation whose cause is almost never treated organically, or localized etiologically in the face; rather, it is overwhelmingly taken up and transferred within a cultural and symbolic network of interpretations which render its material sensation essentially immaterial, or "merely psychological," and carefully translates the priapic exhibitionism of a red face into the socialized and veiling terms: coy, shy, modest, shrinking violet. The idealized "polite society," a society of sensible subjects – which is to say, subjects who have acquired sensibility – depends on some degree of synesthetic acumen in order to organize the appropriate distance between bodies.

34 Kafka cited in Lynd, Op. cit., 164.

35 Eve Kosofsky Sedgwick, "Shame, Theatricality, and Queer Performativity: Henry James's *The Art of the Novel*," in *Touching Feeling: Affect, Pedagogy, Performativity* (London and Durham, NC: Duke University Press, 2003: 35–66), 44.

36 More fully, Foucault says:

> Here, giving an account of your life, your *bios*, is also not to give a narrative of the historical events that have taken place in your life, but rather to demonstrate whether you are able to show that there is a relation between the rational discourse, the *logos*, you are able to use and the way that you live.
>
> Michel Foucault, *Fearless Speech*, ed. Joseph Pearson
> (Los Angeles, CA: Semiotext(e), 2001), 97

37 For example, the scandalous truth-telling of Diogenes the Cynic does not reverberate in the following contemporary scene of public display offered by Sedgwick:

> I used to ask listeners to join in a thought experiment, visualizing an unwashed, half-insane man who would wander into the lecture hall mumbling loudly, his speech increasingly accusatory and disjointed, and publically urinate in the front of the room, then wander out again. I pictured the excruciation of everyone else in the room: each looking down, wishing to be anywhere else yet conscious of the inexorable fate of being exactly there, inside the individual skin of which each was burningly aware; at the same time, though, unable to stanch the hemorrhage of painful identification with the misbehaving man. That's the double movement shame makes: towards painful individuation, toward uncontrollable relationality.
>
> Sedgwick, "Shame, Theatricality, and Queer Performativity," 37

38 In his lectures on "The Courage of Truth," Foucault identifies the transformation of parrhēsia within Christian discourse, wherein, most tellingly, parrhēsia came to mean, as well as critique, a confidence and open heartedness toward God; a "trembling obedience" in the mode of confession. Michel Foucault, *The Courage of Truth: The Government of Self and Others II, Lectures at the Collège de France 1983–1984*, ed. F. Gros and trans. G. Burchell (Basingstoke: Palgrave, 2011), 332–333.

39 See the following Guardian piece from 2015 for a discussion of Knausgaard's conviction that "writing is a way of getting rid of shame": (www.theguardian.com/books/2015/mar/01/karl-ove-knausgaard-interview-shame-dancing-in-the-dark) [accessed 1 October 2017].

40 Karl Ove Knausgaard, *My Struggle, Vol. 1: A Death in the Family*, trans. Don Bartlett (London: Vintage Books, 2013), 24.

41 Karl Ove Knausgaard, *My Struggle, Vol 2: A Man in Love*, trans. by Don Bartlett (London: Vintage Books, 2013): 496–497.

42 Gilles Deleuze, "Literature and Life," trans. Daniel W. Smith and Michael A. Greco. *Critical Inquiry* 23, no. 2 (Winter, 1997: 225–230): 225.

43 Ibid., 225–226.

44 Though we would do well to note that the offending line from Freud's 1933 lecture "Femininity" allows the cultural forces of "convention" to stand alongside anything that could be called feminine essence: "Shame, which is considered to be a feminine characteristic *par excellence* but is far more a matter of convention than might be supposed, has as its purpose, we believe, concealment of genital deficiency." Sigmund Freud, "Femininity," *The Standard Edition of the Complete Psychological Works of Sigmund Freud, Volume XXII (1932–1936): New Introductory Lectures on Psycho-Analysis and Other Works*, 1–182: 132.

45 For recent exploration of gendered shame see *The Female Face of Shame*, eds. Erica L. Johnson and Patricia Moran (Bloomington and Indianapolis: Indiana University Press, 2003).

46 Liz Constable, "Shame," *MLN* 112, no. 4 (1997: 641–665): 643; Christopher Lebron, *The Color of Our Shame: Race and Justice in Our Time* (New York: Oxford University Press, 2013); Jennifer Biddle, "Shame," *Australian Feminist Studies* 12, no. 26 (1997): 227–239; Martha C. Nussbaum, *Hiding from Humanity: Disgust, Shame and the Law* (Princeton, NJ: Princeton University Press, 2004); Jennifer Jacquet, *Is Shame Necessary? New Uses for an Old Tool* (Allen Lane and Penguin Random House, 2015).

47 David M. Halperin and Valerie Traub, "Beyond Gay Pride," in *Gay Shame*, eds. David M. Halperin and Valerie Traub (Chicago, IL: The University of Chicago Press, 2009: 3–40), 3; Francis Broucek, "Shame and Its Relationship to Early Narcissistic Developments," *International Journal of Psycho-Analysis* 63 (1982: 369–378): 369 (cited in Sedgwick and Frank, Op. cit., 6); Thomas Scheff, "Shame in Self and Society," *Symbolic Interaction* 26, no. 2 (2003: 239–262): 239.

48 Timothy Bewes, *The Event of Postcolonial Shame* (Princeton, NJ: Princeton University Press, 2011); Giorgio Agamben, "Shame, or On the Subject," in *Remnants of Auschwitz: The Witness and the Archive*, trans. Daniel Heller-Roazen (New York: Zone Books, 2002), 87–136.

49 Rob Halpern, *Common Place* (Brooklyn, NY and New York: Ugly Duckling Press, 2015). We are grateful to Marc Botha for this connection. See Marc Botha, "Toward a Critical Poetics of Securitization: A response to Anker, Castronovo, Harkins, Masterson, and Williams," *American Literary History*, 28.4, no. 1 (2016: 779–786). Botha also has further work on the subject forthcoming.

50 Halpern, Op. cit., 32.

51 Ibid., 23.

52 Ibid., 31.

53 Ibid., 137–138.

54 Charles Darwin, "Self-attention – Shame – Shyness – Modesty: Blushing," in *The Expression of the Emotions in Man and Animals* (Chicago, IL: The University of Chicago Press, 1965 [1872]: 309–346), 309.

55 Ibid., 313.

56 Sally Munt, *Queer Attachments: The Cultural Politics of Shame* (Aldershot, UK: Ashgate, 2008) 6.

57 Agamben, "Shame, or On the Subject," 103.

58 Ibid., 105.

59 Ibid., 106.

60 Ibid., 134.

61 Though there is an emerging archive of Guantánamo poetry (see, for example, *Poems from Guantánamo: The Detainees Speak*, ed. by Mark Falkoff (University of Iowa Press, 2007); and for critical commentary on such an archive, Judith Butler's *Frames of War: When Is Life Greivable?* (Verson Books, 2009).

62 Ruth Leys, *From Guilt to Shame: Auschwitz and After* (Princeton, NJ: Princeton University Press, 2007).

63 Ibid., 178.

64 Ibid., 176.

65 For the broader contours of Leys's critique, see her "The Turn to Affect: A Critique," *Critical Inquiry* 27, no. 3 (2011): 434–472.

66 Leys, *From Guilt to Shame*, 60.

67 Martin Buber, "Guilt and Guilt Feelings," in *Guilt and Shame*, ed. Herbert Morris (Belmont, CA: Wadsworth Publishing Company, 1971: 59–81), 67.

68 Margaret Mead, "Interpretive Statement," in *Cooperation and Competition among Primitive Peoples*, ed. Margaret Mead (Boston, MA: Beacon Press, 1961: 548–515), 494.

69 Ibid.

70 Eric R. Dodds, *The Greeks and the Irrational* (Los Angeles: University of California Press, 1951).

71 Ukai Satoshi, "The Future of an Affect: The Historicity of Shame," in *Traces: A Multilingual Journal of Cultural Theory*, eds. Naoki Sakai and

Yukiko Hanawa (Ithaca, NY: Cornell University, Distributed by Hong Kong University Press, 2001), 3–36. We are grateful to Geoff Gilbert for bringing this coordinate to our attention.

72 Bernard Williams, *Shame and Necessity* (Berkeley: University of California Press, 2008 [1993]).

73 As Williams puts it, "The mere fact that we have two words does not, in itself, imply that there is any great psychological difference between shame and guilt" (Ibid., 89). It is significant in light of our previous discussion that for Williams shame and guilt are both feelings – or psychological states – and, what's more, feelings that may prove difficult if not impossible to distinguish.

74 Ibid., 90–91.

75 Ibid., 93.

76 Ibid., 222.

77 Williams's claim for the "heteronomy" of shame – shame as produced through situated relations and often through non-intentional acts – shares a strange affinity with Brian Massumi's argument, noted above, for the *autonomy* of affect where all affects including shame are seen to be triggered independently of intentional objects. Both accounts privilege situated, embodied subjects, whilst challenging the primacy of a rationally directed conception of human agency.

78 Lebron, Op. cit., 22.

79 Bewes, *The Event of Postcolonial Shame*, 165–166.

80 Ibid., 20.

81 Ibid., 15.

82 Ibid., 39.

83 Ibid., 46.

84 Sedgwick, "Shame, Theatricality, and Queer Performativity," 37.

85 David M. Halperin and Valerie Traub, eds., *Gay Shame* (Chicago, IL: The University of Chicago Press, 2009).

86 Ibid., 5.

87 Douglas Crimp, "Mario Montez, For Shame," in *Gay Shame*, eds. David M. Halperin and Valerie Traub (Chicago, IL: The University of Chicago Press, 2009: 63–75), 73.

88 Leo Bersani, "Excluding Shame," in *Gay Shame*, eds. David M. Halperin and Valerie Traub (Chicago, IL: The University of Chicago Press, 2009: 176–177), 176.

89 Judith Halberstam, "Shame and White Gay Masculinity," *Social Text* 23, nos. 3–4 (2005: 219–234), 226.

90 Biddle, Op. cit., 232–233.

91 Ibid.

92 Halberstam, Op. cit., 223.

93 Jessica Berman, "Is the Trans in Transnational the Trans in Transgender?," *Modernism/Modernity* 24, no. 2 (2017), 217–244.

94 Famously, de Beauvoir writes,

> One is not born, but rather becomes, a woman. No biological, psychological, or economic fate determines the figure that the human female presents in society; it is civilization as a whole that produces this creature, intermediate between male and eunuch, which is described as feminine.
>
> Simone de Beauvoir, *The Second Sex*, trans. and ed. H. M. Parshley (Harmondsworth, Middlesex: Penguin Books, 1987[1949]), 295

2 Montaigne's Writing

"Honteux Insolent"?

Elizabeth Guild

Michel de Montaigne's "De l'oisiveté" (Of idleness) ends with a memorable description of anxiety, its turmoil and enigmatic self-estrangement. The traces of melancholy in the *Essais* have already been widely, vividly discussed, unlike both this anxiety and the other affect with which the chapter ends. "Esperant avec le temps luy [sc. mon esprit] en faire honte à luy mesmes" (hoping in time to make my mind ashamed of itself) (33/25): shame, to be produced by writing.[1] But if writing will restore both hope and the future, why would shame, that searing sense of inescapable, mortifying overexposure and unacceptability, an affect used to humiliate or exclude, be desired? Even if shame may be a positive index of interrelatedness (that is, as a condition of both ethics and communication), this does not mean that we desire it. Writing – ordering, recording – may well reduce anxiety; however, Montaigne hopes to shame himself, rather than feel free of shame. How he understands his mind's relationship with itself and what this has to do with intersubjectivity, conventionally the dimension of shame, here seems as enigmatic as the "chimères et monstres" (chimeras and monsters) (33/25) of his anxiety.

The relationship between anxiety, shame and writing invites exploration, using a psychoanalytic approach attentive to the dimension beyond conscious intention and knowledge inhabited by the chimeras and monsters, to supplement decisive accounts of shame such as those of Sartrean ontology or Lévinasian ethics.[2] Lévinas insists on shame's intersubjective nature, recalling us to responsibility and fraternity. He offers a more intricate, other-inhabited model of the self than Sartre's, therefore seeming more akin to Montaigne's preoccupations in the *Essais*. However, Lévinas's shame is not hoped for. On the contrary: shame still chains us to our 'identity in a way that forecloses any future that could be otherwise.'[3]

The puzzling hope for shame shares something of the enigma in Montaigne's self-description in "De l'inconstance de nos actions" (Of the inconsistency of our actions) as being "honteux insolent" (ashamed insolent) (335, my translation). In what follows, I shall draw two strands together. On the one hand, how the enigmas just mentioned may be connected in his writing, which is *insolens* (Lat.) in the sense of being beyond what is accustomed or acceptable, and shaming. On the other, that puzzle: ashamed, we prefer concealment, and we also prefer to be shame-free; but Montaigne writes against both. That his writing is intermittently avowedly "confessional" only partly explains this. The orthodox religious apparatus of confession worked to both absolve from and produce shame and the desire to repent; Montaigne's "confession" works otherwise. It is the vehicle for freedom from a repenting relationship with himself, and therefore a different form of both self-relation and self-understanding. In what Montaigne has to say about shame, and in how he risks writing, he hopes for a revalued sense of shame; not overdetermining and corrosive, not yet realized but potentially reachable ("esperant," hoping) as a positive and transforming affect. It belongs to a different epistemology and ethics. To trace this, I shall focus initially on shame and some textual instances of it, then move on to confession and its relation to those enigmatic chimeras and monsters, and what Montaigne dares or risks; last, if we read the chapter as a form of preface, its closing words invite us to wonder what this desire for shame implies for us as readers.

Existing readings of the end of "De l'oisiveté" (Of idleness) elucidate the melancholy Montaigne will write himself out of, the inanition of "oisiveté ennuyeuse" (tedious idleness) (I, 39, 241/215), the ethical concerns, the writing's performativity here and the desire to give form to imagination's boundless flow, which still threatens to exceed articulation, requiring repeated returns to the version of himself he wants to represent. In "De l'inconstance de nos actions" (Of the inconsistency of our actions) he reflects on his turbulent inconsistency, for which his initial focus on "variation et contradiction" cannot altogether account. The "vent des accidens" (wind of accident) (II, 1, 335/293) and his capacity to trouble himself intensify his instability, which is further amplified by his changing perspectives on himself. He declares himself a container of contradictions. "Honteux insolent, chaste luxurieux, bavard taciturne ... menteur veritable, savant ignorant" (ashamed insolent, chaste lascivious, talkative taciturn ... lying truthful, learned ignorant).[4] These contradictions imply a different epistemology and ethics; the subject cannot conform to a logic that presupposes either wholeness or stability, exceeds full knowledge and lacks a perspective from which ethical judgment could be formed. As the Tournon edition's punctuation vividly reminds us, the list is *written* to dramatize how the concept of "contrarietez" (contradictions) (335/294) limits self-understanding: the intriguing contradiction of "honteux, insolent" (ashamed, insolent) (Villey-Saulnier, 335) as "honteux insolent" (ashamed insolent) becomes quite other. What is the continuity between shame, what is shaming and "insolent" – in its historical sense of going beyond acceptable limits? Others have already brilliantly explored the implications for repentance of Montaigne's epistemology of the mobile, inconsistent self; but not for shame.[5] If we never arrive at the point of self-understanding required for true repentance, what of the place of our own shame? And why may writing offer access to this?

Montaigne's writing delights in the most elastic of "rolles" (registers (33/25), an anti-Ciceronian aesthetic of "sauts et gambades" (leaps and gambols) (III, 9, 994/925) which remains "desreglé" (irregular) (I, 26, 172/154)); this is the form of writing's mimesis of oral language, "rouler au vent, ou à le sembler" (tossed in the wind, or seem to be) (994/925). It is unabashedly "bigarré" (motley) (994/925) in its lack of generic conformity, its thematic changeability and volatility, its (impossible) merging of speech and writing and its unconventional rhetorical splore. Montaigne's descriptors of all this include such conventionally shaming words as "si frivole et si vain" (so frivolous and vain) (Au Lecteur/To the reader, 3/2), "vile" (abject) (II, 8, 385, my translation), "bas" (low) (II, 6, 379/333), "fagotage" (heap) (II, 37, 758, my translation), 'flux de caquet' (flow of babble) (III, 5, 897/831) and "excremens" (excrements) (III, 9, 946/876). Striking words for writing that thoroughly engages us: not to be tidied away as instances of knowing irony, but rather, persistently both unsettling and seductive. But Montaigne is neither shame-free, nor is this an aspect of shameless melancholy, with its "almost opposite habit of insistent communicativeness which finds satisfaction in self-exposure" driven by self-loathing;[6] even if Montaigne was melancholy, his self-exposure is not the melancholic's self-accusatory refrain. Despite his pose of wanting to risk self-exposure on the page, he suffers as much conventional genital shame as the next man, and more profoundly dishonorable situations also shame him; he also actively seeks shame, through the act of writing.

Whilst shame's meaning in the text is not yet clear, we might agree that the word declares ethical interests. But ethics per se are no cure for anxiety or melancholy. Perhaps they alleviate shame? The dimension of cure is in the process of writing, rereading, rewriting, etc. and in the commitment to openness: "oser dire tout ce que j'ose faire" (to dare to say all that I dare to do) (III, 5, 845/778), the risky speech that for some makes Montaigne a *parrhēsiast*. I shall return to "oser," and *parrhēsia*; but first, another comment in "Mourning and Melancholia" seems relevant. The melancholic has a "keener eye for the truth than other people who are not melancholics … we only wonder why a man has to be ill before he can be accessible to a truth of this kind" (246) – truth as in disillusioned realizations.

Diagnosing Montaigne is no one's business; but whatever the cause, Montaigne's writing is disillusioned and disillusioning. Melancholy? Or related to love and its loss, and to shame? Love of La Boétie, his death; a qualified love for his father, also lost. These losses, particularly the first, may have been catalysts for the disquiet Montaigne found when he retreated from public life, and thereafter for his writing; no need to dwell on this further here. Instead, let me turn to what Martha Nussbaum calls "love's knowledge," which returns us insightfully to the theme of shame. In an essay on the *Symposium* Nussbaum traces out the discovery of "vulnerability to contingency through love" (174), and pauses (189) on Alcibiades' comment: "and with this man alone I have an experience which no one else would believe was possible for me – the sense of shame" (216A).[7] Alcibiades loves Socrates; through love he encounters the "terrifying and painful awareness of being perceived" (188): shame. This is the existential and ethical cost of being known, and implicitly, philosophy is asked what it thinks about it. Also staged is the contingency known through love – awareness of lack, of dependency on another imperfect being and of vulnerability to our own passions and their capacity to befuddle rational thinking. But through this comes awareness of amplifications of thinking and being; also, that certain things remain unknowable without this experience of contingency and what here is called "shame."

Do Not Betray Your Cause

The unbearable nature of the judgment (imagined as) located in the other's eyes is a staple of discussions of shame as primarily a social phenomenon. However, the shame invoked in "De l'oisiveté" (Of idleness) seems either internal, or suggests that Montaigne thinks of the other as inhabiting him more profoundly than sociological or everyday construction recognizes. That we internalize the other or others, or that it is the Other that makes us who we think we are, are not new ideas. But the othered self most active when shame takes hold needs further analysis. I shall take this in two steps: first, notions of shame inherited but not necessarily shared by Montaigne; second, what his distinctive usage, and what he risks, suggest about shame's place in his writing and self-exploration. A third step, from "do not betray your cause," to "be true to your desire" (for shame) forms my final section.

A shift from concealment to self-disclosure, to a nakedness free of Christian associations, "oser dire tout ce que j'ose faire" (to dare to say all that I dare to do) (III, 5, 845/778), does not adequately account for the shame in question; "dire" and "faire" leave undisclosed the unconscious or prereflective dimension of his being. It is also at odds with the function of Montaigne's "confession." For instance, Montaigne confesses no shame for breaking his promise to the dying La Boétie to publish the *Discours de la servitude volontaire* (*Discourse on Voluntary Servitude*), or his rejection of "toute sorte d'obligation … devoir d'honneur" (any sort of obligation … debt of honor) (III, 9, 966/897). But what about other inherited significances of shame?

Shame appears in the text in a range of Classical examples and anecdotes, and in instances with a more Christian tinge, in often banal reflections on sexuality and the body. Montaigne usually works with *honte*, occasionally *vergogne* (which both translate *aidôs/verecundia*), and only three times *pudeur* (from *aiskhunê/pudor*), each time, mockingly. Key Classical sources at the time were Aristotle, *Nicomachean Ethics* and Plutarch, *Moralia*. What is notable is that Montaigne can use Classical texts to do more interesting thinking than he can Christian culture's, in which shame's ineradicable link with the sexed body and with passionate desires deemed sinful is overdetermining and inhibiting. Shame may be mocked, but is habitual.

The most significant traits of Aristotelian thought for the *Essais* are: its focus on accountability; that shame, while an affect, not a virtue, is nonetheless indicative of the ethical self; that it plays, via memory, between past and anticipated selves; and it concerns honor, for it exercises our capacity to face mortifying realizations or encounters without fear. Not that being free of fear would make one shameless; rather, fearlessness would transform one's way of assuming whatever is shameful.

Greek culture is often regarded as having set great store by public reputation and honor; thus (experience or dread of) loss of esteem, and flaws in one's social presentation, carried weight. The injunction, "do not betray your cause," so fundamental to the ethos Montaigne would have identified as Greek (Athenian or Lacedaemonian, or more singularly, that of Socrates), played its part: it mapped onto courage (attached to reputation, shame's antithesis). Montaigne, by contrast, was skeptical about the significance of reputation, and whilst he asserted the difference between his public identity, "le Maire" (the mayor), and "Montaigne," each gains meaning from the other; he more often reflects on the complex, tense continuity between public and private identities.

One legacy of this focus on esteem, perception and social identity is shame's hold in everyday living – but amplified by a preoccupation with the meaning of one's life set in a longer, though not religious, perspective: shame both inherited and transmitted from one generation to the next. Sin figures so rarely in the *Essais* as to suggest a desire to understand affect, motivation and action – everything to do with ethos – in secular rather than doctrinal terms. Nor are psychologizing versions of shame – whether failure to live up to an idealized version of myself, failure to live up to myself as I see myself from a more abstract place of perfection, or awareness that I am coming too close to an unwanted version of myself, and a fear of others discovering it – central to his reflections. What the social, ethical and psychological emphases seem to need, for greater understanding of the gap that shame occupies, is a way of thinking about the enigmatic and elusive dimension of the relationship between private and public self, inside and outside, self and other. That is, a relationship thrown into chaos, as Montaigne was to discover, when he retired from the life to which he had been fitted by his birth and formation, and to be reordered, by an endless process of writing and reading, which he sometimes calls 'confession.'

"Parler de moy" (to Speak of Myself)[8]

Montaigne's "confession" has recently been discussed via Foucauldian *parrhēsia*, courageously frank self-expression, speaking directly the inner truth of the speaker.[9] Montaigne's – risky – speech is thus viewed as an urgently ethical site and stance, simultaneously an end in itself and a means to a further end, others' well-being. While my interpretation touches on *parrhēsia*, there is a key difference. Foucault's speaker seems confident in the truth (s)he is about to tell, as if it can be spoken unmistakably;[10] neither seems true in Montaigne's case. Risk, however, seems an imperative:[11] "A peine oseroy-je dire la vanité et la foiblesse que je trouve chez moy" (I would hardly dare tell of the vanity and weakness I find in myself) (II, 12, 565/516), but: "j'ose non seulement parler de moy, mais parler seulement de moy; je fourvoye quand j'escry d'autre chose et me desrobe à mon sujet" (I dare not only to speak of myself, but to speak only of myself; I go astray when I write of anything else, and get away from my subject) (III, 8, 942/875). The antithesis, cowardice or cowardly conformity, would be shameful, in both a customary sense and in terms of Montaigne's ethos as writer.

The nobility as well as necessity of the risk of openness is inferred from the cowardice attached to failing this principle: "la pire de mes actions et conditions ne me semble pas si laide comme je trouve laid et lache de ne l'oser avouer" (the worst of my actions and conditions does not seem to me so ugly as the cowardice of not daring to avow it) (III, 5, 845/778). Disavowal and the failure to speak openly are sites of abject shame. Such representation requires reflection on oneself as both subject and object – necessary components of shame also. But if the principle of this writing is "se faire veoir tel qu'on est ... que je me face connoistre tel que je suis" (to show ourselves as we are ... that I make myself known such as I am) (II, 17, 647, 653/596, 603), its condition is recognition of its impossibility, on two grounds. First, the condition of lack of perfect correspondence between words and being; second, lack of arrival at the position from which such correspondence might even be possible, albeit hoped for. Added to which: "je donne à mon ame tantost un visage, tantost un autre, selon le costé où je la couche. Si je parle diversement de moy, c'est que je me regarde diversement" (I give my soul now one face, now another, according to which direction I turn it. If I speak of myself in different ways, that is because I watch myself in different ways) (II, 1, 335/293–4, translation modified). The repetition of "diversement" does not secure coincidence between the look and the word at any given moment, and the difference between the disjunctive instance "parler *de moy*" (to speak about myself) and, in the French original, the grammatical direct object "je *me* regarde" measures their noncoincidence.

Montaigne's statements of position and intent involve acting towards himself; the verb "faire" (do) recurs, together with "oser" (dare, risk), whose link with being shame-free is evident; but "esperer," to hope for what the process of writing might achieve, seems more risk-laden than "faire" does. It relates to a dimension beyond volition and intention, and risks self-deception: is not the project of "speaking of oneself exactly as one is" not only an impossible prospect but already self-deceiving?

In the absence of a chapter entitled "De la honte" (Of shame), instances of the theme are illuminating. Set aside the various commonplace observations about sexuality and body parts, in keeping with Montaigne's ironizing of conventional shame in "Sur des vers de Virgile" (On some verses of Virgil) ("nous avons à l'avanture raison de nous blasmer de faire une si sotte production que l'homme; d'appeller l'action honteuse, et honteuses les parties qui y servent, (asteure sont les miennes proprement honteuses et peneuses)" (perhaps we are right to blame ourselves for making such a stupid production as man, to call the action shameful, and shameful the parts that are used for it) (878/812)) shame as narcissistic wound, self-respect salvaged by comic self-exposure. Set aside, also, the role of the Cynics in the *Essais*, insofar as Montaigne's relationship with shame is not theirs; neither in their mode (a performative nakedness, scandalous behavior), nor for their purpose (to challenge *doxa*); he does this by other means. More revealing of Montaigne's own shame, together with those first person singular instances of "oser" (to dare or risk) mentioned above, are the following: his understanding that fear of shame needs to be surmounted quite as much as shame per se; shame as betrayal of one's cause (I, 16, 70/58), which relates to shame as lack of self-respect (I, 39, 247/221), which in turn is partnered by the shame of living without risk (I, 24, 129/114); and the link between "honte" (shame), pain and death, as all unbearable, undifferentiated states, all tests of one's being (see II, 6, 71/324 and II, 16, 623/574), so much so that intolerable shame, like intolerable pain, is grounds for suicide (II, 3, 350/305). The shamefulness of lying, hypocrisy and disavowal set them as antithetical to the ideal of open speaking, which Montaigne wants to risk: "ne trahir l'histoire de ma vie ... ne desmentir l'image de mes conditions" (I should not betray the story of my life ... not give the lie to the picture of my qualities) (III, 9, 980/910). Shame thus seems key to understanding Montaigne's self-relation – along with death and pain.

According to Montaigne, philosophy provides little protection against both shame and death. The first instance of "honte" in the *Essais* exemplifies both:

> pour un plus notable tesmoignage de l'imbécilité humaine, il a esté remarqué par les anciens que Diodorus le Dialecticien mourut sur le champ espris d'une extreme passion de honte, pour en son eschole et en public ne se pouvoir desvelopper d'un argument qu'on luy avoit faict. Je suis peu en prise de ces violentes passions.
>
> (for a more remarkable testimony of human frailty, it was noted by the ancients that Diodorus the dialectician died on the spot, seized with an extreme passion of shame, for not having been able to shake loose, in his own school and in public, from an argument that had been put to him. I am little subject to these violent passions).
>
> (I, 2, 14/9)

The example questions philosophy's effectiveness, marks shame's power as affect, and proffers Montaigne's claim to exemption. Shame's ethical force is absent. Running through the instances of shame mentioned above is a tension: shame inhibits but also prompts right living, that is, living a courageous version of one's life, ready to have one's sense of self tested, and ready to speak for and of this, in spite of risk. Thus the apparently inner shame sought by writing would be unambiguously the latter: fearless shame, as further examples, drawn from Montaigne's reflections on risky speech; on the relationship between private and public "self"; instances of cultural shame; and what it means to repossess and know how to belong freely to oneself, "r'avoir de soy ... sçavoir estre à soy" (to repossess ourselves ... to know how to belong to oneself) (I, 39, 239, 242/213, 216), will attest.

"De la praesumption" (Of presumption) ruminates on the traps, trappings and lures of social existence, and how cultural or public demands render precarious the individual's "true" relationship with others and self. The subject negotiating the straits of social life is most tested by lying, hypocrisy and self-deception. The cost of lying is dishonor, understood as a painful desubjectification with, potentially, equally painful self-recovery, prompted by (now) ethically charged shame.

> Mon ame, de sa complexion, refuit la menterie et hait mesmes à la penser. J'ay une interne vergongne et un remors piquant, si par fois elle m'eschappe, comme par fois elle m'eschappe, les occasions me surprenant et agitant impremeditéement. Il ne faut pas tousjours dire tout, car ce seroit sottise; mais ce qu'on dit, il faut qu'il soit tel qu'on le pense, autrement c'est meschanceté.
>
> (My soul by nature shuns lying and hates even to think a lie. I feel an inward shame and a stinging remorse if one escapes me, as sometimes it does, for occasions surprise me and move me unpremeditately. We must not always say everything, for that would be folly; but what we say must be what we think; otherwise it is wickedness).
> (648/596–7)

Montaigne acknowledges that he lies; social existence is such that there will be lying "par fois" (sometimes), and self-justifying calculation as to what should remain unsaid, to avoid "meschanceté" (wickedness). But who is to trust his or her own judgement? This is equally pertinent to the intention of writing the principle of which is "se faire veoir tel qu'on est" (to show ourselves as we are) (647/596). The aporia and gaps in both instances claim the reader's attention – presumably as anticipated. A few pages later he continues: "de faillir à mon escient, cela m'est si ordinaire que je ne faux guere d'autre façon: je ne faux jamais fortuitement" (to slip up unknowingly is so common for me that I scarcely ever slip up in any other way; I never slip up accidentally) (653/602).

Is "ne ... guere" (scarcely) scrupulous truth or does it cast doubt on Montaigne's self-knowledge and capacity to correspond to his self-representation? Who knows? The point is that Montaigne's writing ensures that this doubt and ambiguity raise such questions.

Here, as much as the "risk" of speaking openly – "insolently" – about matters beyond those to which his readers were accustomed, Montaigne's writing runs another. Namely, readers' reluctance to follow where he leads: towards the doubt, self-doubt and shame they cannot yet imagine wishing to assume. Not the "interne vergongne et ... remors piquant" (inward shame and ... stinging remorse) (648/596) of this chapter, which, although "interne," is a response to occasions – it occurs primarily between self and external others; a different form of shame, less bound, also, to the suffering from reminiscences that is "remors." We shall find it, perhaps, in "De la solitude" (Of solitude), a chapter which may shed light on the enigmatic shame of "De l'oisiveté" (Of idleness); yet it has its share of enigma. Not least – despite the chapter's many suggestions as to how we may become "our own person" on our own – how those who are "en la danse" (in the midst of the dance) (237/211) but would prefer (like Montaigne) not to be, are ever to disentangle what is "particulier" (private) in themselves from what is 'publicq' (public) (237/211).

"Public" and "private," solitary and active are not distinct (the chapter's first sentence takes point on these); nor are nature and culture. The ideal of the solitary life, "vivre plus à loisir et à son aise" (to live more at leisure and at one's ease) (238/212) seems self-evident. However, the "Mais" (But) that immediately follows requires us to question it. The "*cura*," worries or anxieties, touched on in two quotations from Horace, are worries and moral failings, or in a Christian world, sins, such as "l'avarice ... les concupiscences" (avarice ... lust) (239/213); and it is still not clear what is meant by the "*conditions* populaires qui sont *en* nous" (the gregarious *instincts* that are *inside* us (239/213, my emphases), which possess us and from which it is imperative we repossess ourselves ("il se faut ... r'avoir de soy" (239)). Having been part of the world that is to be left, how exactly do we decontaminate or cure ourselves? Montaigne repeats metaphors of "contagion" and "mal" (disease); the seeker of solitude becomes sick ("malade"), and risks becoming sicker if he is moved. If a "condition" is "instinct" (Frame's translation), can it be shed?

Shortly after, Montaigne will offer the metaphor of the "arriereboutique toute nostre" (back shop all our own), the place of the freedom he seeks in solitude, "nostre vraye liberté" (our real liberty) (241/214). It must be, "faut-il," the place to "prendre nostre ordinaire entretien *de nous à nous mesmes, et si privé que nulle accointance ou communication estrangiere y trouve place*" (have our ordinary conversation *between us and ourselves*, and so private that no outside association or communication can find a place) (241/214–5, my emphasis). This new form of conversation with oneself about oneself suggests hope for self-coincidence; but as written, its impossibility appears on the page, and this imperative is sacrificed to the desire to write. This may seem a place of innermost privacy, but is nonetheless a shop, tied to notions of commerce and the exchange that here is verbal communication. However, ambiguous though this now seems, it has to do with a redefined ethics of shame.

Montaigne's thoughts quickly turn to our misguided "actions accoustumées" (customary actions) (241/215), as if to strengthen the case for retirement into solitude: "de mille il n'en est pas une qui nous regarde" (there is not one in a thousand that concerns ourselves) (241/215). For whom do you risk your life rather than surrender? For what do you study, risking your health? For an indifferent leader, or sterile scholarship, so misled are we by our desire for reputation and glory. The "causes" we will not betray, that bind us to the world, are counterfeit. The discovery that such ideals are "fauce monnoye" (false coin) (241/215) – the economy of exchange still persists – leads to a form of shame that is not explicitly redefined, but emerges over the next page or so. As Montaigne develops his vision of what it means to live for oneself, or "sçavoir estre à soy" (to know how to belong to oneself), as the "plus grande chose du monde" (the greatest thing in the world) (242/216), a new version of shame appears. Freed from the world's values such as reputation, and from confusing what others might expect with what one wants oneself, into a loving and apparently self-sufficient relationship with oneself ("n'espouser rien que soy ... qu'il se flatte et caresse" (be wedded only to ourselves)), shame coincides with self-respect. His injunction is: "respectant et craignant sa raison et sa conscience, si qu'il ne puisse sans honte broncher en leur presence. « *Rarum est enim ut satis se quisque vereatur* »" (respecting and fearing his reason and his conscience, so that he cannot make a false step in their presence. "*For it is rare for anyone to respect himself enough*") (242/216). This will return as an imperative: "ayez honte et respect de vous mesmes" (feel both shame and respect for yourself) (247/221).

This shame is intended to coincide fully with that rare thing, self-respect, imagined as free from the contamination of external values. Utopian? In both instances, the observation is immediately followed by a Latin quotation – first Quintilian, later, Cicero – not as models, or guaranteeing the possibility of this way of living. On the contrary, they reinsert the self into the world of (textual) culture, of others' perspectives and judgements, and are no sooner voiced than undercut. Moreover, by the time Montaigne cites Cicero, he has distanced himself from his ideal, "gloire": "c'est bien loing de mon compte" (it is very far from my reckoning) (246/220). The chapter ends with dismissal of both Cicero's and Pliny's thought as on the side of "gloire" and of an aberrant relationship with language, "une philosophie ostentatrice et parliere" (an ostentatious and talky philosophy) (248/222).

The chapter comes to rest on this antithesis of "comme il faut que vous parliez à vous mesmes" (how you should speak to yourself) (247/221), an "entretien" (conversation) (241/214) aligned with "vraye et naifve philosophie" (true and natural philosophy) (248/222). Its essentials are self-respect and freedom from a desire for "gloire," glory, and from the form of shame that prolongs the power of others not worthy of respect and of imaginary judgement. Let us trace Montaigne's movement towards a way of being in which shame and self-respect coincide productively with writing openly, from the first instance of his own shame in the *Essais*, then working through his other key avowals of it.

The first occurs in "Nos affections s'emportent au-delà de nous" (Our feelings reach out beyond us). Montaigne has just added to a list of exemplars of hapless preoccupation with their own remembrance the case of the Emperor Maximilian, so preternaturally modest that he willed that his cadaver be clothed in underpants: cue a joke at his expense. But Montaigne admits:

> moy qui ay la bouche si effrontée, suis pourtant par complexion touché de cette honte. ... je ne communique guiere aux yeux de personne les membres et actions que nostre coustume ordonne estre couvertes. J'y souffre plus de contrainte, que je n'estime bien seant à un homme, et surtout, à un homme de ma profession.
>
> (I who am so bold-mouthed, am nevertheless by nature affected by this shame. ... I hardly communicate to anyone the members and acts that our custom orders us to cover up. I suffer from more constraint in this than I consider becoming to a man, and especially to a man of my profession).
>
> (I, 3, 18–19/13)

This turns around conventional dynamics of shame and shaming, but also recognizes gaps: between embodiment and gendered sociopolitical identity; between desire for concealment (fear) and to speak out (courage); and moreover, between valid grounds to feel shame, not determined by cultural norms – and a humiliatingly unfree subjection to such norms, unredeemed by having the courage to represent it. The use of the first person singular – that disjunctive "moy" (me) – seems akin to the resolute assertion, "j'ose" (I dare), but is still far from the redefined shame towards which Montaigne will move. The sexual and genital shame and shaming commented on in "Sur des vers de Virgile" (On some verses of Virgil) (see above, p. 11), is comparable. Again, Montaigne concedes the power of cultural norms, already criticized elsewhere in the chapter, but differentiates his own sense of shame through comedy; otherwise, there is only an implied positive alternative, namely, daring to speak openly of it: "confession."

Montaigne frequently insists on his difference from others' expectations and desires for him; if lived as failure, this lack of coincidence would correspond to the gap in which conventional shame would operate. He insists on internal difference also: "je donne à mon ame tantost un visage, tantost un autre" (I give my soul now one face, now another) (335/293–4). The vocabulary of visibility nods to that awareness of personal visibility which shame conventionally patrols. Montaigne is clear, this inconsistency is not shameful but constitutive. He goes on to expand on his own diversities, inconsistencies, discordance – and ashamed-unashamable leads his list, "honteux insolent" (ashamed insolent). There is neither a fully coherent, whole self to govern identity, nor consistent correspondence between one's differing identities, private and public, preferred and expected.

While this absence suggests grounds for unsettling shame's cultural hold, across a wide range of chapters Montaigne offers a different reason for dislodging conventional shame: namely, the realization of the inconsistency of the Other (in whose "eyes" I imagine myself falling short), the "fauce monnoye" (false coin) (241/215) of counterfeit ideals and, implicitly, selves.

The four most significant instances occur in "D'un defaut de nos polices" (Of a lack in our administrations), the "Apologie" (two), and "De mesnager sa volonté" (Of husbanding your will). All relate to the ongoing religious conflicts and their consequences, whether this meant inhumane behavior (Castellio's and Giraldus's starving to death (I, 35, 223/200)); disavowed betrayal of religious cause; behavior which contravened or failed avowed ideals, a charge Montaigne lays on all Christians (II, 12, 442/390); sacrifice of faith to political interest (the English oscillating between Roman Catholicism and Anglicanism (II, 12, 579/531)); or expedient settlements which betrayed both religious doctrine and stated intention – peace (III,10, 1019/949).

The first three are staged in the first person singular or plural: "j'entens, avec une grande honte" (I hear, with great shame) (223/200), "nous devrions avoir honte" (we ought to be ashamed) (442/390), "dequoy j'ay honte" (at which I am shamed) (579/530). The fourth, while less personal, nonetheless speaks of shared responsibility: "la pluspart des accords de nos querelles sont honteux et menteurs; nous ne cherchons qu'à sauver les apparences" (most of the settlements of our quarrels nowadays are shameful and dishonest; we seek only to save appearances) (1019/949). All instance the destructive *absence* of shame in situations in which intersubjectivity has been reduced to a subject-object structure in which self-elected subjects disregard or deny the freedom and future of those they consider other, reducing other subjects to objects. Their lack of shame shames them.

But the lack in the Other is also the source of shame. Not God per se, but God as operant at the time. In the first instance, the persecution and neglect of Castellio and Giraldus, rather than ask, what "Christian" society could behave this way, we experience the shame that surges when we realize that the "God" we had believed still ensured charitable rather than cruel behavior seems not to exist. The second brings a similar, shaming realization: not Christians failing their faith so much as the horror that perhaps the "God" they have assumed as their own does not exist: "si ce rayon de la divinité nous touchoit aucunement, il y paroistroit par tout" (if this ray of divinity touched us at all, it would appear all over) (442/390). The third instance, England's flip-flopping between denominations, from the viewpoint of France where religious differences had led to already protracted wars, is again that of the shameful discovery of the lack in the Other, not divine but man-made: different for each church, therefore lacking consistency. Last, deceitful dealings make manifest the lack in the Other. The shame resulting from this awful realization differs from the conventional shame from which Montaigne distanced himself; it is emphatically assumed, as an ethical perspective with which Montaigne identifies: "j'ay honte" (I am ashamed). Joan Copjec's analysis is illuminating:

> shame is awakened not when one looks at oneself, or those whom one cherishes, through another's eyes, but when one suddenly experiences a lack in the Other. At this moment the subject no longer experiences himself as the fulfilment of the Other's desire, as the center of the world, which now shifts away from her slightly, causing a distance to open up within the subject herself. ... In shame, unlike guilt, one experiences one's visibility, but there is no external Other who sees, since shame is the proof that the Other does not exist.[12]

This comment underscores that the above instances of shame chime with Montaigne's persisting vocabulary of visibility, such as: "c'est un'humeur couarde et servile de s'aller desguiser et cacher sous un masque, et de n'oser se faire veoir tel qu'on est" (it is a craven and servile idea to disguise ourselves and hide under a mask, and not to dare to show ourselves as we are) (II, 17, 647/596). Here is an (impossible) ideal of perfect coincidence between (self-) representation and being, only possible not when one is shame-free, but when one has traversed the limits of conventional shame, to assume this redefined version and, as already suggested in relation to the convergence of shame and self-respect, another alternative shame, which I shall now explore further.

Be True to Your Desire?

If the Other is exposed as lacking or inconsistent, what ethical compass is left? Why not betray your cause if it has already betrayed your belief in it? If one's formative identificatory ideals (one's "name," one's exemplary behavior as a gentleman, the immortalizing power of art such as writing), are not one's own or insufficient, how then to identify an alternative by which to live? Montaigne's elected means include his own ways of writing – writing which celebrates its contingency and impermanence ("j'escris mon livre à peu d'hommes et à peu d'années" (I write my book for few men and for few years) (III, 9, 982/913)). But it is still not quite clear what shame, rather than conventional benefits, is desired.

In "De l'oisiveté" (Of idleness), the context of this unfamiliar, incongruous shame is anxiety. How might shame be a cure for anxiety, and, via writing, what ethical and affective self-relation does it indicate? The focal dimension, that which is enigmatic and alienating, puts in question the nature of the relationship between self and other as well as the nature of the "private" self; psychoanalytic thinking may help us clarify the precise meaning of shame's potentially benign relationship with both anxiety and writing.

For Freud anxiety is objectless – "nameless dread" (as distinct from fear which has an identifiable source) – but for Lacan, it "n'est pas sans objet" (is not without an object);[13] as the litotes suggests, there is excess, particularly in the extraordinary certainty with which it makes its presence felt, while remaining unrepresentable. Such is the quality of Montaigne's anxiety: "tant de chimeres et monstres fantasques les uns sur les autre, sans ordre et sans propos" (so many chimeras and fantastic monsters, one after another, without order or purpose) (33/25). However, though alienating, it is his own: "*m'enfante* tant de chimeres" (bears me so many chimeras, my translation). Anxiety seizes his body, and he acknowledges his close identity with the strange otherness which possesses him. These are his mind's 'profondeurs opaques de ses replis internes' (opaque depths of its innermost folds) (II, 6, 378/331), and also a reminder of his embodiment, of not yet understood connections between body and mind (both agitated, both stuck). In other words, between movement, thinking and affect.

Only a few chapters earlier, Montaigne represented himself as scarcely suffering "violentes passions" (violent passions), unlike Diodorus (the Dialectician) whose shame killed him (I, 2, 14/9). But now, excessive, destructive affect takes hold: anxiety robs him of his capacity to think, alienating him from himself. As a reader, now a writer, he was content to engage with textual others, and to form his own text in constant connection with them; in the early chapters, there are more "others" than "self," without the complexities of the relationship of self and other that will emerge in the course of the *Essais*. They first erupt in this eighth chapter.

Its narrative is of disillusionment; its affects are anxiety and shame; its compass, an inquiry into perception, memory, identity, and desire, in the form of the relationship between self and other, private and public, past and future, affect and thought. It does not fit prevailing epistemological, ontological, or ethical frameworks, particularly in relation to shame.

Montaigne retired, wanting to be free of attachment to others, "toutes les liaisons qui nous attachent à autruy" (all the ties that bind us to others) (I, 39, 240/214), and to live "plus à loisir et à son aise" (more at leisure and at one's ease) (238/212), embracing a Classical contemplative ideal. Instead, he encountered a version of himself that coincided neither with his remembered past self nor with either the self desired by others or the ideals he had retired to embody. Freedom proved elusive; rather, he discovered himself to be bound fast to aspects of his being he could neither assume nor simply reject. That he was bound to what he could not recognize as himself and yet knew to be intimately his own ("m'enfante," bears me) is figured by those chimeras and monsters, "ce où nostre raison ne peut aller" (whatever our reason cannot reach) (I, 27, 179/161): evidence of his being subject to unacknowledged "extreme passion" – not only his grief for La Boétie and for his father, but constitutively, a key locus of his incapacity to understand and represent himself. By the time of writing "Des boyteux" (Of cripples), the monstrous, already defined as that which (only) *seems* beyond rational understanding ("nous appellons monstres ou miracles ce où nostre raison ne peut aller" (we call monsters or miracles whatever our reason cannot reach) (I, 27, 179/161, translation modified), is encompassed by different self-understanding: "je n'ay veu monster et miracle au monde plus expres que moy-mesme" (I have seen no more evident monstrosity and miracle in the world than myself) (1029/958)). But as yet he represents himself flailing in the boundless enigma that is anxiety, willing his rescue by representation, and by converting anxiety into shame. If shame frees from anxiety, it must restore the capacity to think, that is, reestablish some distance between subject and object – but here, counter-culturally, less a space for self-protective privacy than for disillusioned self-representation.

This anxious encounter with himself is with an as-yet unthinkable (monstrous) self, and with the realization that it coincides neither with what he was born or formed for (name, social standing, profession, etc.), his "proper" identities, nor with his ego-ideal, one version of which was that life of contemplative leisure. For Lacan, what is encountered in anxiety is *jouissance*, the excessive, unspeakable underside of all we desire, and from which our ordinary activities screen us. We can live as if we are free of it, or insist that it is external; but our anxiety intimates that it is internal: it is that which "singularizes us, but also doubles and suffocates us" (Copjec, 102). Anxiety is an encounter with what is most "ourself," but experienced as so alien as to threaten our sense of who we are – "chimeres et monstres fantasques" (chimeras and fantastic monsters). Anxiety-free, disillusioned self-knowledge accepts the irreducibly enigmatic nature of our *jouissance* and traces within us of others – witness Montaigne's recognition in "Des boyteux" (Of cripples) of himself as enigma, both the most monstrous and miraculous of beings. In *L'Envers de la psychanalyse*, Lacan calls this "honte," shame;[14] for him, it signals the escape from "ontology's pre-comprehension of the subject" (Copjec, 103). Is this the "honte," shame, which Montaigne hopes writing will lead him to? It is strikingly different to Sartre's with its originating distinction between self and other, and Lévinas's ethically charged, responsibility- and fraternity-prompting shame; it acknowledges the presence of the other in our most intimate, barely representable self, both conscious and unconscious, disillusioned acknowledgement of which radically changes our sense of self.

Moreover, as Montaigne's later partnering of miracles with his inner monsters reminds us, once encountered, they offer us the perspective from which to be true to ourselves with a sense of awe. This enigmatic shame seems to resonate not only with Lacanian "honte," shame, but also Classical Greek *aidôs*: both shame and respect or reverence. Nonetheless, each of these forms of shame is distinctive, embedded in its own culture's temporality, understanding of identity and of the relationship between private and public, ethics and sources of "truth." What particularly marks Montaigne's is evident in his own shame: disillusionment with the Other, that which conventionally propels me to be true to my best self. *Aidôs* seems relevant to a publicly perceptible best self, distinct from the private (although the acts of protagonists such as Antigone suggest otherwise); Lacan, indeed psychoanalysis, insists on the complex interrelatedness of private and public self, and Lacan also redefines the key ethical terms and relations that are at stake; between the two, Montaigne represents himself at the very point of realizing the issue. Classical *aidôs* was an affect which restrained the individual from doing wrong; Montaigne's "honte," shame, enables him to act in ways that others might condemn but do not wrong his sense of himself, and guards him from self-deception; such is the private "honte et respect de vous mesmes" (shame and respect for yourself) (247/221) he urges in "De la solitude" (Of solitude), and which the dispassionate perspective of the writer, for whom self is both subject and object, hopes to convey "en ce corps aërée de la voix" (this airy body of words) (II, 6, 379/332, translation modified), irrespective of risk.

"Honteux insolent," ashamed insolent to the end, Montaigne safeguards the innermost privacy of the "arriereboutique" (back shop), a space protected by shame, self-respect's cognate redefined to fit Montaigne's unsettling of existing epistemologies and ethics of the self, no longer bound up with wrongdoing but preventing him from wronging himself; and he persists in writing, keeping the "arriereboutique" open to the "boutique." "Plusieurs choses que je ne voudroy dire à personne, je les dis aux peuple, et sur mes plus secretes sciences ou pensées renvoye à une boutique de libraire mes amis les plus feaux" (many things that I would not want to tell anyone, I tell the public; and for my most secret knowledge and thoughts, I send my friends to the bookseller's shop) (III, 9, 981/911). His most secret knowledge, perhaps, is that he remains opaque to himself.

And the reader? If the "diligent" reader who engages with this "vile," "vain" writing rethinks what shame means in his or her life, all well and good; but that's for the reader, in private, to decide.

Notes

1 All references are to Michel de Montaigne, *Les Essais*, eds. P. Villey and V.-L. Saulnier (Paris, 2004), and all translations, unless otherwise stated, are from D. M. Frame, *The Complete Works* (New York, London and Toronto, 2003).
2 J.-P. Sartre, *L'Etre et le néant* (Paris, 1943), and E. Lévinas, *Totalité et infini: Essai sur l'extériorité* (The Hague, 1961) and *De l'évasion* (St Clément-la Rivière, 1982).
3 L. Guenther, "Shame and the temporality of social life," *Continental Philosophy Review* 44, no. 1 (2011), 23–39 (30).
4 Here I am using André Tournon's edition of the *Essais* (Paris, 2003), 21; Frame's translation (294) modified.
5 For instance, T. Cave, "Le Récit Montaignien: Un Voyage Sans Répentir," in *Montaigne: Espace, Voyage, Écriture*, ed. Z. Samaras (Paris, 1995), 125–35.
6 S. Freud, "Mourning and Melancholia," in *On the History of the Psycho-Analytic Movement, Papers on Metapsychology and Other Works*, trans. J. Strachey, S. E. XIV (London, 1957), 243–58 (247).
7 M. Nussbaum, "The Speech of Alcibiades: A Reading of the *Symposium*," in *The Fragility of Goodness* (Cambridge, 2001), 165–99.
8 III, 8, 942/875.
9 See for instance R. Leushuis, "Montaigne *Parrhesiastes*: Foucault's Fearless Speech and Truth-Telling in the *Essais*," and V. Krause, "Confession or *Parrhesia*? Foucault after Montaigne," in *Montaigne after Theory, Theory after Montaigne*, ed. Z. Zalloua (Seattle, WA and London, 2009), 100–121 and 142–60.
10 See M. Foucault, *Fearless Speech*, ed. J. Pearson (Los Angeles, 2001).
11 For fuller discussion, see my *Unsettling Montaigne* (Cambridge, 2014), chapter 4.
12 J. Copjec, "The Invention of Crying and the Antitheatrics of the Act," in *Imagine There's No Woman* (Cambridge, MA and London, 2002), 108–31 (128).
13 J. Lacan, *Le Séminaire X: L'Angoisse* (Paris, 2004), 105.
14 J. Lacan, *Le Séminaire XVII: L'envers de la psychanalyse* (Paris, 1991), 223.

3 Shamefulness and Modernity

Remarks on Shakespeare's Sonnet 129

Thomas Osborne

Shame is – unremarkably – historically variable. In classical and in much early modern tragedy the tragic hero is typically confronted with – at the very least – an ambivalence towards his own fate; whether it is less shameful to face up to shame and take arms against it, or to succumb to it – Hamlet's predicament perhaps.[1] Of course, one would never expect tragic fate to be anything but ambivalent. The question is rather what kinds of ambivalence structure tragic experience in our modernity.[2] In taking arms against the prospect of shame, the traditionally tragic hero has to pay the ultimate price with his own life. In other words, shame in tragic literature has what might be described as a basic structure of insurmountability. This is not so with other dramatic forms, even if the level of the fault is severe. In *Two Gentleman of Verona*, Proteus betrays his best friend Valentine and pursues Valentine's mistress, Sylvia, is then discovered in his betrayal, voices his own shame and guilt over the matter, and is promptly forgiven by all the injured parties. Tragic drama aside, there can be ways back from shame – at least in literature – and, indeed, successfully demonstrating one's sense of shame can be one of them. And, of course, shame can hit different literary depths or strengths of intensity, and it can be ambivalent in differing ways – not all of which reach the levels of impossibility proper to traditional tragic discourse. Shakespeare's great Sonnet 129 – which shall be the focus of our remarks here – is a good example of this variability, and perhaps even of a novel, "modern" experience of shame, not least because the experience described appears to be so intense:

> Th'expense of spirit in a waste of shame
> Is lust in action; and till action, lust
> Is perjured, murd'rous, bloody, full of blame,
> Savage, extreme, rude, cruel, not to trust,
> Enjoyed no sooner but despised straight,
> Past reason hunted, and no sooner had
> Past reason hated as a swallowed bait
> On purpose laid to make the taker mad;
> Mad in pursuit, and in possession so,
> Had, having, and in quest to have, extreme;

A bliss in proof and proved, a very woe;
Before, a joy proposed; behind, a dream.
All this the world well knows, yet none knows well
To shun the heaven that leads men to this hell.[3]

An adventurous Freudian reading would no doubt quite aptly note that shame here appears as much as a drive as a reactive emotion retrospective to any action. In any case, the pursuit of lust in action is here specifically presented as an irrational one; past reason hunted, past reason hated. Rationality and irrationality here should of course be understood relatively; "rational" or "irrational" in terms of the agent's conception of their own interests. Sonnet 129 certainly treats irrationality in this sense. Why would anyone pursue such desires in knowledge of the outcome? To lust or not to lust is hardly the question; one has no choice. Yet Sonnet 129 also captures precisely the ambivalent *rationality* of lust in action – or rather lust till action; *till* here (in line 2) signifying a purposiveness towards expenditure not just a period of time – in the sense of a coherent logic of behavior that is inevitably to be pursued again. The sonnet exhibits this kind of rationality even whilst depicting – in what Vendler calls its "frenzied illogic" – the whole process as more or less entirely mad.[4]

I want to argue in what follows that Sonnet 129 exhibits an intriguingly "modern" conception of shame as generalized, impersonal and reflexive. Further, it is interesting to consider whether literary value can itself be assessed at least in part in terms of how well it captures the kind of "rational irrationality" that is presented in the sonnet. There is not much new in this. It is, for instance, the reason that Freud himself turned so often to literature to make his observations of the working of the unconscious in psychic life. But it can also help us see perhaps a little of why some literature works better than other kinds of cognitive activity precisely in exhibiting such phenomena – aesthetically rather than conceptually, but nonetheless accurately for all that.

Sonnet 129 on this argument would not just amount to a vivid descriptive record of an emotive state of shame following on from the pursuit of lust in action, but could be said to capture, in all its contradictions, an active cognitive structure embodying the rational contradictions entailed not just in sexual action but in much purposive action *per se*. Here the measure of literary value would not merely lie in the depiction of the emotional intensity of desire as such, but in the complexity – simultaneously rational and irrational – of the structure proposed. In a piece that is usually taken as a direct precursor to Shakespeare's own efforts in Sonnet 129, Ben Jonson had earlier expressed the intensity of sexual shame as an emotional response:

Doing, a filthy pleasure is, and short;
And done, we straight repent us of the sport:
Let us not then rush blindly on unto it,

> Like lustful beasts, that only know to do it:
> For lust will languish, and that heat decay,
> But thus, thus, keeping endless holiday,
> Let us together closely lie, and kiss,
> There is no labour, nor no shame in this;
> This hath pleased, doth please, and long will please; never
> Can this decay, but is beginning ever.[5]

But Sonnet 129 does more than provide this sort of poetic depiction of a common emotional feeling. In Jonson, we have the emotional intensity of the situation but not the complexity of the emotion. Jonson depicts a way of overcoming the inevitability of sexual shame by injecting it with something like love or affection. But Sonnet 129 gives intelligibility to the structured complexity of the emotional experience of shame in a way that depicts both its rationality and its irrationality – which is really to say its necessity – at the same time. What, then, *is* the shame that is captured here? The word itself appears only once in the sonnet and we need to be careful of the word, or at least sensitive to its semantic complexity in the Elizabethan era, as well as in the Shakespearean lexicon specifically. Here, the invocation of shame in the first line suggests at once "that degraded sex is a shameful spiritual waste; that it wastes or despoils the sense of shame; and that it is a waste of the deterrent of shame as an emotion, since lust is incorrigible."[6] The word denoted most directly, and in a manner that applied almost entirely to women, is a dereliction of modesty or chastity. Here a waste of shame would denote the "wasting" of modesty, the squandering of chastity. A further meaning – closer, no doubt, to current conceptions – would be as a kind of objective moral state, that of disgrace. For instance, the pun on waste as waist here might imply that the pursuer has expended his seed in a disgraced waist – signifying, perhaps, a prostitute. Finally, by adding a subjective dimension we arrive at what is perhaps a more modern conception – the reflexive notion of shame as a general emotion of self-disgust, self-recrimination or shamefulness. And indeed, editorial annotations in most modern editions of the sonnets appear to prioritize this notion; the emotion of shamefulness existing in a kind of waste or wasteland.

Clearly with this last conception it is not just a question of the word "shame." More generally, the whole of Sonnet 129 is surely concerned with depicting not just finite shame (guilt, in effect) but, as it were, on-going *shamefulness* as a reflexive emotional state or complex emotional idea. This is less about the shame of *having done* something so much as a general sense of shamefulness as a kind of ongoing moral experience or predicament. This experience as captured here is presented as being both impersonal and singular; as experienced by a particular person, undoubtedly, yet in an impersonal way that overwhelms subjectivity and autonomy (shame in the sonnet appears to be something that *happens* to a person).

Shame and Heteronomy

For all of the impersonality of Shakespeare's depiction, shame cannot simply be associated here with the powers of external social norms impressed upon the individual – and this departure is, perhaps, not what is least striking about the sonnet. In most of the contemporary secondary literature on shame, for example, it is taken to be a negative emotion that derives from the gaze of the other; one is ashamed before others.[7] Shame here is a social emotion, perhaps *the* social emotion. This is the notion of shame as social heteronomy, the shame of exposure to an external observer, but that is clearly not quite what is at stake here in Sonnet 129. No one has been dramatically exposed to anything or anyone, or at least not to anyone determinate. Exposure to oneself – reflexive shame? – might be another matter, as might be exposure to God.[8] But neither, as the closing couplet seems to register – and in spite of the general atmosphere of self-recrimination – does anyone exactly *repent* of anything in Sonnet 129. The sonnet expresses a general regret perhaps, and certainly much self-disgust, but not finite repentance exactly. And if there is an observer here it is not really external – courtly society, prevailing morality, God – but is at most an internalized other.

Bernard Williams argued that the internalized other in such reflexively generated shame is a watcher or a witness and that seems obviously to be the case here: someone observing their own behavior and finding it wanting from some respect.[9] But from what respect? Williams contended that there is a "primitive" structure to shame but that this is not reducible to exposure to the powers of social heteronomy but to the feeling of one's own loss of power. Freud is perhaps not far away here. Freudian shame typically relates to fear of loss of control or power in various ways; to evacuation, excreta, exposure, ejaculation. Indeed, in his study of Leonardo da Vinci, Freud even suggested ironic surprise that modern "civilized" humans ever engaged in the sexual act at all.[10]

Sexual activity can be experienced as a loss of will in a paradoxical way. The emphasis in the early lines of Sonnet 129 on action is of interest in this context; as if the more that sex is a question of action the less there is of agency in it, a point only underlined albeit with some lexical anachronism – as James Brown has observed – if one finds oneself overhearing "in action" as *inaction*.[11] There is action and then lust in action but all this is maddened action, albeit in its own way purposive, and not autonomous, conscious agency. The pursuer even in a blaze of action is in fact more or less passive before the powers of lust. In this respect lust represents not simply moral degradation but loss of power, an expenditure of spirit not just in the direct sexual sense but in the sense of one's spirit of action, one's ethical autonomy. So what is this shame of? It is surely less shame of the sexual act itself, its animality (as we saw in Jonson's verse), or even simply of the maddened process of lust *till* action, but shame at the perversion *of* action itself. This is the form taken by the loss of power in this case; a loss above all of self-respect – perhaps it could be glossed simply as self-disgust at the loss of autonomy. Which means that, if nothing else, the moral psychology of Sonnet 129 stresses, by implication yet firmly, autonomy of the will as a desirable value, in contrast to the maddened experience it depicts. Again, shame here is, in a sense, more egoistic than socially heteronomous. Self-disgust is, as it were, centrifugal to the self; it takes us ever further inward. This sort of shame is at the opposite pole from the shame of social heteron-omy, the shame that is responding to the gaze of social norms. But the shame in Sonnet 129 is, in a sense, hyper-egoistic. I say this because of course there is a normally egoistic element to all shame; even the shame derived from exposure to the social gaze has an egoistic element as the internalized shame of the gaze of the other. For instance, in Williams's example, Ajax's shame in Homer clearly derives from social norms of martial honor yet it impacts upon the ego – upon Ajax himself. It is so-cially derived and yet the shame *belongs*, so to speak, only to Ajax.[12] In contrast, Sonnet 129 depicts, certainly, a very different sort of shame; but it is not different merely in terms of obvious difference of content – sexual as opposed to martial conduct – but in terms of its relation to the ego. There is no suggestion that the pursuer in Sonnet 129 has actually contravened any social norms, for example, by way of what would have been regarded as any kind of sexual impropriety. In fact, the sense of the sonnet – again, in the final couplet especially – suggests that the pursuer is actually engaging in at least the local social norms of lust for his class in an entirely expected way. So shame here is not derived heteronomi-cally but, on the contrary, is generated from within the ego itself; it is at this basic level narcissistic, better expressed as hyper-egoistic (if we reserve narcissism for its Freudian sense, i.e. in treating one's own body as a sexual object). This, in short, is generalized, reflexive yet impersonal shame; or simply – *shamefulness*.

Shamefulness and Guilt

Generalized shame? After all, one would perhaps expect this hyper-egoistic or narcissistic notion of shame to articulate on the contrary with something finite, for instance the notion of guilt *about* some-thing. We were once famously supposed, as part of our modernity, to have moved from a so-called shame culture (centered on the gaze of others) to a guilt culture (centered on the individual) and perhaps this situation at first view might seem to fit that, however largely discred-ited a view it is.[13] But in Sonnet 129 the pursuer is not exactly "guilty" of anything. Rather all the action is presented in terms of forces that seem to be more or less anonymous and impersonal, beyond anyone's control; something "objective" is happening to the subject of the sonnet. In fact, the speaker is captured by something that is all the more forceful because of its impersonality. What is "full of blame" is not represented as an individual act of fault but as an impersonal force, something that manifests itself in effect as necessity – the expenditure of lustful spirit in the pursuit of sexual gratification. In fact, the sense of a loss of power itself surely derives from the construction of lust in action as an anonymous force which, so to speak, attacks the ego; a fate rather than a choice – hence the prevalence, syntactically, of the passive forms and the impersonal voice throughout the sonnet. Bodily drives here are more a question of *fate* than choice. The shame experienced by the pursuer does not relate so much to acting badly, or – in spite of the theme of lust in action – to the commission or omission of any particular kind of "act," but merely to being human in so far as we all know that this is just how things are – since none know well how to shun this heaven.

Obviously enough, against this apparently gender-blind emphasis on impersonality we might want to observe, again from the literal evidence of the final couplet, that it is specifically men that are led to this hell. One might presume that the woman, the mistress, is another matter. The pursuer is caught in a predicament of which the pursued appears to be liable. She appears to be guilty at the very least of entrapment – "a swallowed bait / On purpose laid." However, although ideologically speaking the sonnet clearly and entirely unsurprisingly inhabits the Elizabethan masculinist world, one can plausibly argue that modern conceptions of sexism actually are of limited relevance here. In fact, there is no internally semantic reason that the pursuer cannot be female. What is presented to us in Sonnet 129, at least, is an anonymous and hence general *structure* of conduct; not a motivated process in terms of gender or anything else – beyond the urge to lust in action itself – but a predicament of agency *per se*.

Now, central to this predicament are two things that are of interest, especially in the light of – that is by way of relatively stark comparison with – Williams's discussion of shame in the ancient world. These are what could be called, on the one hand, a thin conception of both guilt and shame, and on the other, the fact of their relative isolation from each other. To enter into some consideration of these two things, let us for heuristic (not historical) purposes return to the Greek conception of shame adumbrated by Williams. He outlines an ethically thick conception of shame belonging to the Greeks that also includes within it much of what we – "we moderns," perhaps (Williams was, after all, a good Nietzschean) – would categorize as guilt. This shame system has several aspects that contrast it with what Williams associates with the modern morality system (which he denigrates): it has thick ethical content (the ethical self or ego is not merely an abstract, say Kantian, moral agent); it is interactive between self and other in that it does not simply reduce to social norms (heteronomy) nor recourse to irreducibly individualistic senses of necessity (egoism); and it is what we could call reparative in that it involves the possibility of a forward-looking ethical work – the experience of shame, in short, can be the basis of making amends, of improving oneself.

This structure can usefully – heuristically – be contrasted to the picture of shame presented in Sonnet 129. As we have seen, shame here is not based on a thick conception with any recognizable actual content, but comes across merely as a rather one-dimensional form of hyper-egoism. Of course, one might quite legitimately say that it would be impossible to present a thick conception within the fourteen-line convention of a sonnet. The point, however, is that there is no apparent or implied background of shame conventions in relation to lust in action given here, other than the basic fact *of* shame as shamefulness to which the sonnet refers or which it implies. One can say that such thick conceptions could not be included in the space of a sonnet; but perhaps it would be better to say, given the depth of Shakespeare's art, that the sonnet has been chosen as a form precisely so as to obviate the need for thick ethical elaboration.

In any case, there were no doubt reasons why Shakespeare should have chosen the restricted sonnet form precisely because of its limitation in this respect, limitations which, so to speak, served to express precisely the thin, narrow scope of the concept that he wished to capture. So shame here is indeed a general shamefulness rather than, so to speak, a specific shame; it is in essence an empty or abstract category in ethical terms, albeit a highly powerful one: the connotations of thin may not be weakness or insignificance (as Williams's ethical theory often seems to imply) but range, power, adaptability. Thick concepts, we might say, are full but rooted; thin concepts are empty but mobile. Both can be powerful and intense, and worthy objects of complex artistic reflection.

It is also worth noting that what we are calling in shorthand the generalized hyper-egoism of shame in Sonnet 129 is somewhat different from the kinds of egoism that Williams describes as being possible on ancient world conceptions of shame. Williams refuses Dodds's opposition between shame and guilt as being too simplistically synonymous with heteronomy and egoism; and he insists, as we have already noticed, that egoistic shame was a possibility even in the ancient world. The shame of Sophocles's Antigone for example – in insisting that she bury her brother against the will of Creon – was not, argues Williams, governed in the least by the power of social heteronomy.[14] On the contrary, it was entirely egoistic and autonomous, going against social conventions; her sense of necessity was deliberately and entirely her own and was, as Williams suggests, not without an element of self-righteousness and self-indulgence as a result. Antigone's was, in this sense, a genuinely ethical egoism which, since after all her conduct was no doubt admired in its way, also expressed the wide bandwidth of Greek attitudes towards non-heteronomic forms of shame, i.e. towards forms of shame that were not just derivative of the punitive gaze of society. One could feel shame in an egoistic sense, *and* at the same time, if ambivalently, it could meet with social recognition, even approval. The very different case of Sonnet 129 is obviously not narcissistic in *this* sense; its redolence of egoism is not thick enough even to entertain parallels with the case of Antigone – it is rather an empty, abstract narcissism and, in contrast to what Williams calls Antigone's active egoism, we have a sort of passive egoism. Sonnet 129 seems to express a sort of *casually*, passively narcissistic egoism, with shame thinned out to a vague, general, amorphous, if intense and powerful, sense of regret – the waste of shame – but also of inevitability, even of resignation to the forces that have captured the pursuer.

Equally, this has little relation to guilt in any narrow sense. The waste of shame, in any event, is not tied in with a sense of guilt except on the opposing side to it; guilt is not part of the shame structure of the pursuer but an aspect, on the part of the trap laid by the one pursued, of what has brought it about. It is the pursued who should feel mere guilt! The limited semantics of shame as chastity, moreover, would have it that guilt and shame are wholly opposed; if shame is chastity it is conscience-free, but once wasted it is compromised. Guilt in all senses, then, is external to shame in Sonnet 129 and so, in so far as there can be said to be a shame system implied here at all, there is little sense in which shame and guilt could be said to be in a strongly interactive relation with each other. The guilt of the one does not wholly coincide with the shame of the other, or rather with the more generalized sense of shame as simply "there." Nor is there much scope for reparation here, for making amends. The egoism of shame does not conform to any sense of autonomy or self-determination on the part of the pursuer and so no hope of escape or self-improvement by reflective conscience on the shame system is offered; the pursuer is merely sunk in the waste of shame until the spiral of lust in pursuit of lust in action begins all over again.

Impersonality

It is a grim, if brilliant, picture. But of course, as we noted earlier, this is a work of literature – neither a moral tract nor a piece of descriptive psychology – and we need to pay some attention to what this might mean. The literary status of Sonnet 129 has been the object of some iconic debate over which we need to linger just long enough to get more clearly to the issue of impersonality in the sonnet, which is important to my argument. Robert Graves and Laura Riding used Sonnet 129 to argue that the status of a piece of literature is closely dependent upon its authentic typographical rendering, and seemed to assume that there could be such a thing as knowledge of what such an authentic rendering might be.[15] Authenticity here was a derivative of pronunciation and orthography – we should recognize that the sonnet would have sounded in a certain way and would have been spelled in a certain way and that these would have been related. Modern orthographical norms and conventions, Graves and Riding argued, tended to undermine the authenticity of the work in this respect, and to simplify it – thus making Shakespeare easier than he should be for modern readers.

The modern critic who has opposed Graves and Riding with most heat is Stephen Booth; pointing out that we cannot be clear as to how Sonnet 129 would have been pronounced any more than we can be certain of precisely what it would have looked like on the unprinted page to Shakespeare.[16] Roman Jakobson and L.G. Jones had earlier responded to the Graves and Riding position by emphasizing the lexical and syntactic – rather than the merely phonological or typographical – basis of structure. Sonnet 129, they argued, contains "an amazing external and internal structuration."[17] In Jakobson and Jones's reading, Sonnet 129 is the epitome of the creative principles that would later be encapsulated in the terms fullness and parsimony; doing as much syntactic and semantic work as possible over as small a space.[18] Jakobson and Jones listed the various forms of structural relation on which the sonnet is built – binary correspondences of what they labeled alternation, framing and neighborhood – showing that the sonnet, in accomplishing the effect of madness and obsession, is built on a rigid hierarchy and for the most part binary interrelation of lexical and semantic elements.

This analysis became a classic of formalist structural criticism as well as a benchmark in interpretation of the sonnets. Helen Vendler, in a well-known response to Jakobson and Jones, argued that instead of a structural analysis, it was necessary to take into account the progressive movement of the poem as it were diachronically in the course of a reading. Hence we need, she argued, to reconstruct the sonnet as a psychological experience – one which unfolds over time. Subsequently, in her book, *The Art of Shakespeare's Sonnets*, Vendler substantiated this argument by insisting that the sonnet in fact shapes a sort of progressive curve in terms of its assessment of the pursuit and attainment of lust, from being one of dismissal and rejection to being one of – partial – acceptance. Thus the definition of lust in the sonnet, she argues, changes over time as we read the lines – "from disgusting act to dream," from waste of shame to heaven.[19]

Vendler was keen to reject the contention in Jakobson and Jones's analysis that the distinguishing mark of the poem is its structural logic of impersonality – the lack of personal pronouns in particular, but also the preponderance of substantives and transitive verbs. It would be too simplistic to say that Vendler's reading opposed a semantic priority to Jakobson and Jones's syntactical one, but nonetheless the terms of her argument do seem to oppose an interpretive reading that is, so to speak, on the side of the author and the reader to a structural one based purely on objective, formal symmetry in the language; the typical opposition found for so long in debates between humanism and scientism over the philosophy of interpretation.

The interpretive merits of Vendler's own analysis of Sonnet 129 notwithstanding, the argument against this way of looking at things is at least twofold and both are important to our understanding of the sonnet. On the one hand, and as a general point, the terms of that debate have long been superseded. Vendler herself presented what in many ways was a structural – though certainly not formalist – interpretation of the sonnets with her designation of key words and couplet ties in each poem. What is at stake, rather, is Vendler's contention that a structural analysis is by definition incapable of doing justice to the diachronic progress of a poem; a contention more or less entirely undermined by the fact that Jakobson and Jones themselves in their analysis included an analysis, limited certainly, of temporal progression within Sonnet 129, most notably between a kind of centrifugal tendency in the first seven lines and a centripetal one in the latter seven lines.[20] On the other hand, Sonnet 129 does unquestionably have an exceptional structural impersonality; but this is surely – paradoxically? – for a *semantic* reason – to do, as we shall see, with the character of objective, passive shamefulness itself, or at least the character of it that Shakespeare chose to capture and convey. Perhaps, in this sense, Vendler would have had at least a partial point if Jakobson and Jones had analyzed almost any other sonnet in the series in this very particular, brilliantly reductive way. But Sonnet 129 is different. It really *is* impersonal by design – which means, in sum, that Jakobson and Jones were perhaps right if only for Vendlerite reasons. And as Vendler says herself – we need to ask why Shakespeare himself chose to make the particular decisions that he made in composing this sonnet: "There are of course reasons we can imagine for such compositional choices…".[21]

The reason that Vendler herself gives is that what is at stake is of the order of a kind of psychological trial or attempt; an attempt initially to condemn lust as ultimately a miserable, self-defeating enterprise, before acknowledging its attractions, with the couplet ironizing both models.

> [T]he major aesthetic move of the sonnet is to paint over our first impression – the shame and blame of lust – with a second, the joy and sorrow and unreality of lust; and then to paint over that with the ironizing and totalizing third – that no matter how much we know of the aftermath, we will be unable to shun the joy.[22]

It would be unnecessary to attempt to refute this interpretation if only for the simple reason that, in essence, the form of its refutation is obvious – if the attainment and pursuit of lust were not enjoyable then it is difficult to imagine anyone entering upon them, nor of Shakespeare embarking upon his initial quatrain. What is significant is not that the interpretation is wrong but that it entirely bypasses the issue of impersonality in the sonnet, an issue which Vendler acknowledges only to dismiss with her notion of a chronological reading.[23] But the chronological reading does not make the issue of impersonality go away. In fact, it exacerbates it as an issue. If as Vendler insists the final four nouns in the third quatrain – bliss, woe, joy, dream – "refute" the first four nouns of the poem – expense, spirit, waste, shame – then why does the mode of expression remain, in formal terms, impersonal?

As Jakobson and Jones note, Sonnet 129 is the only sonnet in the sequence of 154 containing no personal or corresponding possessive pronouns. Most of the sonnets make much use of the first person, and in three only third-person pronouns appear.[24] Here in Sonnet 129 there are none. This is not to say, however, that other sonnets in the sequence are devoid of abstraction altogether – Brown points, for instance, to number 60 in this context.[25] The difference is that in Sonnet 129, abstraction is motivated or at least it seems to capture a "motivational pressure," as Brown puts it; documenting a motivation, as it were, without a subject – what we might call a sense of motiveless motivation. As Brown observes, similar forms of motivated pressure without obviously determinate forms of narrated or narratable motivation as such may be found in *Hamlet* as well, a kind of pressure without obvious narrative development – an idea that interestingly echoes Stephen Greenblatt's probing towards a conception of Hamlet as being a character without character and *Hamlet* effectively a play without a clearly progressing plot.[26] The way that Sonnet 129 develops also seems to embody aspects of this. Sonnet 129 appears to flow narratologically in a kind of anti-narrative way, as it were, *uphill*, building image upon image relentlessly and indeed with a certain implacable inexorability but without obvious culmination since – given the feeling that the action takes places almost backwards in time – everything appears to be already over and done with even in the pursuit, such that it is difficult to know whether the action consists in the drive towards the expense of spirit or in the expenditure itself or even in the self-disgust – since all are mixed together. In Sonnet 129, everything that happens has *already happened*, as evidenced by the preponderance of past participles, as it were piled one upon the other – enjoyed, despised, hunted, had, hate, swallowed.[27] So the effect overall is not just about abstraction; it is motivated impersonality, if that – as with the notion of a narrative logic that is somehow anti-narratological – is not too much of an oxymoron.

No subject of the action has a role here, not the first person of the poet's voice, not the third person of a lusting subject, nor even of the object of lust – even the laying of the trap is expressed passively, on purpose laid. The subject of the poem, then, is the blind force of expenditure – the expense of spirit – itself; the force of which force, so to speak, being underlined by the implacable work of repetition that occurs in the poem – lexical repetition of key terms (lust, action, extreme, savage, mad), thematic repetition, and, as Jakobson and Jones show, iterated forms of structural contiguity and opposition between and within the four strophes. Such insistent repetition does two things; it reaffirms, as it were, the *intensity* of the force of expenditure and it makes of that force a kind of inescapable circle or spiral always folding back upon itself. Vendler's argument that the poem is not structurally static but does in fact progress from passive to more active voices can still hold within this horizon of interpretation; but if the tone becomes more active – but no less impersonal – in the third quatrain ("in quest to have, extreme"), by the end of the final couplet we have returned to the beginning, from hell to heaven to hell and back. So whereas for Vendler, Sonnet 129 is concerned with the psychological effects of lust on the subject of lust and for Jakobson and Jones it is a question of specifying the aesthetic qualities of its formal symmetry, on this reading its primary object is neither psychological nor aesthetic but, in a sense, cognitive; the capture of a certain kind of objective experience that is only possible through literature.

Intelligibility and Complexity

Of course, what the poem achieves can be stated in relation to several registers; at one extreme (as Jakobson and Jones show so marvelously), it is a kind of syntactic miracle, and at the other, one might even say in the Freudian vein that it foreshadows the idea of the repetition compulsion as a kind of drive. Shakespeare, we might wonder, was perhaps influenced by *Beyond the Pleasure Principle*. The Freudian drive is of course precisely something impersonal, something "there," as it were beyond the "psychological" intentionality of this or that individual captured by it. Freud, in this respect, was no more of a good "psychologist" than Shakespeare: their concerns, in each case, went far deeper than that. More prosaically the poem accomplishes something that is difficult to imagine being accomplished in any other (non-artistic) kind of cognitive activity: to render intelligible – that is as, so to speak, irrationally rational – what in other respects would be regarded simply as self-defeating, irrational behavior. To use a different terminology, complex literature can *exhibit* such irrational rationality. What literature can exhibit – which is not to say that this is all it can achieve – is irrational behavior *as* irrational whilst also rendering it intelligible and hence, in a sense, rational. Sonnet 129 does exactly this; it is a rational reconstruction in that it contains its own peculiar logic of development according to which different emotional states – desire, regret, disgust, self-recognition – are held in parallel rather than simply canceling each other out. Only with the advent of psychoanalysis three centuries later was an intellectual discourse of irrational rationality developed that itself used literature as an extensive source for its reflections. In this sense, it can properly be said that Sonnet 129 is "awaiting" psychoanalysis, but also that the use of literary examples within psychoanalysis from its earliest history was not an incidental feature of it. Literature, with its complexity of association (great literature is never reducible to good "psychology") and its attention, in so many of its forms, to the embodied aspects of rationality as well as the peculiar and often contradictory rationalities of embodiment, represents not just an archive of para-clinical material but, as Freud himself made clear in his very use of concepts such as the Oedipus complex, part – in advance – of the conceptual fabric of psychoanalysis itself. As Freud knew, literature was thinking psychoanalysis well before Freud.

But if, additionally, there is something *modern* about Sonnet 129 and its conception of shame, it surely lies in this characterization of shame as both embodied and generalized, as it were, beyond any particular subject. It is not that modernity is uniquely "shameful," but that works of literature such as Sonnet 129 capture further dimensions and aspects of shame. If modernity is a shame culture in many ways, it is a pluralized one; where there are different kinds and extremes of shame, and in this sense Dodds's dichotomy of shame versus guilt cultures was too simplistic and polarizing. Not least of the originality in what Shakespeare captures, just as Freud was to do later in a wholly different vein, is the *ordinariness* of such rational irrationality in its modern format. Sonnet 129 is of course insistent, hectoring and somewhat insane, but its penultimate line ends with what is more than likely a joke on the poet's name ("… none knows well [Will] / To shun…") and a sort of resigned, ironic humor to the effect that this rather tawdry situation is just how it is (all this the world knows well). If there is weakness of the will here it is normal rather than pathological; a matter of anthropological constitution rather than the happenstance of individual psychology. Shakespeare's summation in the couplet expresses a deflationary effect in relation to what would otherwise be a traumatic progress from the promise of heaven to hell and back again… and endlessly. But this shamefulness is surely secular as well as ordinary. What is anthropologically constitutive about it is different from the kind of constitutional weakness of will that one might associate with, say, original sin.[28] It is a weakness of will governed not by any alienation from the deity but, so to speak, from the forces of the drive. And what we are calling the secularism of Sonnet 129 is only exacerbated by the theological register of the final couplet – heaven and hell – and by the fact, again pointed out by Brown, that this register is subjected there to a deliberate deflation, since hell in Elizabethan argot could also mean "pudenda." At all events, lack of autonomy – lack of self-determination – here seems to be of a particularly worldly order, a normal predicament rather than an inordinate lapse.

In capturing the ordinariness of shamefulness in this way, we have in effect, if not necessarily a novel, then certainly a specific conception of it. Indeed, as has been suggested, we can see Sonnet 129 as conveying something interestingly *modern* in this respect. For example, it is surely obvious that Sonnet 129 would not have been ethically intelligible to the ancient Greeks discussed by Williams, and for at least two reasons. For one thing, the notion of an impersonal yet rather ordinary or everyday kind of shame would have been foreign to them, for whom shame was always about personal if not exactly "psychological" shortcomings as they become visible to others in the wider culture. Then again, the strong linkage to sexuality also seems to be ineluctably modern; or rather, the linkage to a *generalized* sexuality is. For, as noted earlier, the sense of shamefulness in Sonnet 129 is no longer simply what could be called sexist shame – i.e. female shame, as designated by men – but is, as it were, abstracted into a sort of homogeneous predicament, the generalized wasteland of shamefulness. Perhaps, again, there is a Freudian resonance here, and this is perhaps what gives the piece its aura of modernity; the idea of a generalizing and ambivalent libido, a sexuality that exists in a zone of indiscernibility between good and bad, moral and not; where the irrational and rational are fused as to be, separately, meaningless categories. And just as with Freud, this generalization takes us beyond the mere category of the libido or sexuality. Indeed, what is "shameful" in Sonnet 129 is not reducible to sexuality; rather, it concerns irrational action in general, a linkage facilitated in Shakespeare's own time by the fact that to Elizabethans, the very term "action" also signified, quite specifically, sexual action.[29] If action signified sex, we might surmise it a logical reversal that sex might signify action. The shame of the situation derives, as it were, not just from sex but from our constitutional or anthropological weakness of will, our persistent inability to give our conduct purely self-directed rational form. It is our failures of rationality that are shameful, perhaps, but also normal, and even to be treated in a deflationary spirit. On the other hand, there is a peculiarly modern "anxiety" exhibited here as well. The Greeks were not concerned with being or not being rational; from Williams's account it is clear that their conception of autonomy was more to do with outward intelligibility – giving their action intelligible form to others; but rationality as desire, explaining oneself on the basis of the rationality and not just the outer morality of our conduct – this surely is modern, and something constantly registered, as an anxiety as much as a value, across Shakespeare's work, albeit a *normal* anxiety rather than an extremist one.

Of course, it would be entirely absurd to attribute this transformation to Shakespeare; at most a work of verbal art such as Sonnet 129 exhibits it as a possibility. Wider scholarship around this question, however, does lend some credence to the idea of a general shift around this period; or rather, it appears that Shakespeare might best be seen as responding to a general intensification of the problematization of shame during the early modern era. The kinds of enhanced individualism and self-awareness that have been recognized as basic features of the Renaissance since Burckhardt led to an intensification of shame discourse around the individual, including around questions of self-responsibility and blame, that have been documented by a variety of modern cultural historians.[30] Fernie's study, drawing on a wide range of scholarship, indicates that such an intensification increasingly led to a focus on *crises* of shame; as if an individualized shame culture had become deeply problematic, even traumatic, just as it had become more culturally available and prevalent.[31] I think we can argue that Shakespeare's oeuvre offers us a somewhat nuanced angle on this development; on the one hand, the sheer variability of kinds of shame in Shakespeare, well documented by Fernie, indicates the extent to which Shakespeare's contribution was not least in pluralizing notions of shame, precisely in *not* reducing it to one or other particular kind of moral experience; on the other hand, in the specific instance of Sonnet 129 we can see something else happening – a kind of normalization of shame, as if to deflate the exaggerated reactions to it and to integrate it more into the daily features of ordinary, secular life. There are many kinds of shame in Shakespeare; some extreme, some not. The shame of Sonnet 129 is both; it is extreme ("savage, extreme, rude, cruel...") but also, by the closing lines, normal, expected, perhaps in its own way tragic and contradictory but, still, for all that, nothing to get too excited about.

Autonomy and Necessity

This raises a further issue. What is the scope for autonomy and self-responsibility under such conditions? If indeed the closing lines of Sonnet 129 entail a deflationary effect worthy of Montaigne, a plausibly secular non-moralistic type of skepticism about the capabilities of human intentions – broadly to the effect that moderation is always best and lust is madness, but perhaps we should tolerate it as human, if not indulge it – one might think that autonomy (in the broad sense of self-determination) would be an impossibility under these conditions. But what Sonnet 129 shows is that autonomy can consist in or at least be aimed at in a sober, deflationary kind of reflection precisely on necessity. Williams claims of the Greeks that shame and necessity were connected ideas, and that this connection exists in some contradiction with most modern – for which read, Kantian – ideas of shame. Shame for the Greeks was impersonal in that sense that it was simply *fiat* that one should feel shame if one had failed to act in a certain way proper to one's status, or equally even if one had acted "properly" and yet the outcome was not the right outcome. But it did not include the "if" factor proper to Kantian morality; that is the sense that one feels shame in the light of feasible alternatives that one might have pursued but did not.[32] On the one hand, the modern conception tends to dissociate necessity and autonomy, and so necessity and shame; in order to experience shame, to be self-reflecting, autonomous and so on, one must be guided by genuine alternatives, if the choices actually made are to be considered ethical at all. For the Greeks, on the other hand, necessity and ethics were connected; one did what one had to do. Of course, such a connection persisted into the modern era, for instance in Luther's (and Weber's) "Here I stand I can do no other...".

Sonnet 129 discloses a different gloss on this idea, however. It does not presume to transcend necessity – one cannot act as if lust and passion were not like this; but nor does it merely stoop to a brute animality, to the capitulation of a complete acceptance of it. Rather, it discloses a further sense of necessity; regret itself acts as a kind of observation point on who we are, and indeed the poem could be said to work not so much as a blunt statement of moral fate but as a miniature ethical exercise or prompt into what is human – if perhaps, if one insists, overwhelmingly *masculinely* human – about ourselves, to obtain, perhaps, some ironic distance from if hardly control over the forces that direct us and otherwise saturate us. It is in fact itself a little exercise in autonomy, whilst acknowledging the impossibility of complete success in the exercise itself.

All in all, then, we have in Sonnet 129 a very modern notion of reflexive shame, or rather of generalized shamefulness. Or rather, Sonnet 129 has its place in a highly pluralized terrain that hosts our modern conception – or rather conceptions – of shame. This modernity is not, as some conceptions have it, a shift from a shame culture to a guilt culture; but a shift to a different kind of shame culture (that would also include the category of guilt). To sum this up: the heteronomy of shame here is infra-individual rather than derived from clearly external social norms or social forces. This sort of shame, like most conceptions of guilt, is oriented introspectively towards the self, its gaze is internal, but unlike guilt it is, as it were, impersonal and even nonspecific, a matter seemingly of necessity or at least inevitability rather than choice. Shame here, in contrast to guilt, becomes not just related to what we might have done, but to who we *are* and of what we are capable. At the end of this line (and at the beginning of so much else), as has been suggested, is Freud. But such a structure also calls to mind some profound comments of Max Weber, in somewhat Kafkaesque mode, on the concept of modern guilt and shame.

For Weber, the distinctively modern type of shame, the very particularly "godless feeling of sin" that characterizes the moderns, relates not to having done any particular deed, but to the notion that by virtue of what one *is* one is perpetually and residually capable of it; in this sense, we are not so much guilty in the eyes of the law as perpetually shameful *before* it:

> It is that distinctive type of "guilt" and, so to speak, godless feeling
> of sin which characterizes modern secular man precisely because of

its own *Geisnnungsethik*, regardless of its metaphysical basis. Not that he has *done* a particular deed, but that by virtue of his unalterable qualities, acquired without his co-operation, he "is" such that he *could* commit the deed – this is the secret anguish borne by modern man, and this is also what the others, in their "pharasaism" (not turned determinism), blame him for.[33]

Weber goes on to point out that there is a "mercilessness" to this attitude because there is no escape from it; Shakespeare's model – like that of Montaigne and many aspects of Renaissance skepticism more generally – was no doubt more sanguine, more deflationary, but no less modern.

Notes

1 Ewan Fernie, *Shame in Shakespeare* (London: Routledge, 2002), 109ff.
2 Giorgio Agamben, *Remnants of Auschwitz*, trans. Daniel Heller-Roazen (New York: Zone, 1999), 96–97.
3 William Shakespeare, *William Shakespeare: The Complete Works*, eds. Stanley Wells and Gary Taylor (Oxford: Clarendon Press, 1988), 767.
4 Helen Vendler, "Jakobson, Richards, and Sonnet CXXIX," in *I A Richards. Essays in His Honour*, eds. Reuben Brower, Helen Vendler, and John Hollander (New York: Oxford University Press, 1973), 193.
5 Ben Jonson, *The Complete Poems* (Harmondsworth: Penguin, 1975), 251.
6 Fernie, *Shame in Shakespeare*, 92.
7 See for instance Jon Elster, *Alchemies of the Mind: Rationality and the Emotions* (Cambridge: Cambridge University Press, 2008); also Norbert Elias, *The Civilizing Process* (Oxford: Blackwell, 1994), 417–418.
8 James Brown, "Comments on Sonnet 129," unpublished ms, 2014.
9 Bernard Williams, *Shame and Necessity* (Berkeley: University of California Press, 1995), 219–223.
10 Paul Hazard, "Freud's Teaching on Shame," *Laval Théologique et Philosophique*, 25, no. 2 (1969): 253.
11 Brown, "Comments".
12 Williams, *Shame and Necessity*, 84–85.
13 Eric R. Dodds, *The Greeks and the Irrational* (Berkeley: University of California Press, 1951).
14 Williams, *Shame and Necessity*, 85–87.
15 Robert Graves and Laura Riding, "A Study in Original Punctuation and Spelling," in *The Common Asphodel*, ed. Robert Graves (London: Hamish Hamilton, 1949).
16 Stephen Booth, *Shakespeare's Sonnets* (New Haven, CT: Yale University Press, 1997), 447ff.
17 Roman Jakobson and L. G. Jones, "Shakespeare's Verbal Art in *Th'Expence of Spirit*," in *Language in Literature*, ed. Roman Jakobson (Cambridge, MA: Harvard University Press, 1987), 214.
18 For a critique, see Jon Elster, "Fullness and parsimony," in *Explanation and Value in the Arts*, eds. Salim Kemal and Ivan Gaskell (Cambridge: Cambridge University Press, 1993), 146–172; also Thomas Osborne, "Rationality, Creativity and Modernism," *Rationality and Society*, 23, no. 2 (2011): 175–197.
19 Helen Vendler, *The Art of Shakespeare's Sonnets* (Cambridge, MA: Harvard University Press, 1998), 129.

20 Jakobson and Jones, "Shakespeare's Verbal Art," 199.
21 Vendler, 1996, 129.
22 ibid.; Vendler, "Jakobson, Richards, and Sonnet CXXIX," 182.
23 Vendler, *Art of Shakespeare's Sonnets*, 125.
24 Jakobson and Jones, "Shakespeare's Verbal Art," 202.
25 Brown, "Comments."
26 Stephen Greenblatt, *Will in the World* (London. Pimlico, 2005), 305.
27 Cf. Jakobson and Jones, "Shakespeare's Verbal Art," 200.
28 Brown, "Comments."
29 Booth, *Shakespeare's Sonnets*, 443.
30 See Fernie, *Shame in Shakespeare*, 41–73; and, in particular, Werner L. Gunderscheimer, "Renaissance Concepts of Shame and Pocaterra's *Dialogli della vergogni*," *Renaissance Quarterly*, 47 (1994): 34–56.
31 See Fernie, *Shame in Shakespeare*, 71–73.
32 Williams, *Shame and Necessity*, 76.
33 Max Weber, *Economy and Society*, vol. 1 (Berkeley: University of California Press, 1968), 576; also Elster, 2000: 34.

4 Lyric Shame

Denise Riley

> What is the language using us for?
> Said Malcolm Mooney moving away
> Slowly over the white language.
> Where am I going said Malcolm Mooney.
> Certain experiences seem to not
> Want to go into language maybe
> Because of shame or the reader's shame.
> Let us observe Malcolm Mooney.
> —W.S. Graham, "What Is The Language Using Us For?"

We could recall W.H. Auden's assertion that "Art is born of humiliation." I really don't know about this generalization; but I want to mention, briefly, the possibility of "A Song of Shame." My hunch is that
there's something about working in poetry (above all in lyric writing)
which is inherently bound up with shame. Indeed, that shame may act
as a driving "motor" of lyric. I'm thinking – not of the content itself, nor
of the embarrassment for the writer of standing up to perform, nor the
awkwardness of claiming authorship when she may be dimly conscious
of her many debts and influences – but of pure shame as an element in
the very impulse that produces lyric and breaks into song. With lyric
writing, there's something in the very production of song and shame
that's intimately related. What is this something?

   To start with a curiosity: there's a proximity of shame to exhibitionism. An "exhibited" kind of writerly shame can be concealment tangled
with unconcealment. You do need a confident immodesty to display
your own shame. Yet that real confidence could be covering over an
equally real humiliation. Some bold authorial show of shame needn't
cancel out the emotion itself. Why make such a bother about it, though,
when anyone would naturally expect that the sense of shame would simply keep you quiet? That any genuinely ashamed writer would likely be
shamed, by herself, into silence? That line of thought says it's implausi-
ble and perverse to make a noise out of the feeling of shame. However,
if your shame is such that you can't manage to speak, you might be able

to *write,* instead. Literary writing may function, for some, exactly as a means of *not* speaking – of avoiding face-to-face speech altogether. A way of "finding" not your spoken voice, but your read-onscreen or on-paper voice.

I'm not thinking so much about the shame of some actual occasion for song, and which could speak about itself defensively, as with W.B. Yeats' late poem, "The Spur":

> You think it horrible that lust and rage
> Should dance attention upon my old age;
> They were not such a plague when I was young;
> What else have I to spur me into song?

I mean, rather, that the shame inherent in lyric writing isn't merely to do with the act of enunciation as drawing attention to yourself and so risking your dread of standing out, or your fear of the sin of pride. Nor is it to do with the content itself, as in that Yeats verse. It's not the guilt of ostentation, but some fundamental state of shame embedded in being a lyric writer at all. I do recognize that this sounds bizarre and counterintuitive; I'm putting it forward only tentatively, not as some grand thesis.

Why might there be such a founding shame? In part, because if you think about how you'd acknowledge your place in a language that's "held in common," that would entail avoiding the biography-boasting that's now demanded of authors. And to avoid it as part of recognizing the pragmatic nature of writing – because you are necessarily speaking into an in-between area where it's not you who is solely in charge of the speaking, since your awareness of potential listeners and readers has a powerful effect on how you'll speak, yet where you can't know who is receiving it, your personal authorship is truly not pertinent. In how it is transmitted and how it is received, there's something incalculable and properly anonymous about writing. This has nothing at all to do with the sum of your biography and your private attitudes. Your whole existence is, of course, an accident; your writing is a different kind of accident. And *you* can't take credit for either. A feeling of shame appears when this is not understood, and the biographical demand intrudes; you are asked, in effect, to subscribe to a misapprehension about your part as a writer. You, an author, are being given too much credit for something which isn't of your own making, in the way that biographical assessment supposes it is. Hence your possible shame.

For the fact you experience through writing is this: it's the voice of language itself which is trying to speak. This isn't some aesthetic mystification, but is the felt practical condition of lyric writing in particular. So part of the lyric shame, perhaps most of the shame, is to do with being regarded as the source of the writing; being hailed as its author in the strong sense of that word. Whereas you know very well that you are ot the source. The language is. The history of lyric has worked its way into the present-day lyric. That lyric has needed to be released from you, as its author; its elements of personal confession may well have been scoured and simplified. But I don't mean that the presence of the author is a contamination – just that, if language gets close to its truest point of becoming a pure "speaking out," the private accidents of your authorship fall away, as far as they may. And then this speaking out of language itself might emerge from a residue of what's been "burnt away." The "fire" in question certainly isn't anything to do with martyrdom, or with a trial of the writer. But it is the free burning of language itself.

Here is William Blake's "The Clod and the Pebble," from his *Songs of Innocence and Experience*, published in 1794:

> Love seeketh not itself to please,
> Nor for itself hath any care,
> But for another gives its ease,
> And builds a Heaven in Hell's despair.
>
> So sung a little Clod of Clay
> Trodden with the cattle's feet,
> But a Pebble of the brook
> Warbled out these metres meet:
>
> Love seeketh only self to please,
> To bind another to its delight,
> Joys in another's loss of ease,
> And builds a Hell in Heaven's despite.

So some forms of song, like the hard pebble's darkly self-centred warbling, can endure; but other kinds of song, like the clod's, live perilously close to a state of dissolution. Made, like humans, of clay, it crumbles into a melody of sacrificial altruism which is washed away. Such a song would dissolve, or liquefy, or would be trampled like the clod into muddied waters. This short lyric of mine has drawn on Blake's disintegrating "clod," as it wonders about achieving clarity, and about abasement, hopeful need and possible dissolution:

Maybe; maybe not

> When I was a child I spoke as a clod, I
> Understood as a stone, I thought as a thrush
> But when I became a man I put away
> Plain things for lustrous, yet to this day
> Squat under hooves for kindness where

Fetlocks stream with mud; shall I never
Get it clear, down in the soily waters.

There's a terrific and cheerfully direct statement of this intimacy between shame and song, voiced by one of Fyodor Dostoevsky's characters
in *The Brothers Karamazov*:

> When I fall into the abyss, I go straight into it, head down and heels
> up, and I'm even pleased that I'm falling in just such a humiliating
> position, and for me I find it beautiful. And so in that very shame I
> suddenly begin a hymn.

This speaker's song stems, he thinks, straight from the comical mortification of the flesh; Dmitri (or Mitya) says that he's fallen in love with a
"low woman."[1] This falling, as the abasement from which a sounding
appeal may rise, also harks back to that long tradition of "De Profundis,"
out of the depths. Psalm 130 begins:

> Out of the depths have I cried unto thee, O LORD.
> Lord, hear my voice: let thine ears be attentive to the voice of my
> supplications.

Job's lamentations are in the mode of raising your voice only from the
very depths. Such "singing in distress" is rather like the behavior of
plants; flowering itself is a sign of distress, in that a plant starved of
nutrients will produce flowers but not leaves, in its desperate attempt to
make seeds, its own future. Birds sing, not from pure joy but to mark
and defend their territory. We can also think of the hydraulic pressure
that results in sound – like the whistling kettle surging to the boil (even
the despised "hydraulic metaphor" has its uses). Song can be the outcome of some intense inward pressure, like an exhalation of breath following inner exertion. Such a pressure might include the song of shame;
a shame at making a noise which must become bearable – in that both
the shame and its transforming noise can be borne. A final short piece:

Another lyric

It sits with itself in its arms. Out of
the depth of its shame it starts singing
a hymn of pure shame, surging in the throat.
To hold a true note could be everything.
Getting the hang of itself would undo it.

For me, it's a question of moving from *shame* (in so far as that's not rational; I mean, in so far as it's in excess of the conditions of authorship

I've mentioned) to *sorrow*. Which, of course, is rational – sorrow at the trials of life and at the state of this world is, to put it mildly, reasonable. In short, my own aim is to finally convert "shame" into a bearable sadness. When the pressure of shame itself can become a productive force, the lyric poem might sometimes just be one way of enacting and demonstrating this conversion from private shame to acknowledged sorrow.

Note

1 Book III of *Karamazov*; *The Sensualists*, Chapter 3, "The Confession of a Passionate Heart."

5 Writing to Spare One's Blushes

Jean Jacques Rousseau's *Confessions* and the Automation of Confidence

Christopher John Müller

> I am made unlike any one I have ever met; I will even venture to say that I am like no one in the whole world. I may be no better, but at least I am different.
>
> —Jean-Jacques Rousseau, *The Confessions*[1]

Shame has a tendency to catch us out, to emerge as if out of nowhere. The feeling can suddenly appear, making us feel put on the spot, isolated and alone. A word, a glance or clumsy gesture suffices to ossify the ground underfoot, fluster the body and affect the flow of words through an involuntary silence or an undignified torrent of excuses. Even though experience has taught us in which situations we are likely to feel shame, this foreknowledge offers little defense. For in such anticipation of a potentially embarrassing or awkward situation, shame already makes us feel singled out in a manner that orients our thoughts and commands our actions.

In *Impersonal Passion*, Denise Riley recounts one of the complicated social encounters in which shame can erupt. Having suddenly fallen ill before a party, a guest feels the need to phone the host to excuse her absence. The situation, as Riley elaborates, produces the "feeling of emitting an aura of lying, and the corresponding fear of not being believed," even though the truth will be told.[2] The prospect of truthfully communicating a simple fact that was not her fault – the would-be guest did not, after all, choose to fall ill – leads to racing thoughts, an intensification of the original symptoms of the illness and panicked indecision. What to say? How to say it? Turn up ill and leave again, just to prove that she is not lying? In my case at least it is likely, that, depending who is at the other end of the line, the eventual phone call would either not happen at all or would result in awkward overcompensations and fumbled excuses, inevitably amplifying the impression that the other must take the illness to be fictitious. Upon ending the call, an impression of narcissistic arrogance (why did I assume my absence to be such a big deal?) is likely to mingle with the momentary pathos of existential solitude – why does this always happen to me, why did I get myself ill, why am I so awkward?[3] What is experienced here, I suggest, is what Günther Anders calls the "pain of unfreedom," a pain in which he recognizes the basic, fateful motif of shame. For Anders, whose multifaceted phenomenological observations of the workings of shame have been overlooked for too long in the English-speaking world, "to be ashamed means: *not being able to do anything about the fact that it is not one's fault.*"[4] Today, of course, the scenario Riley evokes has found a convenient solution, one which disarms and sanitizes the situation by seemingly offering protection from existential grief as well as the contingencies of a conversation that might well make one feel exposed: be generously impolite, save the other and yourself from an awkward situation beyond your control, pick up your phone, shudder at the thought of calling, send a text message.

This turn to artifice and writing, this turn to a machine to maintain a semblance of freedom and self-determination, this act of sending a text in one's place and making oneself known from a secure distance is the focus of this essay. As I conceive of it here, the act of writing is entwined with a feeling of exposure that coincides with the irrepressible bodily agitations with which shame amplifies one's self-awareness the very moment it undermines one's presence of mind. This peculiar nakedness visits us when we feel the pull of a silence that makes our words vanish down a knotted throat to a place and physiological reality that cannot be accessed; it affects us also when physiological excitement seems to take over speaking, when we hear ourselves rambling on, voicing the indistinct mutterings of a body losing composure and self-control. I mobilize Jean-Jacques Rousseau's *Confessions* and aspects of Günther Anders's mostly undiscovered work on shame to flesh out and contemplate some poststructuralist notions of language that are at times being too easily (and impulsively) dismissed.[5] To do so, I focus on this inaccessibly private self, which is so powerfully exposed to us, the very moment shame hijacks speech to make one feel embarrassingly singular and unable to reach out to others. It is this feeling of involuntary exposure that Jean-Luc Nancy describes in a beautifully rendered definition of nakedness that captures the intensity of the feeling of singularity that can befall one, for example, when one finds oneself emitting 'an aura of lying' despite telling the truth:

> to be naked is, first and foremost, to be undressed, to be without any covering that could present or signify a state or a function. It is to reveal everything but, at the same time, to show that there is nothing more to see.[6]

Nancy's words can help distinguish between two modes of self-presence that cannot simply be opposed to one another: involuntary exposure and the more composed presence that collected speech and writing seems to offer. Nancy's description of nakedness suggests that, rather than revealing a presence behind the cover, the intensity of the feeling of exposure merely reveals an absence, an abandonment to a situation that can be paralytic, distressing but also blissfully exciting. The moment I find myself baring all and presenting the "naked truth," is also the moment I have nothing more to show that could substantiate who or what I am. Amidst the intense nervous activity the situation commands, I am reduced to passivity, have lost access to the resources with which "I" usually present myself. My confused words grappling for sense and conviction make me feel like a spectacle, dispossessing me of myself the moment I am so inescapably there.[7] This very absent mindedness, then, this indecision when being reduced to being "me precisely" (as Anders puts it), that is, to a me stripped of everything that is usually at "my" disposal (*my* ability to present myself to others, *my* confidence, *my* words, *my* bodily composure, etc.) is the focus of this chapter. I hasten to add that the "exaggerated" descriptions I have offered so far are entirely theoretical and idealized, for any account of the feeling of exposure inevitably recovers a self-presence where it was once missing.[8] The retrospective act of describing such a situation inevitably signals that one has found an escape from this passivity and thus escaped the uninvited feeling of scrutiny to sufficiently collect one's thoughts, choose one's words and regain a persona one cannot simply choose to undress from. The moment one writes in composed sentences, one is, to use Anders's words, no longer caught in a situation in which one is reduced to being "me precisely" – someone one "has not chosen" to be – but has found a retreat in the cover of writing and the edited, more composed presence this seems to promise.[9]

I open with this protracted reflection to signal that combining the words *shame* and *is* to offer a definition in writing inevitably posits the danger of catching one out, leaving one red faced and speechless at the very moment when the feeling itself imposes a tangible reminder of its being. Rather than merely offering itself to definition and rationalization, shame announces its presence by autonomously "de-fining" – that is, encircling and delimiting – one's ability to grab hold of oneself in articulation. Shame announces its presence by catching one out. Yet the threat constituted by this involuntary exhibition does not inhibit speech, or even writing. The fact that the feeling interrupts and inhibits us, and this often in an unwelcome manner, also emphasizes that one has already found routes to less unsettled, more composed ways of being. The longed-for escape from exposure that has us reach out for artifice and "signifying covers" we are momentarily stripped of, involves a retreat into spaces opened by the trickery of what Jacques Derrida calls "supplements" (clothing, writing, explanatory words, stereotypes and social conventions, but also "smarter" devices). These give us a limited agency, by allowing us to maintain our distance and act as the wirepuller behind a mask we don't necessarily realize that we are wearing – until, of course, we are caught out and stripped of our comforting agency. This play of cover and exposure points to a generative relationship with artifice that expatiates beyond cognition, and that is at work *before* we can feel exposed in shame. The grip of silence blocking access to words can only be felt because we already have words to share, we only feel naked and exposed because we are normally dressed, no longer covered by the unfelt nakedness that adorned our bodies at birth.[10] Shame, as I conceive of it here, can be read as the mark of an entanglement in arti- fice, which does not make the feeling less real or binding. Rather, this entanglement is part of the reality of the feeling. For in shame one finds oneself stripped and uncovered, unfreely dispossessed of the means by which one has inevitably (and unwittingly) found an escape from the uncomfortable feeling of being precisely oneself.

The challenge when thinking about shame, as I understand it, and in particular when considering its status as a feeling that gives us scruple, moderation and other forms of openness toward others (but also disre- gard and disrespect), is how to conceptualize the feeling of irreducible singularity to which one finds oneself exposed when singled out in shame. In "On Escape," Emmanuel Levinas elaborates on the "pain of unfree- dom" that Anders isolates, by suggesting that "what appears in shame is *precisely* the fact of being riveted to oneself, the radical impossibility of fleeing oneself to hide from oneself, the unalterably binding presence of the I to itself."[11] It is this *precise existence* that I wish to contemplate by turning to Jean-Jacques Rousseau's *Confessions*. By offering an exagger- ated, over-sentimentalized description of absolute singularity, Rousseau's text anticipates and stages several twentieth century phenomenological and existential treatments of shame that hinge on the feeling of absolute singularity. These treatments of shame are, to varying degrees, related to or reimaginations of Martin Heidegger's dismissal of purely "anthropo- logical," "psychological" and "physiological" conceptualizations of the human "built around a notion of a generally binding *Biology*," which proposes that an inescapable experience of singularity is constitutive of human existence.[12] The general trait of human existence, as Anders puts this, unfolds through a felt singularity that is accentuated by a bodily weight, for in shame we are reminded of a paradoxical freedom:

> *I cannot get out of my skin, even though I can conceive of it as such,* which I meet in the freedom of the experience of myself – but as non- free. Shame is not born of this incongruity; this incongruity is itself already shame. In shame the self wants to free itself, in so far as it feels definitively and irrevocably delivered to itself.

In this desire, however, it remains in a "deadlock," for it remains at the "mercy of the irrevocable, and thus of itself."[13] For Anders, this contradictory freedom to experience oneself as being unfree points to the formative power of artifice, and Rousseau's text can offer an illustration of why the singularity of shame can be read as neither an exclusively biological nor merely sociocultural phenomenon, but one that is rooted in "artificial additions" which the body begins to naturalize after birth. Put otherwise, Rousseau's text begins to *"inanimate"* shame, to use David Wills' term, and to see in it not an authentic mark of what it means to be human, but a mark of the human's inauthenticity and lack of essence, its entanglement with prosthetic additions, narratives and artifice operative beyond cognition.[14] I draw on Rousseau's text to distinguish two modes of confession: the involuntary revelation of finding precisely oneself exposed in shame, and the voluntary gesture of revealing oneself in writing. This will set the basis for some thoughts on how consideration of the "artificial" dimension of shame alters our understanding of the play of agency and inhibition which the feeling of shame coincides with. As the example of "'lying' when you aren't" has illustrated, being singled out in this manner does not point to a detached solipsism and selfishness, it is rather the mark of an irreducible (if highly selective) openness to others. As Riley points out, the anxieties of canceling at short notice are directly related to who is on the other end of the phone.

Denise Riley's reflections on "'lying' when you aren't" have a precursor in a famous scene of Jean-Jacques Rousseau's *Confessions*. The text, which opens with the elaborate declaration of the author's absolute singularity given in the epigraph, records the first 53 years of Rousseau's life, starting with his childhood memories. In Book 1, Rousseau "trace[s his] nature back ... to its earliest manifestation" (28), to an incident that is presented as the origin of this feeling of being absolutely singular. We learn how as a young child he was wrongly accused of breaking a comb whilst studying unsupervised in a kitchen. In a perfect example of "emitting an aura of lying" when telling the truth, Rousseau relates how his stubborn professions of innocence merely made the consequences more severe. He is punished not only for the broken comb, but also for the far more serious crime of lying and hiding behind fraudulent words. "It is now nearly fifty years since this occurrence," Rousseau informs his reader,

> but I declare before Heaven that I was not guilty ... Imagine a person timid and docile in ordinary life, but proud, fiery, and inflexible when roused ... a creature without a thought of injustice, now for the first time suffering a most grave one at the hands of the people he loves best and mostly deeply respects. Imagine the revolution in his ideas, the violent change of his feelings, the confusion in his heart and brain, in his small intellectual being! I say, imagine all this if you can. For myself I do not feel capable of unravelling the strands, or even remotely following all that happened at that time within me.
> (29)

This crucial scene is narrated as a rift – "imagine if you can, I cannot" – as a fall from a naive innocence and harmonious unity to an irredeemable experience of singleness. As Jean Starobinski outlines in a highly influential reading, Rousseau is here forced to experience, for the first time, both the "power and impotence of words."[15] The moment he is forced to realize that he cannot turn to anything else but words to profess his innocence, a dependence on language is revealed that has the capacity to leave him exposed. Because his words fail to sway his accusers, 'the child' (Rousseau does not deploy his all-knowing 'I') is reduced to a state in which he has "nothing" to show in his defense, and is left naked "without any covering that could present or signify a state or a function." The knowledge of his innocence hence does not prevent shame, but rather coincides with its expression and condemns him further in the eyes of his accusers.[16] Singularity is here presented as something passive, something that *happened to him because* of an artificial medium into which Rousseau is ignorantly born. Still a child, he lacked the experience to recognize that his words might be read as the mark of dissimulation. The false accusation is equated to a second birth, for the experience of nakedness also animates his impulse to reach out for covers and mobilize the power of artifice. Afraid of being forced to show "that there is nothing more to see," he begins to ensure that he can provide memory supports, and surfaces that are cultivated so that there is something to show.

As Starobinski and later Derrida point out, Rousseau uses the motif of the broken comb to explain how "evil" and "separation" enters the world through innocence and union. The episode is narrated, as Starobinski explains, in a manner that ensures that both the accusers and the accused remain free of guilt: "There is only an accusation and an apparently guilty party thrust forward as if by chance and *automatically* offered up for punishment."[17] The contingent circumstances surrounding the broken comb have culminated into a situation in which shared words generate a feeling of separation, because they single out the speaker and embolden the more powerful accuser. In Rousseau's inability to communicate his innocence, language loses its transparency and is recognized as an artificial cover that opens us to others only by also keeping us in reserve, *automatically*, all by itself. Here the real tragedy begins. Speaking for himself and his cousin (who had also been falsely accused of a transgression), Rousseau narrates this fall from the transparency of language as follows:

> No longer were we young people bound by ties of respect, intimacy and confidence to our guardians; we no longer looked on them as gods who read our hearts; we were less ashamed of wrongdoing, and more afraid of being caught; we began to be secretive, to rebel, and to lie.

(30)

Being taken for a liar when he was not gives Rousseau first-hand experience of the power, fact and existence of artifice, as well as an intuitive sense of how to begin to use this power. The realization that people do not "read our hearts," but respond to appearances and surfaces mediating on our behalf, is here presented as effecting a marked shift in the attitude towards language. His inability to share the secret of his innocence has opened the possibility of secrecy, a form of solitude and singleness that actively excludes others (*I* will not share, *I* will act *as if*). His passive exposure into painful isolation animates the ability to retreat behind a cover, with this "the act of writing" begins, even before he has learned to shape letters. The pain of not being himself, that is the pain of being identified as a liar and being reduced to a precise existence without any means to substantiate and manipulate his presence, begins to animate words in a new way. In its singular pain, the body has also found access to a source of confidence and composure. It has begun to learn to trick itself out of the inhibition to act, and overcomes the binding ties of respect. It begins to do what it once did not dare. A process of self-fashioning is animated with this exposure to and by artifice. Cast out into the world, Rousseau learns to create and live in his own. Yet this newfound agency and freedom remains unfreely bound to a precise existence that can only be escaped provisionally. For the body tricked out of inhibition and the feeling of being limited can always begin to announce its return. Its confidence can waver and begin to pull him in the direction of a precise existence in which he finds himself indetermined again, and in need of a renewed cover and grappling for new ways to substantiate and "show himself." In the face of the scrutiny and attention of others, through the consequences of actions, or changing circumstances, the covers that have been naturalized and woven into the intuitive fabric of the self can suddenly begin to feel like an uncomfortable fit – they can seem alien and inappropriate, make us feel exposed or animate our passions against a world into which we do not seem to fit.

It is this tension between finding composure and losing it that *The Confessions* stages in an exaggerated manner. A striking aspect of Rousseau's account is that it habitually fails to dramatize shame when it narrates transgressive acts and intimate secrets that are the results of deliberate acts. The unfelt inhibition that enabled him to do the thing recorded seems to lead to a factual style. In stark contrast to this, however, the text records, in at times obsessive detail, instances in which the author felt socially awkward, was unable to maintain composure and lost the confidence required to counter the disempowering sting of shame.[18] Put otherwise, the text records in great detail moments of indecision and indetermination, moments in which he would like to substantiate his being and make an impression but finds himself unable to do so. This inability threatens especially when he is forced to face others and speak:

> So much am I a slave to fears and shames that I long to vanish from
> mortal sight. If action is necessary I do not know what to do; If I
> must speak I do not know what to say; If anyone looks at me I drop
> my eyes. When roused by passion, I can sometimes find the right
> words to say, but in ordinary conversation I can find none, none at
> all. I find conversation unbearable owing to the very fact that I am
> obliged to speak.
>
> (44)

This passage, the first of many like it in the text, in effect restages the
incident of the broken comb.[19] For what is revisited here is a feeling
of impotency that he cannot fully escape as it is also the source of his
power. This impotency is an indelible reminder that he has only a limited command over artifice, for the cover of appearance does not only
open an interior retreat, it also subjects him to judgments that happen
"in his absence," when "he" is not there, unable to show himself and
emerge from behind the mask. The social fears the text records are
moments in which Rousseau is stripped back to being "me precisely"
and finds himself unable to present the "secret," "actual" self that
addresses us in writing, the one being worked out through the cover
of appearances. And it is here that writing offers a further arsenal, for
it offers the possibility to compile a script and a reminder of who he
is. It can work on the minds of others the moment he cannot. In *The
Confessions*, writing in a very concrete sense becomes a tool that helps
him maintain composure. In a memorable passage, Rousseau recounts
how he was forced into an awkward silence during a dinner invitation
because the hosts "talked the fashionable Paris jargon, full of diminu-
tives and subtle little allusions, which afforded poor Jean-Jacques little
chance of shining" (272). "Distressed of [his] own dullness" he saves
face by pulling from his pocket "an epistle in verse" that he had written at a prior date. The piece, we learn, was "not without fire" and this
gives him the opportunity to read it "in an exaggerated manner," thus
moving the dinner party to tears, and awakening the feelings that his
presence was failing to excite (273). Writing here offers a short cut to
composure and intimacy, it allows him a way of being present whilst
retaining his distance, and it enables him to force the social encounter
to unfold in a manner he is comfortable with, for the unsettling presence of others can be transformed into an affirmation that he could not
otherwise attain.

In the course of documenting his "fears and shames," Rousseau arrives
at some images that translate with uncanny accuracy into the digital age.
During one of his protracted self-portrayals, Rousseau reflects on how
his feelings and his intellect are two "almost irreconcilable characteristics": "feelings come quicker than lighting and fill my soul, but they
bring me no illumination; they burn and dazzle me … I am excited but

stupid; If I want to think I must be cool." Because this excitability means that his "thoughts arise slowly and confusedly, and are never ready till too late," he imparts how he could "conduct a delightful conversation by post" because this would force others to "wait" until he has attained the composure that he so often lacks in the spur of the moment (113). This passage strongly resonates with some of the conclusions that Sherry Turkle draws in *Alone Together,* a text that contemplates the shifting patterns of communications configuring themselves around digital devices. She tracks the manner in which e-mail, text and instant messages are making us "flee the telephone," fearful that impromptu conversations might "reveal too much." Her text especially focuses on teenagers who have grown up with such devices. Turkle cites an interview with seventeen-year-old Elaine, who explains her antipathy for calling along similar lines to Rousseau. In fact, Elaine's account corresponds to *The Confessions* almost *verbatim*: "When you can think about what you're going to say, you can talk to someone you'd have trouble talking to. And it doesn't seem weird that you pause for two minutes to think about what you're going to say."[20] The advantage of onscreen communication is that it is "a place to reflect, retype, and edit." It is, as Turkle cites Elaine, "a place to hide."[21]

Rousseau's *Confessions* acts as a reminder that the dynamic Turkle isolates as being a particular effect of digital media is merely an amplification of a tendency that is already always at work, as soon as the body has been exposed to (and by) the power of artifice. The reflection on writing with which Rousseau explains his fantasy of conducting a "conversation by post" culminates into a definition of writing. I will cite this definition with Jean Starobinski's framing questions, as these lucidly draw out the dynamic tensions between self-presence and absence / absentmindedness and composed presence that Rousseau's text stages at every turn:

> How to overcome the misunderstanding that prevents [Rousseau] from expressing himself according to his true value? How to escape the risks of improvised speech? To what other mode of communication can he turn? By what other means manifest himself? Jean-Jacques chooses to be *absent* and to *write*. Paradoxically, he will hide himself to show himself better, and he will confide in written speech: "I would love society like others, if I were not sure of showing myself not only at a disadvantage, but as completely different from what I am. The part that I have taken of *writing and hiding myself* is precisely the one that suits me. If I were present, one would never know what I was worth" (*Confessions*). The admission is singular and merits emphasis: Jean-Jacques breaks with others, only to present himself to them in written speech. Protected by solitude, he will turn and re-turn his sentences at leisure.[22]

The dream of composure, self-mastery and protection from contingency that writing offers is presented as being intrinsically connected to, and a symptom of, the *fact and fear of being caught out*, of losing hold of oneself in the instant of an encounter, of finding oneself stripped and scattered, debarred from access to oneself the very moment the weight of one's presence is most ardently felt. In order to spare his blushes and show himself "better," Rousseau hides by inscribing himself in exteriorized words. He presents himself through an abstraction of self that can be rearranged, retained and edited. Rather than merely presenting himself, he presents for scrutiny silent words in his place. Rousseau hides himself through visibility. He only shows himself so as not to be caught out and seen; in doing so, he attains a "presentable" self where previously there was nothing to be shown that could have substantiated his being. Writing here touches on the living presence of the body by covering it through rationalization and exteriorization, by adding to it an inanimate substrate that replaces its presence and has already dislocated it from its "proper" place in the here and now of the "lived moment," a moment that can be overwhelming, dazzling, filled with flashing emotions and impulses that interfere or threaten to hijack speech. By enabling him to "break" with the moment and with others, writing grants time and distance. It promises full self-presence and full composure because it allows the writer to fully absent himself in person. The incessant play of maintaining composure and losing it that is the mark of the lived experience of the body is here pushed to (a farcical) extreme, for Rousseau escapes the singularizing feeling of inadvertently "revealing too much," only by also condemning himself to solitude and not showing himself at all.

In *Of Grammatology*, Jacques Derrida cites the passage from *Transparency and Obstruction* just quoted to begin to introduce the "profound law" of supplementation. For it is only the addition of the exteriorizing medium that brings that which is seemingly interior to the fore. As such, the supplement arrives as if to fill a void, for it is only its addition that retroactively reveals the presence it seemingly merely adds itself to. Hiding in writing, as Rousseau (and Elaine) impart, affords time. But it cannot definitively break with the intensity of being "me precisely," it merely grants the space to conceal the struggle to gain composure. It makes the time it takes to work out what this "me" might be in this particular instance. The privacy and autonomy gained thus cannot escape the feeling of exposure, or even the confusion and perturbation to which Rousseau attests, but this struggle for composure now emphatically plays itself out between the writer and the medium that offers the promise of substantiating a felt presence and passion in such a way that it can be shown to others (and oneself). Derrida calls the "battle" that starts the moment "I wish to raise myself above my life even while I retain it, in order to enjoy recognition" *writing*.[23] And *The Confessions* records the debris of this more hidden struggle unfolding "within" in some detail.

The following description with which Rousseau illustrates the "extreme difficulties" he has in writing, is especially productive:

> Have you ever been to the opera in Italy? During changes of scenery wild and prolonged disorder reigns in their great theatres. The furniture is higgledy-piggledy; on all sides things are being shifted and everything seems upside down; it is as if they were bent on universal destruction; but little by little everything falls into place, nothing is missing, and, to one's surprise, all the long tumult is succeeded by a delightful spectacle. That is almost exactly the process that takes place in my brain when I want to write.
>
> (113)

The elaborate nature of the metaphor is radically at odds with the chaos it seeks to capture. It represents disorder in an orderly fashion, elevates an "I" into the role of a narrator narrating his own struggle to articulate himself. The act of writing thus stages and covers a precise existence that Rousseau cannot bring himself to show – not merely because he is too proud to reveal it, but because it is impossible to translate the intensity of feeling into writing, he has to lose his precision to find it. The "precise existence," therefore, might be understood as an indelible impulse to edit in view of felt contingency and indeterminacy, an impulse to seek form and determination, to cover the exposure of being left "without any covering that could present or signify a state or a function" in order to arrive at steady ground on which one can stand. The act of writing here amounts to a waiting game that persists until coherence and sense arrives, *as if by surprise*. Through the painful reedits and attempts to arrive at sense and meaning a presence begins to emerge on the stage of visibility. An actor retroactively emerges who is now narrated as having been at work, all along, pushing everything into place. The moment this harmony is achieved a "delightful spectacle" can be enjoyed. The more this "I" takes on shape in writing, the more coherent its words become, the more Rousseau becomes part of the audience he imagines, the more he is able to see meaning, substance, presence. He attains a self he can begin to enact. The written text thus supplements an "absence." Out of writer's block, indecision and isolation a body has composed itself in solitude to begin to address others and bridge the gap that has forced it into this solitary retreat.

By now, of course, the contradiction is quite out in the open. To commune with others in this manner, Rousseau needs to concentrate, write, worry, talk to himself – motions that seek to shift gears until sufficient drive is found to confidently reach out to others. In doing so, however, he exposes himself to the agonies of finding and rehearsing a role he hopes will please. Rousseau's description of the act of writing, his quest for autonomy through composure, I suggest, can serve as an illustration that shame is intrinsically connected to mediating covers and artificial registers. For the substantiation of self that happens via exteriorization and supplementation starts to unfold long before Rousseau reaches out for a pen. In *The Confessions*, it begins with the idealized account of the broken comb, a moment in which, as he realizes in retrospect, he "emitted an aura of lying" because appearances were against him. Denise Riley ends her incisive intervention on this involuntary ruse by evoking a telephone answering machine, which, as she puts it, "lies professionally on our behalf, whether or not we are in."[24] If we cast our eyes back to the scene of the broken comb, then we might see a parallel. For Rousseau falls victim to just such a machine. His words are taken to be lying on his behalf, they act without him and against his wishes. Although he is *in* he finds no means to pick up the phone and speak to the caller. He is fully laid bare, stripped of signifying covers, is reduced to a state in which he has nothing more to show or say. This is the moment he is forced to realize that his words merely act on his behalf, that they retain a life of their own. A rift is accentuated that is not a lack, for it gives him a self-awareness and self-consciousness that makes him look for means to turn them into trusty allies. This exposure does not just give us a self, but also each other, for it opens the space we need to commune.

Günther Anders, whose engagements with shame have oriented this piece, reminds us that this turn to artifice is not the tragic fall Rousseau would have us believe, but rather the condition of intimacy. As Anders puts it in a diary entry from May 10 1949:

> the story recounted in Genesis presents everything the wrong way round. Adam and Eve could only discover (*entdecken*) their nudity, because they had already covered themselves up (*bedecken*) prior to this. It is only now, with the discovery of nudity, that the gates to Paradise open themselves.[25]

With this at times blissful and at times painful entrapment by artifice, however, the hot puff of "a blushing machine" is also animated, one that cannot simply be switched off.[26] David Wills deploys this evocative term in response to Jacques Derrida's *The Animal That Therefore I Am* to suggest that shame points to the workings of "a machine set in motion by itself, always already on," and writing, as Rousseau conceives of it, is such a machine.[27] The body finding itself ignorantly born into speech can only begin to take hold of words because it is already enveloped by their cover. It can participate in their speaking, but never fully command it. To exercise this power, we need to forget the agency of words. By doing so, we expose ourselves to recurring, occasionally painful reminders that "our" words have the power to catch us out, come back to haunt us and remind us that we cannot get out of our skin. An overused set-phrase, a mindless remark can leave the impression that nobody is "in" (to refer back to Riley's image of an answering machine), words that escape, can also suddenly show us in an inopportune light, or worse, they can let something slip that ends up acting against us, sours a relationship or ties us into a commitment, thus determining the course of our lives in unanticipated ways, awakening a desire to go back, say things differently, escape an unplanned contingency. Speaking thus automatically leads to self-entrapment, but we must not forget that we call this entrapment: "I," "the self," "the ego," "singularity" or any other term we might use to name this experience.

What Rousseau's text accentuates, therefore, is that this exposure and involuntary retrospection is the product of what Wills calls *inanimation*, the originary entanglement of life (not just human life) in inanimate artifice, an entanglement that "quickens" life by interrupting it with a self-distancing mechanism and a spontaneous automaticity.[28] Whilst this may give us "a self" and limited agency, this act of inanimation also lends words and things a life entirely of their own. We turn to supplements, words, social roles, but also smarter machines with a desire to trick the feeling of involuntary exposure by finding ever more artful covers, ever more helpful agents that offer retreats from contingency, and powerful means to achieve and maintain composure. This impulse is neither good nor bad, for the impulse to reach out for cover happens all by itself and beyond cognition, but Rousseau's text (and Turkle's observations) point out that this quest for autonomy can lead to painful isolation. Rousseau, to use Turkle's title, ends up *alone together*, rehearsing a role in solitude whilst yearning for recognition. The stage of writing is populated by phantoms he is unable to face. Moreover, the limelight he imagines threatens to put him on the spot. In writing his *Confessions* and revealing everything, he might have attained composure, but he also creates a substance that can find itself under attack. By lamenting the fact that he cannot make himself known, he voluntarily breaches his own privacy, gives others ammunition that may turn against him.[29]

Besides leading to a script that is overly fixed and a persona one can no longer escape, the process of self-fashioning that unfolds via artifice also creates potentially limiting dependences. Naturalized covers can no longer simply be removed, for doing so leaves one naked. By acting on our behalf, artifice can also trick the body out of inhibitions and inabilities that might better be left intact. Composure can correspond with shamelessness, coolness with a callous or unregistered cruelty (not to mention the power-structures of race, class and gender that shape our embodied experience and sense of self).[30] The desire for freedom and self-determination has a pathological tendency, as Anders puts this, because by its very nature freedom knows no limit: "to be partially free is not enough. The self (*das Ich*) does not only want to be itself now and again; the individual does not only want to be individual as an attribute," but in this quest it will inevitably entrap itself and be entrapped, it will collide with limitations from which the power of artifice promises an escape only by tying our dangerously absentminded hands and unfeeling hearts.[31]

Shame, as I hope this reading of Rousseau has begun to illustrate, cannot simply be traced back to a single body or even an animated corporeal process, for it attains its dynamic from the play of cover and exposure which necessarily involves some sort of addition that exposes and ties us to one another as much as it exposes and ties us to ourselves. Shame attains its dynamic from *bodies*, apart from which a body finds itself singled out and stripped of cover. What transpires, therefore, is that the "I" written onto the page is a product of the continuity of editing and not a continuity of the editor, and this complicates the notion that there is "an I" awaiting expression beneath the cover. The dream of agency, composure, self-mastery and protection from contingency that processes of self-fashioning offer, is intrinsically connected to, and a symptom of, the *fact and fear of being caught-out* (a fear that is, in itself, rooted in a generative relationship to artifice). The idealized space of the self is opened the very moment one loses hold of oneself in the instant of an encounter, when one finds oneself stripped and scattered, debarred from access to oneself at the very moment the weight of one's presence is most ardently felt.

For this exposure to be possible, however, the addition of a medium of exteriorization (be it language or clothing, or "smarter" devices) already has to have become so natural and immediate that its intimate working is forgotten. By armoring himself against the contingencies and hostilities of the social world with a pen, Rousseau hence enacts one of the innumerable untold gestures by the means of which technological supplements are involved in "manufacturing," "manipulating" and "shaping" this bodily feeling, a circumstance, or so I suggest, that forces us to be all the more cautious when defining shame (which is an irrepressible, "automatic" bodily feeling) as a strictly bodily phenomenon. The body offering itself to examination in shame is riveted to chains of supplementation and representation that generate the feeling of exposure, or put another way, a mediating cover (writing, for instance) is "essential" to the bodily apprehension of shame. I will give the final word to Anders, who captures life's originary tangle with artifice by offering us a reminder that constellations of power and scrutiny are necessarily provisional, although our self-entrapment in artifice makes this feel otherwise:

> the thousand forms of hypocrisy, of disguise, and of comedy positively exemplify the negative proof of shame and disgust: the instability of man in relation to himself, his vagueness. The self succeeds only provisionally at abandoning its precise existence as such and thus at taking the form of an another and making itself, as it were the occasion and the matter of multiple personifications. The provisional is itself conclusive: among all the species, man is the one who has the least character.[32]

Notes

1 Jean-Jacques Rousseau, *The Confessions of Jean-Jacques Rousseau*, trans. J. M. Cohen (London: Penguin, 1973), 17. All future references are from this edition and are given in the text.
2 Denise Riley, "'Lying' When You Aren't," in *Impersonal Passion* (Durham and London: Duke UP, 2005), 85–96, 85.
3 On this existential moment see Denise Riley, "Some WHYS and why mes," in *Impersonal Passion*, 59–70.
4 Günther Anders, "On Promethean Shame," trans. C. J. Müller, in *Prometheanism: Technology, Digital Culture and Human Obsolescence* (London: Rowman & Littlefield, 2016), 28–95, 67.
5 Most famously and influentially, perhaps, this dismissal was carried forward by Eve Kosofsky Sedgwick and Adam Frank, in their landmark essay "Shame in the Cybernetic Fold: Reading Silvan Tomkins," *Critical Inquiry* 21, no. 2 (1995): 496–522. Whereas I agree with the important critique of rhetoric, jargon, argumentative strategies and moralism that "Shame in the Cybernetic Fold" equates to "applied theory" in the humanities, by which the authors mean "theory after Foucault and Greenblatt, after Freud and Lacan, after Levi-Strauss, after Derrida, after feminism" (496), I wish to begin to outline here that this turn on theory (or rather, certain theorists) risks losing out on some crucial resources to think and politicize affect.
6 Jean-Luc Nancy, "Concealed Thinking," trans. by James Gilbert-Walsh, in *A Finite Thinking*, ed. Simon Sparks (Stanford, CA: Stanford University Press, 2003), 31–47, 39.
7 Charles Darwin and Martin Heidegger, a decidedly odd coupling, both see in uncontrolled, headless speech an indelible marker that one is caught in the moment of a violent singularization. In *What is Metaphysics*, for example, Heidegger suggests that

> anxiety shatters the word for us. Because the existent as a whole slips away and the nothing presses us, all utterance of the "is" falls silent in the face of the nothing. That in the uncanniness [*unheimlichkeit*] of anxiety we often seek to break the empty silence with random talk only proves the presence of the nothing.

See Martin Heidegger, *Was ist Metaphysik?* (Frankfurt am Main: Vittorio Klostermann, 2007), 35; my translation. Although there is inevitably a degree of incommensurability here, Darwin depicts a similar scene to illustrate the paradoxically heightened self-awareness that blushing coincides with the very moment it disables one's "presence" of mind:

> Most persons, whilst blushing intensely, have their mental powers confused. ... Persons in this condition lose their presence of mind, and utter singularly inappropriate remarks. ... I have been informed by a young lady, who blushes excessively, that at such times she does not even know what she is saying.

See Charles Darwin, *The Expression of the Emotions in Man and Animals*, ed. Paul Ekman (Oxford: Oxford University Press 1998), 321.
8 I am here following the lead of Günther Anders, who in an essay on shame and contingency first contemplated that basing an analysis of human existence on "exceptional" experiences leaves the impression that their importance is exaggerated. See Günther Anders, "The Pathology of Freedom: An Essay on Non-Identification," trans. Katharine Wolfe, *Deleuze Studies* 3 (2009): 278–310, 284–285.

9 Anders, "The Pathology of Freedom," 280.
10 As Jacques Derrida elaborates on our *felt* nakedness in *The Animal that Therefore I Am*:

> there is no nudity "in nature" ... because it *is* naked, without *existing* in nakedness, the animal neither feels nor sees itself naked. And it therefore is not naked. At least that is what is thought. For man it would be the opposite, and clothing derives from technics.

The Animal That Therefore I Am, trans. David Wills (New York: Fordham University Press, 2008), 5.
11 Emmanuel Levinas, *On Escape*, trans. Bettina Bergo (Stanford, CA: Stanford University Press, 2003), 49–73.
12 See Martin Heidegger, *Being and Time*, trans. John Macquarrie and Edward Robinson (Oxford: Basil Blackwell, 1985), 75. When inquiring into what the human is, as Heidegger famously elaborates, one ought to employ the ambiguous, necessarily self-reflexive question "who?" and not the systematic "what is?" of empiricism. Because each "human" life shares the character of *being each time its own to bear* (*Jemeinigkeit*), Heidegger stipulates that "one must always also say the *personal* pronoun when addressing it: 'I am,' 'you are'" (*Being and Time*, 68). For Heidegger, it is hence the experience of singularity and distinctness that constitutes the in each case singular existence through which the question "who?" plays itself out. The experience of singularity, as this might be put in the wake of Derrida and Wills, is produced and shaped by processes of supplementation that retroactively affect and mechanize life.
13 Günther Anders, "The Pathology of Freedom," p. 288. As Jean Khalfa highlights in "Fanon and Psychiatry," Anders's discussion of the experience of freedom is an important influence on Frantz Fanon's work on the psychopathologies induced by colonization (See "Fanon and Psychiatry," *Nottingham French Studies*, Vol. 54 No. 1 (2015), 52–71. I mention this here to signal that the experience of singularity ("I cannot get out of my skin") is fundamentally shaped by history, race, gender and the power relations into which a given individual finds itself bound (see also note 30 below). These questions of cultural politics are kept in the margins here, because the principle aim of this essay is to outline the crucial role "technological artifice" plays in the expression of shame.
14 See David Wills, *Inanimation: Theories of Inorganic Life* (Minneapolis: University of Minnesota Press, 2016). I briefly return to Wills' discussion of blushing below, which he primarily develops in the chapters "Automatic Life, So Life: Descartes" (pp. 31–54) and "The Blushing Machine: Derrida" (pp. 81–110).
15 See Jean Starobinski, *Jean-Jacques Rousseau: Transparency and Obstruction*, trans. Arthur Goldhammer (Chicago, IL: University of Chicago Press, 1988), 8–11. Starobinski's reading underpins Jacques Derrida's treatment of Rousseau in *Of Grammatology*.
16 Günther Anders discusses this shame despite being innocent at length in "On Promethean Shame": "The conventional assumption that shame occurs especially or even only when something 'was one's fault' clearly inverts the true state of affairs. This assumption is a symptom of the immoderate pretensions we have about freedom ... whereby humans attempt to appropriate the pain of unfreedom (which shame represents) in order to present it as a 'pain of punishment' and employ it as such. ... How little it is actual guilt and responsibility that generates shame is evident in the fact that one is also ashamed when wrongly accused, yes, especially then. In this instance, one

is not ashamed because one is hurtfully believed to be capable of this or that misdeed – this would be far too subtle to be true. No, one is ashamed because in the eyes of others, that is, socially, one actually *is* guilty. In brief: one is not ashamed of guilt; on the contrary, that of which one is ashamed often turns into guilt. *I am ashamed – therefore I am guilty is more* valid than *I am guilty – therefore I am ashamed*". This foregrounds the central role that power relations play in the expression and physical manifestation of shame, for it is easy to make someone feel guilty by shaming them. See Anders, "On Promethean Shame," 93.

17 Starobinski, *Jean-Jacques Rousseau*, 9.

18 Even in the famous incident with the ribbon, in which Rousseau unashamedly mobilizes the power of his class status and accuses a maid of a theft he had committed, and thus makes her undergo the very injustice he suffered with the comb, he absolves himself by blaming his

> invincible sense of shame that prevailed over everything. ... It was my shame that made me impudent, and the more wickedly I behaved the bolder my fear of confession made me. I saw nothing but the horror of being found out, of being publicly proclaimed, to my face, as a thief, a liar, and a slanderer.
>
> (pp. 88–89)

Rather than being ashamed of the act, Rousseau is thus "ashamed of his shame," and uses this to distance himself from his act. On this point see Anders, "On Promethean Shame," 35.

19 Some notable examples include (this is by no means an exhaustive list): "The mere thought of all the conventions, of which I am sure to forget at least one, is enough to frighten me. I cannot understand how a man can have the confidence to speak in company" (p. 114); "for one so shy, to speak not only in public ... was enough to have to put an end to me" (p. 152); "I was restrained by the fear of offending or displeasing (p. 239); I tried to speak but the words died on my lips" (p. 274); "What would become of me...if in my confusion one of my usual inanities were to escape my lips?" (p. 354); "Appearances were so much against me that the invincible feeling of shame which always dominated me made me appear like a guilty person in his presence, and he often took an unfair advantage of this in order to humiliate me" (p. 430); "I found myself in the most terrible embarrassment that I have ever known in my life" (p. 452).

20 Sherry Turkle, *Alone Together* (New York: Basic Book, 2012), 187.

21 Ibid. On this point see also Vincent Miller, *The Crisis of Presence in Contemporary Culture: Ethics, Privacy and Speech in Mediated Social Life* (London: Sage, 2016), especially, "Chapter 4: 'Going to Africa': the Problem of Speech in a World Where We Write Instead of Talk," pp. 84–101.

22 Starobinski as cited in Jacques Derrida, *Of Grammatology*, trans. Gayatri Chakravorty Spivak (Baltimore, MD: Johns Hopkins University Press, 1997), 142. See p. 116 of *The Confessions* for the passage in question.

23 Derrida, *Of Grammatology*, 142.

24 Riley, "'Lying' When You Aren't," 94.

25 Günther Anders, *Tagesnotizen* (Frankfurt am Main: Suhrkamp, 2006), 65.

26 See David Wills, "The Blushing Machine: Animal Shame and Technological Life," *Parrhesia* 8 (2009): 34–42. An extended version of the essay is part of *Inanimation* (see note xiv above).

27 Ibid., 40.

28 The Profound implications of Wills's recently published book length discussion of inorganic life cannot be done justice here. Wills uses the neologism "to inanimate" to sublate the meaning of the obsolete verb "to inanimate," "to

enliven, quicken" and the familiar meaning of lifelessness. In doing so, he shows that "the inanimate does not simply fall away ... into the category of nonlife but continues to operate as an uncanny force across the divide that supposedly protects and defines life" (p. 6). See *Textual Practice* 30, no. 7 (2016): 1365–1376 for Mareile Pfannebecker and my joint review of *Inanimation* that also gives a brief account of Wills' treatment of blushing.

29 For incisive, wide ranging expositions of the power relations that are at stake when disclosing a private self, either voluntarily, or through the use of machines that automatically gather data to offer a continuous confession on our behalf, I would like to refer the reader to Josh Cohen's incisive *The Private Life: Why We Remain in the Dark* (London: Granata, 2013), to Lauren Berlant's "The Subject of True Feeling," in *Cultural Pluralism, Identity Politics and the Law*, eds. Austin Sarat and Thomas R. Kearns (Ann Arbor: University of Michigan Press, 1999), 49–84, and to my translation of Anders's brilliant 1958 essay, "The Obsolescence of Privacy," *ConterText: A Journal for the Study of the Post-Literary* 3, no. 1 (2017): 20–46.

30 In view of recent developments in Europe and the USA, it seems important to spell out more openly that the recognition of the inanimating mechanism at work in shame discussed in this chapter can offer resources to the cultural politics of shame and empathy. The processes discussed offer further ways to recognize and contemplate that the irrepressible singularity of "painful feeling," to use Lauren Berlant's term, is "systemic" (53), tied into a "national rhetoric" and a wide range of historical, legal, political, economic and technological determinants. All of these affect the intimately singular feelings of self-worth, dignity and validation that Rousseau begins to lay bare. We are currently witnessing how populism is highly effectively mobilizing and concentrating this pain by feeding it simplistic, digitally amplified covers that are going viral, thus opening violently divisive routes toward confidence, feelings of belonging and agency.

31 Anders, "On Promethean Shame," 66.

32 Anders, "Pathology of Freedom," 289. I should add that my use of the term "human" in this essay did not seek to imply that shame and inauthenticity is a quintessentially human phenomenon, far from it. Writing in 1956, Anders reproaches himself for the lingering traces of anthropocentrism of "The Pathology of Freedom" that come to the fore here, with words that are worth repeating: "The idea that the single species 'human' can be opposed to the thousands upon thousands of immensely different animal species and types is simply an anthropocentric delusion of grandeur. As a warning against this cosmic immodesty, each textbook of "Philosophical Anthropology" should have "the Fable of the Ants" as a preface. This fable recounts how, at their universities, ants learn to distinguish between "plants, animals, and ants." See "On Promethean Shame," 89.

6 Between Shame and Guilt

Lord Jim and the
Confounding of Distinctions

James Brown

The distinction between shame and guilt is widely invoked. In psychology, especially in psychotherapeutic disciplines, a particular version of the distinction between shame and guilt has become almost an orthodoxy: shame passes judgement on the self as a whole and its characteristic expression is self-removal (hiding, suicide), whereas guilt passes judgement on a particular act, and its characteristic impulse is towards reparation and moving on. In anthropology and other disciplines, the distinction between shame cultures and guilt cultures is applied across history: to the ancient Greeks, to the mediaeval English, to the Japanese confronting their American conquerors in 1945, etc.[1] Both these versions – the psychological and the anthropological – of the shame/guilt distinction are apt to encourage, or be understood as implying, a preference for one term over another. The implication is often that guilt is somehow more modern or advanced than shame. If the shame-/guilt-culture distinction is often applied to various cultures and histories, the psychological distinction is often invoked as if it were a permanent truth about the human condition. And yet it is difficult to find any version of the distinction being drawn explicitly prior to Margaret Mead in 1937, when she distinguishes between societies based on the sanctions of shame and guilt, and it only appears to become widespread in anthropology with Benedict's *The Chrysanthemum and the Sword* (1946).[2] In psychology, the distinction becomes something of a topos in the 1950s, but in certain respects it doesn't assume its current form until Helen Block Lewis's 1971 book, *Shame and Guilt in Neurosis*.[3]

There's something suggestive and yet also unsatisfactory in the way in which this distinction has become embedded in various kinds of discourse, and in ways that obscure its own historical specificity. Of course, it can happen that general or even eternal truths may be discovered only at a specific moment in history. DNA took the form of a double helix for countless millions of years before Franklin, Wilkins, Watson and Crick established the double helix as its molecular shape. In a matter as reflexive as guilt or shame, this seems unlikely. Yet there's something striking in the way in which a distinction of relatively recent date has become embedded in various discourses as a general, transhistorical, transcultural truth – so deeply embedded for some that, notwithstanding the contradictory evidence of everyday usage, they will insist on their version as the only true one, not merely within a specialist discourse but in general (though it has also been subject to criticism).[4]

The gist of this chapter is that Conrad's novel *Lord Jim* in effect reveals the preconditions for the emergence of the guilt/shame distinction – and that it also confounds it. Even before the distinction comes explicitly into existence, Conrad has intuited it and overthrown it. One of the ways in which it accomplishes this seemingly anachronistic feat is through its fascination with oral and written language. Therein lies another of the dualisms which the novel invokes and confounds. Questions of guilt and shame come to be entangled with the relation between writing and speech.

As a cadet, training to be an officer in the merchant navy, Jim dreams of glory. Yet even then he chokes at the moment of action partly because of his book-fueled imagination. Later, he becomes first mate of the SS *Patna*, which is carrying 800 pilgrims to Mecca, when the ship is holed below the line. Water gushes in, and is stopped only by a thin, rusty bulkhead which must surely give way. Jim is certain he sees it bulging. Or is that an illusion conjured by his imagination? The other officers decide to leave the *Patna*, its crew and the pilgrims to their fate (an incident based on real events concerning the SS *Jeddah*).[5] Then, at a weird moment while they yell to "George" to jump and join them in the lifeboat, Jim jumps, seemingly in response to a name other than his own (69).[6] This falsification of himself will resonate through the book in other meetings, and other jumpings from one world to another. In fact, the *Patna* doesn't sink: it is found and towed to port. When the officers come ashore having abandoned their ship, they find themselves notorious. The captain disappears. Two others drink so much they have to be hospitalized. Only Jim presents himself before the court of inquiry, though he is offered money not to show his face. But having presented himself for judgment and punishment, Jim then proceeds to hide: the narrator, Marlow, finds him working as a chandler's clerk, but every time the story of the *Patna* catches up with him, Jim quits and moves on, until there's virtually nowhere else to go. Marlow again intervenes, and arranges with the merchant and butterfly collector Stein for Jim to go to Patusan, a remote trading station, to replace a Portuguese man called Cornelius as Stein's representative. At this point, curiously, Jim's luck appears to change, and he becomes virtually the ruler of the place, bringing peace to a situation in which rival groups had been fighting inconclusively but destructively. His fortunes appear to change, yet he brings with him into Patusan an unshareable knowledge of his own fallibility – a knowledge that raises the possibility of his possessing what we might now speak of as guilt rather than shame. Yet it's a moot point whether he has quite the kind of inner life that a capacity for guilt might imply. For most of the novel, his sense of failure exhibits many of the traits that would later be ascribed to shame, especially his sense of total failure implicating his entire self and his impulse to concealment.

However, one needs to be wary in invoking later versions of the guilt/shame distinction in relation to *Lord Jim* – versions of the distinction that could only emerge once guilt had become, among other things, an emotion, which wasn't its primary meaning or possibly even a proper meaning *c.* 1900. For Johnson (1785) in the eighteenth century "guilt" had signified two things: "the state of a man justly charged with a crime; the contrary to innocence" and "A crime; an offence." The possibility of that state being an *emotional* state is not dwelt upon: there were other words for that: shame, remorse, regret, reproach and so on.[7] In 1897, the *Century Dictionary* confirms Johnson's two definitions, with some elaboration, and adds a third. Its three definitions are (a) "A fault: an offense; a guilty action; a crime," (b) "That state of a moral agent which results from his commission of a crime or an offense wilfully or by consent; culpability arising from conscious violation of moral or penal law, either by positive act or by neglect of known duty; criminality; wickedness," and (c) "Technical or constructive criminality; exposure to forfeiture or other penalty."[8] Only in 1901 in the *New English Dictionary* (i.e. the first edition of the OED) is it acknowledged that "guilt" might be used to signify the subjective experience of being guilty.[9] This is in the context of a painstaking definition of guilt as a noun, which distinguishes seven senses, the fifth of which it subdivides into four. The emphasis in the definition as a whole falls on objective facts (guilt as offense or crime, or as the fact of having committed a crime) and publicly acknowledged responsibility and legal liability to punishment. The fifth definition, however, is slightly different. Its first variation is "The state (meriting condemnation and reproach of conscience) of having wilfully committed crime or heinous moral offence; criminality, great culpability." An element of emotion intrudes here, but only as a *response* to the fact of guilt. Only in the final variant of this definition does guilt itself acquire this subjective, emotional dimension: "Misused for 'sense of guilt'." Even here there is ambiguity, given how many things "sense" can signify.

The judgemental insistence that to speak of guilt as signifying a subjective experience is to misuse the word is reflected in much of the evidence of the word's use in formal discourse – yet with the possibility of the emotional sense that has since become strong pressing towards the surface. Thus in Darwin's *The Expression of the Emotions in Man and Animals*, Chapter 11 addresses disdain, contempt, disgust, guilt, pride, etc., and Darwin lists guilt among "Jealousy, Envy, Avarice, Revenge, Suspicion, Deceit, Slyness, Guilt, Vanity, Conceit, Ambition, Pride, Humility, &c." as one of several "complex states of mind," and a moment later he speaks of them as "feelings."[10] On the next page, he speaks of the "expression of guilt" and of having noted "guilty expressions" in his own children.[11] That subtle slippage marks the ways in which guilt can shift from being an objective fact (of wrongdoing) which may occasion the expression of some emotion to being something much closer to the emotion itself ("guilty expressions"). Yet when he discusses the causes of blushing later in the book, Darwin observes what the OED would later insist on as the proper way to use "guilt": "It is not the sense of guilt, but the thought that others think or know us to be guilty which crimsons the face."[12] In Darwin's text, the word "guilt" seems poised to acquire a newly powerful emotional meaning, but this hasn't yet happened. The word "shame" occurs more frequently in the book, and the word "anger" much more frequently, for instance. If some uncertainty attaches to the correct way to use "guilt" that may have something to do with the way in which the larger vocabulary of emotion is in flux in the nineteenth century. Back in 1828, *Webster's Dictionary* had sought to define "emotion" in a way that distinguished it from "passion" and gave the word a specific meaning in relation to an already sophisticated vocabulary for dealing with what we would now speak of as emotions tout court.[13] Its second definition runs: "In a philosophical sense, an internal motion or agitation of the mind which passes away without desire; when desire follows, the motion or agitation is called a passion." However, its catchall first definition was more indicative of the way things were going: "…any agitation of mind or excitement of sensibility." As Thomas Dixon has argued, the emergence of "emotion" as a general category during the nineteenth century marked the loss of some valuable distinctions, such as those between passions and affections.[14] It's common to speak of *Lord Jim* as a psychological novel and even as a *bildungsroman*.[15] In some ways, this is a misleading label: *Lord Jim* could equally be deemed a kind of anti-*bildungsroman*, and considered correspondingly anti-psychological. Yet it is preoccupied with subjective experience, and it's of some significance that some of the language for describing that experience had been and continued to be in flux when Conrad wrote. Perhaps that's a general truth: maybe that kind of language is always on the turn. Conrad may have intuited something elusive about certain key ideas, among them what we've since sought to stabilize as shame and guilt.

In some ways *Lord Jim* conforms to the OED's strictures regarding the proper way to use "guilt." Jim alone of the deserters from the *Patna* presents himself for judgement and punishment before an official Inquiry, which happens to be held before a magistrate in a Police Court. It's natural, therefore, for the novel to speak of Jim's guilt as an established fact. That's one of the meanings that informs the narrator, Marlow's, comment that "still, the idea obtrudes itself that he made so much of his disgrace while it is the guilt alone that matters" (107). Jim does, indeed, find it impossible to bear the knowledge that others know of his failure, of his guilt. This is as close as the novel comes to drawing a distinction between shame and guilt: disgrace is a term that belongs with ideas of public honor (as opposed to private virtue), and thus with what would later come to be spoken of as a shame-culture. Yet Marlow evinces skepticism about matters of fact. He remarks of the judges at the Inquiry that "They wanted facts. Facts! They demanded facts from him, as if facts could explain anything!" (22). As confidence falters in a publicly shared, knowable world of facts in which subjects' actions may be known and judged in such a way that they may be held accountable for them, other senses of guilt start to stir within the text, even if they're not explicitly acknowledged.

On the eve of sentencing, Marlow may insist that "The respectable sword of his country's law was suspended over his head" and that Jim "was guilty too. He was guilty – as I had told myself repeatedly, guilty and done for" (93). Yet by this point Conrad has already made us aware of the suicide shortly after the Inquiry of one of the judges. Captain Brierly

> had never in his life made a mistake, never had an accident, never a mishap, never a check in his steady rise, and he seemed to be one of those lucky fellows who know nothing of indecision, much less of self-mistrust.
>
> (38)

Yet a week after the Inquiry, Brierly very deliberately leapt from his ship to his death. Thinking back to Brierly's attitude to Jim, Marlow reflects that

> while I thought with something akin to fear of the immensity of his contempt for the young man under examination, he was probably holding silent inquiry into his own case. The verdict must have been of unmitigated guilt, and he took the secret of the evidence with him in that leap into the sea.
>
> (39)

The context makes the guilt that Marlow supposes Brierly to have found in himself sound just like the legal finding of guilt that Brierly, sitting with the magistrate, establishes in Jim's case. Yet it's nothing of the sort. It's a kind of guilt that moves into stranger territory: not guilt occasioned by anything one has actually done, but guilt arising merely from an apprehension of what one *might* do. The self-administered punishment feels almost preventative, rather than a payment or retribution for a crime. Indeed, inasmuch as Brierly jumping to his death repeats Jim's crime of leaping off the *Patna* and abandoning his duty, Brierly only commits a fault in the same moment as he punishes himself for it. Under the circumstances, what Marlow takes to be Brierly's finding of guilt in his own case starts to assume paradoxical and Freudian dimensions. Even though the early English translations of Freud often strive to observe "correct" usage by speaking repeatedly of "sense of guilt" where now we might simply say "guilt" (e.g. Brill's 1918 translation of *Totem and Taboo*, which was especially insistent on this), it's arguably partly because of Freud that guilt comes to signify a state of mind in which cause and effect can be reversed, in which a subjective sense of guilt or guilt-worthiness can exist independently of objective evidence, and in which one is not necessarily guilty because one has committed a fault, but one may commit a fault because of a prior sense of guilt. But, though Freud had been developing his system of psychoanalysis for a decade by the time *Lord Jim* was published, he had been working, in his own phrase, in "splendid isolation," and only after 1900 would he begin to acquire a European following.[16]

Once the inquiry has found him guilty, Jim has his certificate canceled, and then the narrator, the older seaman Marlow, fearing what will happen if Jim is left alone, invites Jim to his room. But Marlow also hesitates to inflict his potentially shaming presence on Jim, so he sits down to write. Writing here becomes a way of partially disengaging from the present moment so as to save the other man some loss of face. As Marlow writes (and, of course, from our point of view as readers also speaks and narrates), he reflects on speech and writing, which is a preoccupation in Conrad, and also contemplates the offer the disreputable Chester and Robinson wish him to put to Jim regarding a guano island:

> There is a weird power in a spoken word. And why the devil not? I was asking myself persistently while I drove on with my writing. All at once, on the blank page, under the very point of the pen, the two figures of Chester and his antique partner, very distinct and complete, would dodge into view with stride and gestures, as if reproduced in the field of some optical toy. I would watch them for a while. No! They were too phantasmal and extravagant to enter into any one's fate. And a word carries far – very far – deals destruction through time as the bullets go flying through space. I said nothing; and he, out there with his back to the light, as if bound and gagged by all the invisible foes of man, made no stir and made no sound.
>
> (106)

Yet the act of writing is, in societies of near universal literacy, potentially *more* public than speech. One might therefore expect it to have some potential for incurring or mobilizing shame. It is also an act by which one may objectify a version or aspect of oneself. Conrad has Marlow say that a word "deals destruction through time as the bullets go flying through space," and in the context, it's unclear whether he means the written or the spoken word. As it happens, for Jim in the next few chapters, as he starts shifting from job to job, moving on every time someone reminds him of the *Patna* incident, the spoken word is, as one might expect, the means for effecting a shaming confrontation between himself and the judgement of others.

However, the novel as a whole explores and enacts the relations between textuality and orality. The first four chapters present themselves in third-person narration as a text to be read. The bulk of the book, from Chapter 5 to Chapter 36, is presented as the oral narration of Marlow (however improbably: it would take about ten hours to utter, as some of Conrad's earliest critics complained – see Conrad's "Author's Note," 5). Then, after the brief appearance of a seemingly omniscient third-person narrator at the beginning of Chapter 36, the remainder of the book (just under 10 chapters) is presented in four texts sent by Marlow to the "privileged man" – the only one of his listeners to whom Marlow communicates the remainder of the tale: a fragment by Jim himself; a letter to Jim from his father, a priest; Marlow's covering letter; and a narrative pieced together by Marlow from various sources. Early in their acquaintance, Marlow privately rebukes himself for his confidence in the power of words (109), but then goes on to write a letter of introduction for him, making himself "unreservedly responsible" for Jim (111) – a letter which could, depending on Jim's conduct, embarrass or shame Marlow. Jim greets this as being given "...in a measure ... yes ... a clean slate" (112). Marlow reflects: "A clean slate, did he say? As if the initial word of each our destiny were not graven in imperishable characters upon the face of a rock" (112). Lurking behind Jim and Marlow's interest in face-to-face communication (and Jim in Patusan will make much of showing himself, and speaking face-to-face with friend and foe, and will meet his death that way), are the various writings and letters of the novel. And behind them lies the idea of a permanent text: the kind of law, perhaps, before which one may be found wanting, or the kind of law that blindly dictates destinies, according to which a life's seemingly open, indeterminate face-to-face encounters may accumulate into something closed and determinate – and thus implicitly textual.

The novel most often attaches the word *guilt* to Jim's dereliction of duty in jumping from the *Patna*, though it does also speak of *shame* in other contexts, and Jim's reaction to being found guilty by the court of inquiry strongly suggests some of the elements often associated with shame, and throughout the novel he is described as being prone to blushing or coloring (150, 175). He moves from job to job, and cannot bear to have the story of his misdeed known. In the end, there's virtually nowhere for him to hide within a 3000-mile radius, since he has made himself notorious. On one occasion, instead of simply hiding, he resorts to violence against a Danish lieutenant in the Royal Siamese Navy, who has lost several games of billiards to Jim, and then insults him.

Jim throws him into the Menam River. Marlow records, having seen him afterwards, that:

> ...what dismayed him was to find the nature of his burden as well known to everybody as though he had gone about all that time carrying it on his shoulders. Naturally after this he couldn't remain in the place.
>
> (120)

So even his attempt to vindicate his honor by demonstrating a kind of personal courage ends in what Marlow calls one of a "lamentable species of bar-room scuffles."

In a text in which orality and textuality interact all the time, to some extent the different kinds of culpability or burden carried by Jim correlate to textual, codified systems of rules on the one hand, and a different kind of code, an unwritten code, on the other. The inquiry, on the face of it, approaches Jim's actions in terms of a framework of writing. It applies written rules, and the punishment it imposes is the cancellation of the certificate that entitles Jim to serve as an officer in the Merchant Navy. Yet Jim's sense of forfeited honor, his quest for a kind of redemption, propels him beyond the logic of printed, rationalized regulations. For much of the middle part of the novel, he finds himself suffering from a sense of shame to which many around him are indifferent. One employer, whom he deserts when his story catches up with him, asks,

> 'And who the devil cares about that?' 'I daresay no one,' I began... 'And what the devil is he – anyhow – for to go on like this?' He stuffed suddenly his left whisker into his mouth and stood amazed. 'Jee!' he exclaimed, 'I told him the earth wouldn't be big enough to hold his caper.'
>
> (118)

Among the things that complicate a simple sense of guilt as belonging within a textually organized world, while shame, such as Jim feels, relates to something other, especially to looking others in the face (or failing to do so), and thus to personal contact and orality, two have a bearing here. One is that Jim's sense of honor and thus of shame derive from what various people in the book (especially Marlow and the gnomic merchant, Stein) speak of as his excessively romantic nature, and that in turn has been fed precisely by books. As a cadet, Jim likes to imagine himself being "as unflinching as a hero in a book" (9). This pointedly fails to equip him to act when a schooner and a coaster collide, and the other cadets rush to the rescue. So there's also a question here about how action is motivated, and thus about the role that shame or guilt play as normative influences. Then, beyond that, there's a question about how social order of the kind that might possibly come to produce regulations and courts of inquiry and all the apparatus of print-rationality can be produced in the first place.

Conrad is at pains to suggest that what might be called print-rationality (a product of what Marlow describes to the "privileged man" as "the morality of an ethical progress") doesn't get much of a purchase on a complex world whose sense of reality is often called into question, often by strange transferences or mirrorings. The way Capt. Brierly finds Jim guilty and then executes himself is one such, and anticipates Jim's encounter at the end of the novel with his nemesis, the pirate "Gentleman" Brown. He will see in this vicious man, so different from himself, a reflection of himself. Similarly, the episode on the *Patna* appears quite different from the peculiar greatness Jim achieves when Stein sends him to Patusan, when, after an inauspicious start when he's imprisoned for three days, he becomes virtually the arbiter of the whole place, and, more than that, almost its founder, who aspires to constitute order and justice. Yet the names *Patna* and Patusan are echoes of each other (to change one to the other, one has to do little more than add "us," which is a key word in the novel, especially in Marlow's reiteration that Jim is "one of us": 30, 50, 59, 67, 136, 193, 196, 214, 246). The shame or guilt of the first phase of the story haunts the peculiar kind of glory Jim achieves in the second, when he is hailed as Tuan or Lord Jim.

I mentioned earlier the way in which Conrad seems drawn to the possibility of collapsing opposites into each other – opposites such as the stories of the *Patna* and of Patusan – and suggested that this is one of the reasons why guilt and shame seem (albeit anachronistically and implicitly) to emerge as distinct and yet, in the end, collapse back into each other. Perhaps another reason for this, or maybe just another way of coming at the same reason, has to do with the way Conrad's imagination seems drawn to what one might call founding or constitutive moments – admittedly, less to create stories of the founding and origins of things (though the myth that quickens around Jim in Patusan flirts with that idea) than to create a story in which achievements collapse back upon themselves, including, at the largest scale, the achievements of "civilization" or "progress" as such. This concern emerges especially in the collision between the allegedly civilized European world and the allegedly backward worlds into which Europeans such as Jim and Marlow move. In Conrad's account, the assertion of western superiority does not stand. The civilized world gives rise to such horrors as "Gentleman" Brown and "Holy-Terror Robinson," who seem to be (or, in Robinson's case, to have been, since he's now doddering) intent on rolling "civilization" back to savagery – Brown in his appetite for destruction and inability to endure Jim's air of superiority, and Robinson in the legend of his cannibalism. Civilization can also appear to consist in a kind of evasiveness. It produces figures who seek refuge in the consoling fictions of civilization or progress, such as the "privileged man" to whom Marlow communicates the end of the tale, and who has evidently asserted to Marlow the necessity for any white man who lives among others to be sustained by "a firm conviction in the truth of ideas racially our own, in whose name are established the order, the morality of an ethical progress" (201). Marlow's letter immediately calls the notion into doubt, by raising "the question" of "whether at the last [Jim] had not confessed to a faith mightier than the laws of order and progress." Earlier, in his oral narration Marlow had dismissed "the haggard utilitarian lies of our civilization" (168), and, confronted with Jewel's account of her mother's death and momentarily lost for words, Marlow opines that "words also belong to the sheltering conception of light and order which is our refuge" – a shelter we seek at moments of difficulty just as "a tortoise withdraws within its shell," and what it affords is not just shelter, but an illusion of progress: that the world "is as sunny an arrangement of small conveniences as the mind of man can conceive" (186). Scarcely less deluded are those who passively accept the place granted to them – at least in Marlow's view. These include Jim's father, whom (on the basis of his last letter sent to Jim just before he embarked on the *Patna*) Marlow represents as peddling "easy morality" and "equably trusting Providence and the order of the universe" (202). The criticism is implicitly amplified as Marlow imagines him

> grey-haired and serene in the inviolable shelter of his book-lined, faded, and comfortable study, where for forty years he had conscientiously gone over and over again the round of his little thoughts about faith and virtue, about the conduct of life and the only proper manner of dying.

The novel tempts us with the possibility that, in going to his death, Jim settles accounts with himself. Yet Conrad never quite asserts such a reckoning. It's moot whether Jim possesses the psychological depth that would make such a reckoning with himself believable – the kind of depth that Forster had in mind in distinguishing "round" from "flat" characters.[17] The hallmark of a "round" character for Forster is the ability to change convincingly, if surprisingly. It's the result of their actions and utterances seeming to flow from an inner depth. In one sense, as he goes from the disgrace of the *Patna* incident to glory in Patusan, Jim undergoes an astonishing transformation. Yet even in Patusan he continues to speak with what Watt aptly terms "a schoolboy banality of diction," his speech peppered with "Jove" and "bally," which makes him sound like the hero of a boys' adventure story (Biggles, perhaps).[18] The transformation he achieves is, in the first instance, less of himself than of Patusan. Thanks to his extraordinary status in Patusan, Jim, in effect, inverts the way in which he had been shamed by the presence of anyone who knew the story of the *Patna*. Having inspired the local population to conjure a legend around him, he can then draw upon their belief in him. As Jim points out to Marlow, if his self-belief falters, "I've got to look only at the face of the first man that comes along to regain my confidence" (182). This is at once childlike (it's Cornelius's refrain that Jim is a "little child"), and a kind of inversion of the way in which shame (especially as it would later come to be distinguished in psychology from guilt) is deemed to be a reaction to the gaze of another. Jim, even in his glory, lives in some ways only as others see him, as if his being were molded by the perception of others – a kind of subjection of oneself to the spectatorship of others that Rousseau saw as the taint inflicted on humanity by our loss of a pure, unselfconscious existence in the state of nature.[19] This reflects the side of him that appears to be bound by an honor code, in which shame is the key inner sanction. A sentence of Bourdieu's about the Kabyle of northern Algeria describes this side of Jim uncannily well:

> The point of honour is the basis of a moral code of an individual who sees himself always through the eyes of others, who has need of others for his existence, because the image he has of himself is indistinguishable from that presented to him by other people.[20]

By comparison, when Adam Smith proposed a model for the way in which we are motivated to act ethically, he internalized the spectator so that "the man within the breast" became "the great judge and arbiter of their conduct."[21]

However, Jim takes with him into Patusan a nagging knowledge of his own lapse and fallibility. Jewel realizes that "There is something he can never forget" (187), what he himself speaks of over-emphatically as the "real, real truth" (181) and as "the bally thing at the back of my head." This unquiet self-knowledge (if that's quite what it is; one might equally think of it as a mental itch that marks the refusal of self-knowledge) both fits and unfits him for the role he plays in Patusan.

He enters Patusan almost like a being from another sphere, as if newborn or fallen from the sky. When Marlow sees him with Rajah Allah (a local leader, who had initially imprisoned Jim but is now wary of him), it strikes him that "He appeared like a creature not only of another kind but of another essence," and, but for their having seen him enter their world in a canoe, "they might have thought he had descended upon them from the clouds" (138). This is especially true of his second leap (after the leap from the *Patna*), when, shortly after his arrival, he leaps over Rajah Allah's stockade to escape imprisonment, and plunges into primaeval mud which almost refuses to let go of him, so for a moment he seems to be "burying himself alive" (153). It's a leap made without forethought: no second thoughts prompted by imaginings and fears can snare him, because he had no thoughts at all.

Conrad contrives a situation in which various mythic patterns are invoked, but none is endorsed, and these are especially to do with the founding and beginning of things. As Daphna Erdinast-Vulcan notes, several features of Patusan recall Eden – not least, Cornelius's reptilian nature which casts him as the serpent and betrayer (501). Yet there are other patterns. It's also, less idyllically, akin to a Hobbesian state of nature: as Jim extricates himself from the mud, Marlow notes "there wasn't a week without some fight in Patusan at that time" (153). At the very moment when Jim denies to Marlow the legend that ascribes supernatural powers to him, he bursts "into a Homeric peal of laughter" (160), which takes us from Christian to classical founding myths. Marlow had previously ascribed to him an "Arcadian happiness" (106). However, the novel most insistently invokes the classical past in the idea of tragedy. Even before he knows of Jim's end, Marlow declares of Jewel and Jim that "They had mastered their fates. They were tragic" (188).

In some respects, Conrad is making a familiar move in bringing classical and Christian traditions into collision with each other. It's a collision with obvious implications for what one means by "guilt." Christianity's combination of an obligation to forgive with a doctrine of original sin may make salvation seem elusive and mysterious, but a Christian must, nevertheless, believe in the possibility of it. By comparison, though the flaw of the classical tragic hero may be expressed in what a Christian might recognize as sin, sin isn't essential to tragedy. Even Oedipus's horrific crimes strain against modern Christian conceptions of sin, inasmuch as they were unwitting and unintended. His disappearance at the end of *Oedipus at Colonus* may resemble the ascension, but the fact that it's Oedipus, who has killed his father and fathered children with his own mother, who is singled out for this extraordinary treatment fits awkwardly within a framework which expects only supreme and sacred virtue to be so acknowledged. In *Antigone,* even if one can persuade oneself that Creon is justly punished for his inflexibility, it's harder to see that death is meted out to Antigone and Haemon according to a rational principle of justice: one might see it (following Hegel) as resulting from a clash of irreconcilable, but (so far as they go) valid principles. In Sophocles' *Electra*, even if Clytemnestra deserves to die and her children are obliged to seek justice for Agamemnon's death, there is an obvious and visceral problem in having her die at her children's hands. Christian humanism and neoclassicism would seek to assimilate tragedy to Christian teaching by, for example, imposing on it a doctrine of poetic justice, or by shifting tragedy towards a sentimentalized and consumable pathos. Yet that is not what Greek tragedy affords.

Conrad brings to his treatment of the tragic in *Lord Jim* a reinterpretation of it that finally frees it from the dictates of poetic justice and other such doctrines. It's a reinterpretation that owes much to the terms in which tragedy is reconceived in German thought, especially by German romantic thinkers, as, for example, a confrontation between freedom and necessity, or between will and contingency.[22] For Hegel, for instance, a certain kind of modern tragedy expresses a response to and a repudiation of contingency.[23] Though Hegel would not have approved of this, one might extrapolate from such a view of tragedy to envisage a situation in which one chooses the burden of tragedy, and even a kind of tragic guilt, for the sake of asserting one's being.[24] In a later development of this tradition of thought about tragedy, Nietzsche will explicitly reject Christian conceptions of sin and punishment, with a corresponding repudiation of guilt, and, instead of seeking to reconcile tragedy with Christianity, he delights in regrounding it in pagan ritual.[25] Conrad's repeated allusions in *Lord Jim* to the "dark powers" (sometimes capitalized, sometimes not) may suggest a malign intelligence, intent on inflicting suffering. But one might also see them as "dark" in the sense of being blind, rather in the way "will" for Nietzsche and for Schopenhauer (whom Conrad had read attentively) signifies blind impulse or force. The point of Conrad's allusions to the "dark powers" may be less to replace a benign, single, Christian supreme judge with malign, pagan persecutors, than to step aside from the idea of the universe being presided over by *any* intelligence, thus throwing human minds back upon themselves, with radical implications for what we mean by guilt, since this conception eliminates the possibility of supernatural law-giver before whom we might be found guilty and by whom we might be punished. To render suffering meaningful by construing it as just punishment becomes impossible, and the meaning of tragedy shifts from the ethical to the metaphysical. This tradition of German thinking about tragedy as an assertion of isolated will against contingency furnishes at least one way of interpreting Jim's resolve, when he hears of "Gentleman" Brown's betrayal and his killing of Dain Waris, to present himself before his dead friend's father, Doramin, to die: "There was nothing left to fight for. He was going to prove his power another way and conquer fatal destiny itself" (242). That seems also to be what Marlow is intimating when he writes to the "privileged man":

> The story of the last events you will find in the few pages enclosed here. You must admit that it is romantic beyond the wildest dreams of his boyhood, and yet there is to my mind a sort of profound and terrifying logic in it, as if it were our imagination alone that could set loose upon us the might of an overwhelming destiny.
>
> (203)

Marlow has already alerted his solitary reader to an essential solipsism in Jim that, along with repeated allusions to his romantic imagination, make him, in effect, a type of the romantic artist: "The point, however, is that of all mankind Jim had no dealings but with himself, and the question is whether at the last he had not confessed to a faith mightier than the laws of order and progress" (201).

The romantic imagination is what Stein identifies in Jim, and is a strong candidate for being the "destructive element" in which he recommends immersion. Yet it is, for its proponents, a generative faculty. What Jim makes of Patusan has been likened to a work of art, and Jim himself, who goes into Patusan with little besides an empty revolver and three books (one of them a complete Shakespeare) (143), speaks of the people he finds there as being "like people in a book" (156), even as the story of Stein's ring, with which Jim can claim Doramin's friendship, strikes Jim as being "like something you read of in books" (141).[26] Jim's "gift of finding a special meaning in everything that happened to him" (181) confirms a sense of his being a kind of romantic artist, and thus the product of a recent phase of western civilization and, as Marlow says repeatedly, "one of us." Yet his powers are also expressed in the collective creation of a polity of which he becomes virtually the ruler, and in that regard, he plays a role governed by a different kind of imagination: the sort of collectively exercised and culture-generating imagination that nineteenth-century anthropology charted. A sense of his being engaged in a kind of primal, socially generative moment is registered repeatedly. We're told Stein has seen various places in "the original dusk of their being, before light (and even electric light) had been carried into them for the sake of better morality and – and – well – the greater profit, too" (132), and Jim appears to see Patusan in the same way. In contemplating Jim and Dain Waris, Marlow observes "I seemed to behold the very origin of friendship" – not just the origins of their friendship, but of friendship and thus society as such (157). Jim finds himself hedged about by protective restrictions: "The land, the people, the friendship, the love, were like the jealous guardians of his body. Every day added a link to the fetters of that strange freedom" (157). This is later expanded on in relation to Jewel's love for Jim and his follower, Tamb' Itam's attitude to him:

> He was jealously loved, but why she should be jealous, and of what, I could not tell. The land, the people, the forests were her accomplices, guarding him with vigilant accord, with an air of seclusion, of mystery, of invincible possession. There was no appeal, as it were; he was imprisoned within the very freedom of his power, and she, though ready to make a footstool of her head for his feet, guarded her conquest inflexibly – as though he were hard to keep. The very Tamb' Itam, marching on our journeys upon the heels of his white lord, with his head thrown back, truculent and be-weaponed like a janissary, with kriss, chopper, and lance (besides carrying Jim's gun); even Tamb' Itam allowed himself to put on the airs of uncompromising guardianship, like a surly devoted jailer ready to lay down his life for his captive.
>
> (169)

This sense of Jim being hedged about in his power by special restrictions recalls Frazer's account in *The Golden Bough* (the first edition of which appeared in 1890) of the special taboos that attend the person of the priest-king: "He is the point of support on which hangs the balance of the world" and therefore "his whole life, down to its minutest details, must be so regulated that no act of his, voluntary or involuntary, may disarrange or upset the established order of nature."[27] As John B. Vickery explains, in Frazer's account "The taboos which regulate the life of the priest-king are imposed on him by his people rather than demanded by him out of an obsessive regard for his own welfare."[28] Indeed, the priest-king's "responsibility also involves him in punishment – beatings, banishment, and even death – if drought and pestilence should spoil the crops upon which the people depend for survival."[29] One of the odd things about this system to a modern mind is the way it establishes certain distinctions and overrides others. As Frazer notes, "the rules of ceremonial purity" for kings, chiefs and priests are similar to those observed by "homicides, mourners, women in childbed, girls at puberty, hunters and fishermen, and so on."[30] As Vickery explains, the distinction between the holy and the unclean isn't what matters here; what does matter is the distinction between things that possess an extraordinary power (for good or ill) and those that are merely ordinary: a distinction between the sacred and the profane. For Mary Douglas, socially marginal or unclassifiable figures are often the objects of special concern, so that an unborn baby (whose sex is not yet known, whose status as a person is ambiguous) may be seen as both vulnerable *and* dangerous.[31] Like the other two people in his household, Jim is an outsider. One might say of him what Douglas says of initiates undergoing ritual dying and rebirth: that they go through a phase of having "no place in society," during which their position is marginal, and yet "To have been in the margins is to have been in contact with danger, to have been at a source of power," which Douglas frames in terms of an interplay between form and formlessness, in which the latter is a threat but also presents material that can potentially be molded into the kind of form a society needs.[32] Thus one can find curious fusions and seeming reversals. This way of conceiving and engaging with dangers and powers helps to explain the way in which Oedipus, outcast and taboo at the end of *Oedipus the King*, comes in *Oedipus at Colonus* to possess a sacred power, such that the place where his bones lie will be blessed. Certain violations of a purely ethical code may come to be associated with the possession of extraordinary power. Curses and blessings can change places, in the same way that under certain ritual circumstances (as Durkheim and others noted) the forbidden and taboo can become obligatory. Jim as an outcast from the larger world outside Patusan, and as one that carries an inner vulnerability as exposed by his conduct on the *Patna*, emerges as one possessed of extraordinary powers in Patusan.

Conrad explores related inversions in the way in which he sets up moments of jumping over or crossing boundaries, and parallel or mirroring moments both within Jim's life and also between Jim and others, especially between Jim and "Gentleman" Brown. Brown is another white outcast, another seeking refuge in Patusan, but he is hell-bent on primal destruction, whereas Jim achieves a kind of founding. In the same way that Jim is something more than just a scapegrace son of a parsonage, "Gentleman" Brown is more than just a self-interested plunderer. Marlow, who speaks with him when he's gasping his last from asthma, describes him as a "thwarted autocrat." One expression of this larger or at any rate not merely self-interested impulse in Brown is an impulse to humiliate and shame others. The rest of his men "were merely vulgar and greedy brutes," but Brown was moved by a "complex intention":

> He would rob a man as if only to demonstrate his poor opinion of the creature, and he would bring to the shooting or maiming of some quiet, unoffending stranger a savage and vengeful earnestness fit to terrify the most reckless of desperadoes.
>
> (209)

He speaks of himself as the Scourge of God, as if he were Genghis Khan or Attila the Hun – some primal horde-leader (Conrad speaks of his few men as a horde). Marlow is struck by an odd sense of this villain possessing "a blind belief in the righteousness of his will against all mankind" (219). When Jim aspires to create a new peace or order, Brown has a primal impulse to destruction: "what he had really desired, almost in spite of himself, was to play havoc with that jungle town which had defied him, to see it strewn over with corpses and enveloped in flames." In the face of this threat, "The social fabric of orderly, peaceful life, when every man was sure of to-morrow, the edifice raised by Jim's hands, seemed on that evening ready to collapse into a ruin reeking with blood" (221), though even Brown is spoken of, in the very act of treachery and destruction, as asserting a kind of "right – an abstract thing" (239).

The other figure in the book who invokes the righteousness of his will, and, because of his charismatic authority, can invoke this to get others to act against their own better judgement is Jim. In his interview with Brown, Jim is discomfited by the other seeming to allude to shameful facts in Jim's past (though Brown has no specific knowledge of them). For example, he asks Brown what made him come there, and Brown replies, "Hunger. And what made you?" and Jim starts (226). Moments later, Brown exclaims, "... by God, I am not the sort to jump out of trouble and leave [my men] in a d – d lurch" (227). So Jim, troubled by Brown's "sickening suggestion of a common guilt, of secret knowledge that was like a bond of their minds and of their hearts" (229), allows Brown and his men to leave with their weapons. Brown has elicited in Jim something like the guilt that Jim had elicited in Brierly. Led by Cornelius, the man Jim ousted, Brown and his crew creep by a hidden channel upon Jim's friend Dain Waris and his men, who are stationed to ensure Brown departs. Dain Waris is the son of the chief of the Bugis in Patusan. Dain Waris is killed. Jim has staked his authority and his life to get people in Patusan to allow Brown to leave. Each and every one of "his" people is under his protection.

When news of Waris's death reaches him, Jim does two things. He sits down and tries to write. At least, Marlow says that's when he believes Jim wrote the unfinished document that is later among those sent to the "privileged man":

> What thoughts passed through his head – what memories? Who can tell? Everything was gone, and he who had been once unfaithful to his trust had lost again all men's confidence. It was then, I believe, he tried to write – to somebody – and gave it up. Loneliness was closing on him. People had trusted him with their lives – only for that; and yet they could never, as he had said, never be made to understand him. Those without did not hear him make a sound ....
>
> (242)

He then goes to Doramin, pausing only to look at the corpse of his friend. He announces that he has come in sorrow, and that he is ready and unarmed. And the chief raises himself, claims the price Jim had offered, and shoots him dead.

The moment is routinely spoken of as a sacrifice – less routinely compared to ideas of sacrificial kingship or located in the context of kinds of social theory of that time which override the modern/premodern distinction, notably Durkheim's speculative anthropology. If this echoes the kind of sacrifice of the king which Frazer did much to explore, and which René Girard has since reinterpreted (especially in terms of mimesis and desire, which might shed light on mirroring in the novel), then it starts to raise questions about the ways in which guilt or shame may lose their fixed meanings, especially at a constitutive, founding or unfounding moment, when the frameworks that might determine codes and laws and norms falter, or have yet to be fashioned. In a way which flatters European imperialism, Jim in Patusan presents an image of founding or refounding hero, and his liminal position, poised at moments of founding or undoing, caught between two worlds, jumping from one to another, helps to create the peculiar framework in which Conrad invites us to judge the character as a whole and thus, implicitly, among other things, the question of his guilt or shame.

Turning back to German romanticism with Jim's situation in Patusan in mind, it's notable that certain key terms in Conrad's description of Jim's specially prescribed relation with "his" people, which I related earlier to Frazer's account of the restrictions that hedge a priest-king, recall key terms for thinking about tragedy, especially a dialectical interplay between freedom and imprisonment. Which is the master and which the slave? One might see a relation between what Frazer presents as a form of "primitive" thinking and Stein's vatic prescription for Jim, which has occasioned endless speculation: "In the destructive element immerse" (129–130). The crucial thing about those sacred things that attract taboos and rituals in *The Golden Bough* isn't that they're good or progressive, but that they're powerful – whether generative or destructive. Similarly, the romantic imagination, liberated from an obligation to uphold a particular code of ethics or to serve anything other than itself, is primarily a kind of power. One possible way of understanding the logic of the novel, then, is to see Stein invoking the kind of rationale that Frazer saw at work in various non-western cultures, which could mean that dangerous, threatening things might possess a kind of power that one might seek to appropriate, but Stein applies that rationale to a distinctive product of the west: romantic imagination.

To turn to Jim's death with this way of interpreting the novel in mind is to encounter radical ambiguity. If one sees Patusan as Edenic, it's a Patusan with too many candidates for the role of Satan. I've already noted the way Cornelius's reptilian traits link him with the serpent. Even in the way in which Conrad toned down his portrayal of Brown to downplay the sense of his being the agent of supernatural dark powers, Brown smacks of the Satanic: he has "a satanic gift of finding out the best and the weakest spot in his victims" (229).[33] Yet Jim also brings a taint with himself into this Eden. If he's Adamic, he's an Adam already fallen. He brings with him a kind of guilt as well as his personal sense of shame. The guilt that he brings is at once his weakness and his strength: it motivates him to see going to Patusan not simply as being got safely "out of the way" (134) (which is how Marlow thought of it), but as a redemptive opportunity. In a sense, it's the making of him. Yet Jim's guilt is also what makes him vulnerable, as his mirroring conversation with "Gentleman" Brown reveals. Brown as "thwarted autocrat" has something of Tamburlaine or Genghis Khan about him – an almost primal destroyer, who creates an empire, save that in the modern world outside Patusan he creates nothing. But in confronting Jim he confronts a fulfilled autocrat.

As soon as one thinks of Jim's death at Doramin's hand with *The Golden Bough* in mind, the question arises of whether this isn't a kind of ritual sacrifice that confirms his special status. The possibility of it being expiatory and settling a debt and thus clearing one kind of guilt is clearly enough raised. But Conrad sets against the temptation to read it in redemptive terms Jewel's absolute refusal of pathos and forgiveness. She is defined by her refusal to follow her mother's example, and it's a refusal grounded in what feels almost like a kind of primal scene: the scene of her mother's death. Cornelius is battering on the door, Jewel braced against it, denying him entry. Her mother expires in tears. Jewel takes from her mother two resolutions: not "to die weeping" (186) and never to forgive desertion by her man: "My mother had forgiven – but I, never!" (187). That refusal helps to shape interpretation of the novel's final pages.

It's one of the ironies of Jim's death that, if it figures as a sacrifice in the etymological sense of that word for anyone, it's not for the community over which he ruled. He wasn't propitiating their god or gods by choosing death, and still less was he ascending to be amongst those gods. The myth of his invulnerability is, presumably, destroyed by his death. It is, instead, only for the novel's reader, assembled in a ritual (albeit imagined) community, that the possibility exists of seeing Jim's death as both failure and affirmation, overthrow and assertion, an acceptance of mortality and a transcendence of it, albeit not to an afterlife.

It becomes impossible to place Jim. Marlow says he sees him "under a cloud," which may mean shamed, but also suggests ascension (and not necessarily a Christian one: in *Oedipus at Colonus*, Oedipus finally vanishes miraculously and mysteriously in the middle of a storm). He is impossible to place, because his final act is undecidable, except by us. Jewel and Tamb' Itam blame him for not defending himself. With Jewel's refusal of forgiveness in mind, one might see Jim's dying as one more running away from shame. But the moment of his death, the unflinching paying of the price for his dead friend tempts one to see it quite differently – in ways that moral-psychological readings don't fathom. It's a moment prepared for by Jim's abortive piece of writing, which implicitly raises questions about it. Does he really confront and come to a reckoning with himself in his death in the way that he might have done in a confession or a testament?

> ...They say that the white man sent right and left at all those faces a proud and unflinching glance. Then with his hand over his lips he fell forward, dead.
>
> And that's the end. He passes away under a cloud, inscrutable at heart, forgotten, unforgiven, and excessively romantic.
>
> (246)

Does his proud gaze betoken an end to the blushing concealments of shame? Or does raising his hand to his mouth in death gesture towards a repetition of such concealment? Is this a moment of shame cleared or confronted; or a moment of founding, sacrificial and tragic guilt? It's a moment at once writerly and ritualistic, in which different senses of shame and guilt, which the novel has in some respects imaginatively explored and distinguished, refuse finally to stabilize or separate.

Notes

My thanks to members of the Guilt Group at Birkbeck and particularly to Sam Ashenden, to whom this essay owes a good deal.

1 Eric R. Dodds, *The Greeks and the Irrational* (Berkeley: University of California Press, 1951); April E. Cook, "Honor and Transgression: The Poetics and Politics of Shame and Guilt in *Sir Gawain and the Green Knight*," *Universitas* 4.1 (2008): 1–7; Ruth Benedict, *The Chrysanthemum and the Sword: Patterns of Japanese Culture* (London: Secker and Warburg, 1947 [1946]).

2 Margaret Mead, "Interpretive Statement," in *Cooperation and Competition among Primitive Peoples*, ed. Margaret Mead (New York: McGraw Hill, 1937), 493–495.

3 June Price Tangney and Ronda L. Dearing, *Shame and Guilt* (New York: The Guilford Press, 2004), 12–13, 18–20.

4 See, for example, Ewan Fernie, *Shame in Shakespeare* (London: Routledge, 2002), 15–16; Douglas Cairns, *Aidôs: The Psychology and Ethics of Honour and Shame in Ancient Greek Literature* (Oxford: Oxford University Press, 1993), chapter 1; Christopher Gill, *Greek Thought* (Oxford: Classical Association / Oxford University Press, 1995), 24–26; and Thomas Osborne, "Desperate Equilibrium: On Guilt, Law and Rationality," *Economy and Society* 43.1 (2014): 40–54. The latter proposes an alternative way of distinguishing shame and guilt.

5 See Norma Sherry, "The Pilgrim-Ship Episode," in Joseph Conrad, *Lord Jim*, by Joseph Conrad, 2nd edition, ed. by Thomas C. Moser (New York: W.W. Norton & Co, 1996), 319–358.

6 Joseph Conrad, *Lord Jim*, 2nd edition, ed. by Thomas C. Moser (New York: W.W. Norton & Co). All subsequent references to *Lord Jim* give just the page number for this edition.

7 Samuel Johnson, *Dictionary of the English Language*, 6th edition (London: J.F. & C. Rivington et al., 1785).

8 William Dwight Whitney, ed., *The Century Dictionary and Cyclopedia*, vol. 7 (New York: Century Co., 1897).

9 James A. H. Murray and Henry Bradley, eds., *A New English Dictionary on Historical Principles: Founded Mainly on the Materials Collected by the Philological Society*, vol. 4 (Oxford: Clarendon Press, 1901).

10 Charles Darwin, *The Expression of the Emotions in Man and Animals*, 2nd edition (London: John Murray, 1890), 274.

11 Darwin, *Expression*, 275.

12 Ibid., 352.

13 *Webster's Dictionary* (1828 & 1913). Accessed on March 26, 2017, http://machaut.uchicago.edu/websters (online edition of the 1828 and 1913 editions of Webster's).

14 Thomas Dixon, *From Passions to Emotions: The Creation of a Secular Psychological Category* (Cambridge: Cambridge University Press, 2003), 1–4.

15 J. H. Stape, "Lord Jim," in *The Cambridge Companion to Joseph Conrad*, ed. J. H. Stape (Cambridge: Cambridge University Press, 1996), 64–66.

16 Raymond E. Fancher, Introduction to "The Origin and Development of Psychoanalysis," by Sigmund Freud. Classics in the History of Psychology – An internet resource developed by Christopher D. Green. Accessed on March 26, 2017, http://psychclassics.yorku.ca/Freud/Origin/intro.htm.

17 E. M. Forster, *Aspects of the Novel*, Revised edition, ed. Oliver Stallybrass, introduced by Frank Kermode (London: Penguin, [1927] 2005), chapters 3–4.

18 Ian Watt, *Conrad in the Nineteenth Century* (London: Chatto and Windus, 1980), 430.
19 Jean-Jacques Rousseau, "Discourse on the Origin and Foundations of Inequality among Men," in *The Discourses and Other Early Political Writings*, ed. Victor Gourevitch (Cambridge: Cambridge University Press, [1754] 1997), 187.
20 Pierre Bourdieu, "The Sentiment of Honour in Kabyle Society," in *Honour and Shame: The Values of Mediterranean Society*, ed. J. G. Peristiany (London: Weidenfeld and Nicolson, 1966), 211.
21 Adam Smith, *The Theory of Moral Sentiments*, ed. D. D. Raphael and A. L. Macfie (Oxford: Oxford University Press [1759] 1976), 3.1.39.
22 Marvin Carlson, *Theories of the Theatre* (Ithaca, NY: Cornell University Press, 1984), chapter 11.
23 Simon Critchley, "The Tragedy of Misrecognition: The Desire for a Catholic Shakespeare and Hegel's *Hamlet*," in *Tragedy and the Idea of Modernity*, ed. Joshua Billings and Miriam Leonard (Oxford: Oxford University Press, 2015), 258–259.
24 Cf. Samantha Ashenden and James Brown, "Romantic guilt and identity," *Economy and Society* 43.1 (2014): 83–102.
25 Friedrich Nietzsche, *On the Genealogy of Morality*, trans. Maudmarie Clark and Alan J. Swenson (Indianapolis, IN: Hackett Publishing Company, [1887] 1998); and *The Birth of Tragedy* in *The Birth of Tragedy and The Case of Wagner*, trans. Walter Kaufmann, 15–144 (New York: Vintage Books, [1872] 1967).
26 Daphna Erdinast-Vulcan, "The Failure of Myth: *Lord Jim*," in Conrad, *Lord Jim*, 503.
27 James Frazer, *The Golden Bough: A Study in Comparative Religion*, vol. 1 (New York: Macmillan, [1890] 1894), 110.
28 John B. Vickery, *The Literary Impact of The Golden Bough* (Princeton, NJ: Princeton University Press, 1973), 49.
29 Vickery, *Literary Impact*, 50.
30 Frazer, *The Golden Bough*, 171.
31 Mary Douglas, *Purity and Danger: An Analysis of the Concepts of Pollution and Taboo* (Harmondsworth: Penguin, [1966] 1970), 115.
32 Douglas, *Purity and Danger*, 117.
33 See Ernest W. Sullivan, "The Several Endings of Joseph Conrad's *Lord Jim*," in Conrad, *Lord Jim*.

7   Black and Ashamed

Deconstructing Race in Ralph Ellison's *Invisible Man*

Zlatan Filipovic

In *The Souls of Black Folk*, W. E. B. Du Bois writes of "a peculiar sensation" in the affective life of the oppressed that pits the subject against itself: "It is a peculiar sensation, this sense of always looking at one's self through the eyes of others, of measuring one's soul by the tape of a world that looks on in amused contempt and pity."[1] The constitution of subjectivity taken hostage by the white gaze that Du Bois describes is further exposed as a structure of abiding ambiguity that reveals the Ego's inability to assume its contradictions. "One ever feels his two-ness," he continues, "an American, a Negro; two souls, two thoughts, two unreconciled strivings; two warring ideals in one dark body, whose dogged strength alone keeps it from being torn asunder."[2] This divided black soul, for Du Bois, constitutes both the living center of the American narrative and its unlivable margins at the same time. It is eminently American in the very possibility of its resistance to the objective racial myths within which it is determined, but it is also America's constitutive outside, the excluded threshold of its identity.

The ambiguity of "double consciousness,"[3] that in Du Bois' writing powers the heteronomous constitution of the black subject and that I will argue is affectively articulated as racial shame, is what seesaws the nameless narrator in Ralph Ellison's *Invisible Man* (1952) between different stages of racial displacement.[4] The first stage, identified by Foucault as the process of subjectivization,[5] is characterized by the introjection of the white gaze and its fantasies of racial difference, while the second is represented by its refusal, articulated in self-valorizing metaphysics of black nationalism and identity politics. Both are, however, revealed as displacements of subjectivity, determined within the narrow orbit of racial shame, and as reductive mystifications of partial and contradictory structures of difference that participate in the subject formation. Both reproduce violence and reinforce the structures of invisibility that in the novel force black subjectivity underground. Continually at war with itself, as Du Bois suggests, the black psyche either assumes the objective structures of its own oppression or, summoned back by the contorted cries of history forced out of its lashed, black skin, it resists its own inevitable interpellation in the white narrative.[6] Either way, it remains fixed in the strict binarism of the white gaze and powerlessly consigned to its normative regimes of subject constitution.

Having no field for disclosure in the racialized metaphysics of power relations that dominates Ellison's world, any slippage of identity over and beyond its hegemonic articulations carries an affective cost for the black subject, a "psychic uncertainty" in Ellison's terms, that "he yearns to avoid."[7] This cost, that I will argue acquires its most significant tenor when considered within the economy of racial shame, is what breaks open a third, heterotopic space characterized by invisibility in the novel. For Ellison, shame is irremissibly tied to the normative violence of the white disavowal and what he consequently calls "the pathologies of the democratic process"[8] that plot the painful narratives of black America. Emancipation that, like a stab of epiphany finally descends on the narrator towards the end of the novel, represents not only a metaphoric escape of subjectivity from the tightening embrace of objective racial binaries that trace the limits of black lives, but it also constitutes an affirmation of fragmented social identities that slip through the totalizing assignations of their subject positions. The "cost of insight," as Ellison observes when considering the politics of difference as the watershed of American experience, "is an uncertainty that threatens our already unstable sense of order and requires a constant questioning of accepted assumptions."[9]

In light of this, I intend to consider the implications of racial shame for the theoretical strategies that map out the underlying syntax of subject formation in its relation to power and further develop its significance for our reading of invisibility in Ellison's novel. Although not explicitly concerned with shame, Foucault's structuralist analytic of power and its normalizing regimes that participate in subject formation imply a coextensive terrain of affective structures through which the normative spatialities that regulate our social existence are maintained. Subject formation, for Foucault, is an effect of disciplinary procedures tied to the "totalization of modern power structures"[10] and their individualizing strategies that reduce and subject our multiplicities to unified regimes of identification. It is a cornering of my differences and a binding of my attachments to an identity that I cannot and yet must assume, since it constitutes the sign and cipher of my social visibility. The word "subject" articulates subjection in two ways, according to Foucault: "subject to someone else by control or dependence, *and tied to his own identity by a conscience or self-knowledge.* Both meanings suggest a form of power which subjugates and makes subject to."[11] Although ostensibly exclusive in terms of heteronomy/autonomy of the subject formation, the experience of racial shame integrates both significations of subjection in a temporal order where the white disavowal imposed as extrinsic to black identity is interiorized and exposed as intrinsic to its constitution. Racial shame could thus be seen as an affective hinge that enables the articulation of the objective structures of power by the subjects themselves. As the elision of outside and inside, the becoming of outside inside or the inside outside, the affective experience of shame makes the structures of disavowal immanent to the social terrain. Through racial shame, black lives are thus authored for from within, fatally "tied to [their] own identity by a conscience or self-knowledge."[12]

However, the process of subjectivization does not disable agency. As Aurelia Armstrong suggests, the possibility of resistance in Foucault "is grounded in an agency that precedes disciplinarity and can never be fully colonized by it."[13] Power, as Foucault maintains, is founded on the irrepressibility of freedom and its continuous "refusal to submit,"[14] the fact that "'the other' (the one over whom power is exercised) be thoroughly recognized and maintained to the very end as a person who acts."[15] Power only emerges against the depths of the other's resistance, in a relation of force that defines the vitalism of its oppression. "At the very heart of the power relationship, and constantly provoking it, are the recalcitrance of the will and the intransigence of freedom."[16] And yet, the "will" of the other, for Foucault, is considered *agonistic* and subject to discursive procedures and technologies of power, rather than constituting an "essential antagonism."[17] It is less, he explains, "a face-to-face confrontation which paralyzes both sides than a permanent provocation."[18] This implies that the immanence of resistance to power does not reside in a subjectivity whose autonomy precedes its articulation by the discursive terrain, but in an unmasterable excess produced by the totalizing procedures of power that slips through the interstices of its articulated binaries. This ambiguity and "complicated interplay"[19] of power and resistance that cannot be accommodated by the pendulum of the Hegelian dialectic is represented in the novel by the narrator's abeyant differential position in the hierarchies of power and identity that belies the binary orthodoxies of racial absolutism and identity politics through which his visibility is established. The epiphany of the novel, as we shall see, is the epiphany of *différance* that reveals racialized identities in the first two stages of subject formation as displacements of subjectivity's constitutive multiplicities whose suppression is articulated in the affective experience of racial shame. Subject formation, as Rancière argues, taking Foucault a step further, is not the formation of "a one" that is a self, "but is the *relation* of a self to an other."[20] For Rancière, the process of subjectivization is the political, emancipatory process of deconstruction, of "disidentification or declassification"[21] of identities to which we are consigned by the modalities of power. Subject, he writes, is

> the name of anyone, the name of the outcast: those who do not belong to the order of castes, indeed, those who are pleased to undo this order (the class that dissolves classes, as Marx said). In this way, a process of subjectivization is a process of disidentification

or declassification. Let me rephrase this: a subject is an outsider or, more, an *in-between* ... between several names, statuses, and identities... Political subjectivization is the enactment of equality... It is a crossing of identities... In sum, the logic of political subjectivization, of emancipation, is a heterology, a logic of the other ... it is never the simple assertion of an identity; it is always, at the same time, the denial of an identity given by an other, given by the ruling order of policy.[22]

Rancière's emancipatory heterology of subject formation constitutes resistance precisely to the extent that it is not simply a refusal of subjection that articulates political agency but a refusal of the binary orders of identifications within which that agency is inscribed. To destabilize the strategies of power and its rules of formation, "we could act as political subjects in the interval or the gap between two identities, neither of which we could assume."[23] In this active slippage of identificatory signifiers that Rancière refers to as a "demonstration of equality," the structural binarism that determines for social visibility is deeply "intertwined with the paratactic logic of a 'we are *and* are not,'"[24] which, for Ellison, in fact, constitutes the insuperable condition of our democratic existence, "our oneness-in-manyness."[25]

The differential excess produced by the process of subjectivization that legislates for an unassumable identification and where "the life of *political* subjectivization" or resistance "is made out of the *difference* between the voice and the body, the interval between identities"[26] is revealed in Ellison's novel as a prophetic intervention in the racial imaginary of his time, and an exigent call for the transformation of political structures that will allow for the emergence of new forms of subjectivities and cultural enunciations from the threshold of social visibility. Deconstruction of identity structures, the enactment of equality in the rip currents of difference is, however, what renders the narrator truly invisible in a regime of truth that reduces all social life to a skein Du Bois claims defines our age: "the problem of the color-line."[27] Ellison's nameless narrator is driven underground not because of his initial appropriation of the racial hierarchies that constitute him as invisible, as "a phantom in other people's minds" (*IM* 4), nor because of his subsequent fetishization of black identity in essentialisms of racial difference, but finally due to his rejection of both. At the same time, this invisibility, as we shall see, opens up a heterotopic space for the narrator with unsuspected emancipatory energies that invert the order of truth and detach it from the restrictive regimes within which its effects are disseminated. The hierarchies of power which regulate the forms within which we are able to recognize ourselves as subjects are effectively undermined in Ellison's writing by an inscription of alterity that, as yet, has no political constituency and cannot be articulated within the oppositions that structure the terrain of social visibility in the novel. Ellison is thus looking beyond the blockages of his present, anticipating alternate forms of enunciation that have yet to be realized.

Two Stages of Displacement: Shame and the Boomerang

There is always "a brooding strangeness," Ellison writes, "in our intergroup familiarity" and "in our underlying sense of alienation a poignant – although distrusted – sense of fraternity."[28] Addressing the rearguard work of cultural ambiguity that challenges the totalizing forms of America's national narratives, Ellison's essay, "The Little Man at Chehaw Station,"[29] further extends the concerns articulated two decades earlier in the novel that marked a turning point in Black American fiction. "Black writing," as Early points out, "became [now] less concerned with merely protesting racism or in asserting the humanity of blacks and more interested in delineating African American characters as individuals engaged in distinct battles for meaning and unique struggles against the caprices of fate."[30] However, what underlies the apparent existentialist topography of Ellison's novel is perhaps not the concern with the constituent subject, but with the process of its constitution within a historical schema where racial formulas legislate for identity. While the possibility of being black and being American at the same time powers the political rhetoric of the hour, *Invisible Man* does not only register its contradictions but wears away at any phantasmatic centering of the heterogeneous play of forces that participate in the formation of the American subject. The novel traces the narrator's emerging sense of displacement in the political terrain of radicalized racial attachments, leading to an exposure of subjectivity that exceeds unitary assignations to consistent social positions.

Trapped in a system of binary racial schemas that dominate the social and political realities of pre-Civil Rights America, the narrator's subject formation is negotiated through a narrative succession of identity displacements that provide the implicit structure of the novel. As a young and unsuspecting student backed up against the racial myths of the outside gaze, the narrator initially identifies with the phobic fantasies of whiteness and its normative demands as the legitimate carriers of agency, "show[ing] that humility was the secret, indeed, the very essence of progress," for which he "was considered an example of desirable conduct..." (*IM* 16–17). However, repeatedly disillusioned by the white disavowal of his initiatives upon his arrival to New York, he then reclaims his black skin, discovering a sense of self-identity in the very origins of his shame, but he does it by assuming the compensatory mask of Southern regionalism and by accommodating the historically determined representations of his black identity. The rhetoricity of subject formation represented by the first two stages of displacement is then finally revealed by the end of the novel with the narrator's recognition of identity as a residual effect of racialized historical structures.

"Free of illusions" and "through [with] running" (569), the process of subjectivization for the narrator is finally unhinged by new forms of subjectivity that disarticulate visible identificatory schemas but force him underground. What emerges underground, in the invisible basement section of a white-only apartment building where he finds his home, is a new temporality with no social space to accommodate its epiphany, as the vision of America, "woven of many strands" (577), coincides with the realization that identity is "one, and yet many" (569), subject to movement that resists conclusive representations of social existence. "This is not prophecy," the narrator insists, "but description" (577), a reality beyond the politics of the imaginary that fixes its representation in visible oppositions. It is as yet invisible to history and literally consigned to its basement but it is "warm and full of light" (6), lit up by the narrator using "exactly 1,369 lights" (7) to manifest its blinding truth. Thus, "one of the greatest jokes in the world," as he states in the Epilogue, "is the spectacle of the whites busy escaping blackness and becoming blacker every day, and the blacks striving toward whiteness, becoming quite dull and gray" (577). Ellison's novel is an attestation to the fact that subjectivity is constituted in the interstices of identity categories and structural hierarchies that articulate the imperatives of our social life and the fact that we only ever exist at their limits at which we are exposed to one another.

Ironically, however, the first two stages are accommodated by the public space, but the third drives him underground since the overlays of difference that (dis)articulate identity have no field for disclosure in the social structure claustrophobically defined by fixed racial binaries. His claim for differential structure of identity and for the slippage of its signification as constitutively American is suppressed, or literally "clubbed" (572) down, by a reality produced through the racial imperatives that dictate social practice and totalize identity across its field of differences. Confiding in the reader as "an invisible man," which "placed ... [him] in a hole," the narrator concedes that "[o]nce you get used to it, the reality is as irresistible as a club, and I was clubbed into the cellar before I caught the hint. Perhaps that's the way that it had to be..." (572).

What is "clubbed" underground, however, is the narrator's challenge to the regulatory law within which identity is constructed. It is a challenge that Bhabha, in different but related terms, argues still lies ahead of us

in conceiving of the time of political action and understanding as opening up a space that can accept and regulate the differential structure of the moment of intervention without rushing to produce a unity of the social antagonism and contradiction.[31]

The ambiguity of subject positions reveled in Ellison's novel and the ambivalence that belies their enunciation tear a hole in the racial fabric of American history, "a hole in the ground" (*IM* 6), and upset the relations of force that determine the narrator's present. Ellison's novel is emancipatory in Rancière's sense since it *intervenes* in the process of subjectivization to expose the unseen records of subjectivity that the discursive order, which legislates for visibility, for what can be seen, for what constitutes the thresholds of public space, cannot yet register but has to accommodate in order to account for the historical transformation of its own limits. "This is a sign," in Bhabha's terms, "that history is *happening*."[32]

In his collection of essays *White Man, Listen!*, Richard Wright argues that the "differences between the groups we know as races are associated with the repression of differences within those races."[33] Totalizing binary structures that in the process of subjectivization rely on racial representativeness arrest the play of these differences and, by the same token, produce affective economies in which subjectivity is constrained to assume the burden of the oppositional logic within which it is articulated. One of the primary expressions of this burden is racial shame.

In both stages of the narrator's displacement, shame is present as the very exposure of his blackness to the normativizing knowledge of the white gaze. Structural racialization and its production of legitimate social bodies through valorizing practices and normative constraints of racial laws produces shame in the black subject by the very materialization of those laws and the compulsory identification with its normative demands. Internalized racial normativity corners the black psyche and mobilizes its last-ditch defenses to reclaim and emancipate itself in the stratagems of identification. In the absence of political defense, as Du Bois argues, "there is a patent defense at hand, – the defense of deception and flattery, of cajoling and lying."[34] The appropriation of the white disavowal and the artifice of identifying with the attitudes and sensibilities imposed by the white hegemony offer the privilege of social mobility for the black subject: "Patience, humility, and adroitness, must, in these growing black youth, replace impulse, manliness, and courage. With this sacrifice there is an economic opening, and perhaps peace and some prosperity. Without this there is riot, migration, or crime."[35] Hypocrisy and opportunism of the oppressed, however, are not in any sense particular to the American South for Du Bois; "is it not rather the only method," he asks rhetorically, "by which undeveloped races have gained the right to share modern culture?"[36] What remains unconsidered in this respect is the fact that the interiorized racial oppression also offers a fantasy of self-approval. The desire for whiteness, for "lactification"[37] in Fanon's terms, in a society where "color ... settle[s] a man's conviction,"[38] is a desire for self-approval.

However, racial shame is not only related to the introjection of the white imaginary by the black subject, but is also deeply implicated in the opposite malaise of self-valorizing investments in racial difference where it is reclaimed as pride in order to reconstitute the narrative of black identity. The violence of black nationalism and the myopia of identity fetishism that the black psyche can leverage in order to contest the identificatory processes of internalized oppression share the same basic assumptions with the essentialist fantasies of white power. The mystifying representations of black otherness are reclaimed and fundamentally reaffirmed in what Ellison regards as the glorification of "blood thinking" and "ethnic (and genetic) insularity."[39] Idolizing the commonality of slavery that provides the connective tissue for the heterogeneity of black experience does, however, confer legitimacy and provide historical continuity for broken and disavowed black lives. It enables the emergence of much needed self-consciousness, racial identification and political leverage, but it also totalizes identity and arrests the play of differences internal to it.

Black nationalism is mobilized and represented in *Invisible Man* by Ras the Exhorter, a "wild man" (364), a visionary and a rival leader of radical black separatism whose "hoodlums would attack and denounce the white meat of a roasted chicken" (365). Propelled into violence by the overwhelming historical forces, Ras is the inevitable effect of racial articulations of power. His charismatic, sectarian rhetoric, "wrong but justified, crazy and yet coldly sane" (564), only reflects the opposite end of the never-ending pendulum of racial politics that tears through the social terrain of America. After an attempt by the narrator to wrestle Harlem and its community leaders from Ras to support the more conciliatory and racially integrative cause of the Brotherhood, Ras's poignant appeal quickly exposes the double consciousness of the black subject and the inherent complicity of the Brotherhood in the continuing oppression of black lives:

> You *my* brother mahn! Brothers are the same color; how the hell you call these white men *brother*?... We sons of Mama Africa, you done forgot? You black, BLACK!... You got bahd *hair*! You got thick *lips*! They say you *stink*! They hate you mahn. You African. AFRICAN! Why you with them?... They enslave us – you forget that?... What you trying to deny by betraying the black people?... In Africa this mahn be a chief, a black king! Here they say he rape them godhahm women with no blood in their veins... What kind of foolishness is it? Kick him ass from cradle to grave then call him *brother*?... Is that sanity? Is that consciousness ... the modern black mahn of the twentieth century? Hell, mahn!... He got you so you don't trust your black intelligence... Don't deny you'self!... It's three hundred years of black blood to build this white mahn's civilization and wahn't be

wiped out in a minute. Blood calls for blood! You remember that.
And remember that I'm not like you. Ras recognizes the true issues
and he is not afraid to be black. Nor is he a traitor for white men.

(370–71, 372, 373, 376)

Ras sees "the true issues" in the open relation of forces unmystified by
the protean forms of racial discrimination. For Ras, the black subject can
only emerge in the positive expression of real antagonism that reconsti-
tutes agency through an absolute rejection of the white narrative within
which it has been determined. This "boomerang" moment, in Sartre's
terms,[40] of racial disavowal that finds legitimacy in the self-valorizing
rhetoric of the Négritude movement and pan-African essentialisms is
necessary, according to Fanon, since it rehabilitates the past from the
black pit of shame where it has been buried alive and triggers a fundamental change in the "psycho-affective equilibrium"[41] of the oppressed.
Indeed, Ras could be seen as part of the counterhegemonic struggle over
representation and meaning of the black past that has been scandalized
within the racial schema upon which the white subject founds its prerogatives. When racial riots, instigated by Ras the Exhorter – who by the
end of the novel becomes Ras the Destroyer – finally take possession of
Harlem, he appears on

a great black horse. A new Ras of a haughty, vulgar dignity, dressed
in the costume of an Abyssinian chieftain [with] a fur cap upon his
head, his arm bearing a shield [and with] a cape made of the skin of
some wild animal around his shoulders.

(*IM* 556)

"A figure," the narrator continues, "more out of a *dream* than out of
Harlem ... yet real, alive, alarming" (556, emphasis added). Making
visible the suppressed black past uncannily claiming ownership of the
present, Ras seems to stagger reason itself, but that is only because the
history of *reason* is white.

Ras, however, does not only expose the brutal residues of racial shame
no longer blushing for its indiscretions, but also represents the narrator's
own cresting ambivalence between his formal pledge to the organized
cause of the Brotherhood and his affective pledge to the suffering of
the black community. The two do not coincide, "[t]he Brotherhood isn't
the Negro people" (468), and, with its overbearing, teleological abstractions, the Brotherhood runs aground against the throb of Harlem, its
"raw materials" (472), its "gin mills and the barber shops and the juke
joints and the churches ... the beauty parlors on Saturdays when they're
frying hair ... and a cheap tenement at night ... [where a] whole unre-
corded history is spoken..." (471). To the Brotherhood and its cyclopean,
one-eyed leader Jack, they are only "the mistaken and infantile notions

of the man in the street" (473), whose suffering is martyred for yet another historical narrative of white redemption.

The narrator's desire for whiteness, which characterizes the first stage of his displacement, is ultimately based on the process of subjectivization that articulates the demands for his social existence.[42] In the racialized terrain of white America, the narrator can emerge as visible only by assuming the shame for his own visibility. This is reflected in the naïve enthusiasm of his formative years for Booker T. Washington's conciliatory strategies to accommodate white interests, rather than challenge their racial oppression.[43] The narrator's inability to see the trenchant ambiguity of his grandfather's last words, urging his son to '"[l]ive with … [his] head in the lion's mouth … [and] overcome 'em with yeses, undermine 'em with grins, agree 'em to death and destruction, let 'em swoller you till they vomit or bust wide open'" (16), reveals the extent of his interpellation by the racial myths that produce a fixed geography of power within which black agency is scripted:

> His words caused so much anxiety … he had spoken of meekness as a dangerous activity… And whenever things went well for me I … felt guilty and uncomfortable… When I was praised for my conduct I felt a guilt that in some way I was doing something that was really against the wishes of the white folks… The old man's words were like a curse. On my graduation day, I delivered an oration in which I showed that humility was the secret, indeed, the very essence of progress… I was praised by most lily-white men of the town … considered an example of desirable conduct … [and] was invited to give the speech at a gathering of the town's leading white citizens. It was a triumph for our whole community.
>
> (16, 17)

The interiorized racial binaries and the universal white narratives, seemingly motivating the narrator's guilt for breaking his normative contract, are, in fact, embedded in deeper, ontological structures of shame. The white gaze interiorized by the narrator as the self-policing agency of the Ego-ideal consigns black subjectivity to assume the burden for the signification and visibility of its own skin that one cannot expiate for. No matter what one *does*, the fact of blackness remains fixed, renegrifying every attempt to escape the airtight cage of its imperatives. Shame persists over and beyond guilt, which remains inherently excusable, which one can be forgiven for through acts of self-abnegation, humility or punishment. We forgive only what we can punish. Shame, however, carves out a subjectivity that has no recourse against itself. Subject formation for the narrator is thus inevitably tied to shame because it is related to the body and its inscription within the productive constraints of the regulatory schemas that articulate its meaning. But there is no body outside its racial

inscription. In fact, body or the fantasy of the unraced body is the first
effect of racism. What this means is that the political structures that produce race cannot be dissociated from the materiality of the body that is
only ever articulated within them, as "the inscribed surface of events,"[44]
and the narrator's discomfort at his grandfather's dying plea is only the
growing recognition of this fact. The "curse" of his grandfather's ambiguous words is the birth of racial awareness for the narrator who is
just beginning to realize that race legislates for subjectivity through an
essentialist splitting of body and meaning.

In racial shame, I am *for myself* a refused me. The ambivalence of identification for the black subject resides in the fact that its skin is both the
point of irremissible attachment and the point of regulatory detachment, it
is both "a scene of fear and desire,"[45] in Bhabha's terms. My skin *exposes*
me – both reveals me and determines me outside myself. And to me, its
black dirt is visible by means of the heteronomy I have assumed since,
in racial shame, my subjectivity holds out against itself. I *am* black but,
having interiorized the racial myths of the white imaginary, I see myself
as white seeing myself black. And the racial schema, abrogating all others, betrays all my pretenses and nails me fixed in *being-despite-myself*,
which characterizes the affective structure of shame.

The 'boomerang' for the narrator, however, comes during his "first
northern winter" (*IM* 260), just before he witnesses the eviction of an
old black couple whose shame of dispossession, including the "FREE
PAPERS" from 1859 (272), was exposed in Harlem snow by the white
authorities. Passing a store window, displaying "ointments guaranteed
to produce the miracle of whitening black skin" and signs proclaiming,
"[y]ou too can be truly beautiful … [and w]in greater happiness with
whiter complexion," he seizes sight of a yam stand, glowing black in the
biting white air, "bringing a stab of swift nostalgia" (262). Not being
able to resist the "savage urge" (262) through what he had earlier referred to as "an act of discipline,"[46] he buys and "wolfs down the yam"
(266) while walking,

> suddenly overcome by an intense feeling of freedom… It was ex-
> hilarating. I no longer had to worry about who saw me or about
> what was proper. To hell with all that… If only someone who had
> known me at school or at home would come along and see me now.
> How shocked they'd be… What a group of people we were … you
> could cause us the greatest humiliation simply by confronting us
> with something we liked. No more of that for me… They're my
> birthmark… *I yam what I yam.*
>
> (264, 266, emphasis added)

In the second stage of displacement, signified by the emancipatory return
of the repressed black ontology, the body yet again carries the burden of

affective investments. This time, it is fixed in a new symbolic attachment that seemingly reclaims the prerogatives of its history. In a boomerang of the repressed, the black body now becomes a source of identification: "I yam what I yam" (266). Since there is no escape from under its unbearable weight and since it persists beyond all initiatives to transcend it, the body also becomes the only refuge left for the black subject. For the narrator, it now opens up a new relation to the past which suspends the identificatory strategies of racial pragmatism, "of what works" (17), that determines his relation to the present. The "yams" and their explicit relation to prohibited pleasure, somaticism and hunger, signifying the break-out, the "intense feeling of freedom" (264), of the black body from the prison of its scripted determinations, mark the birth of the narrator as a racial subject.[47] Denying the very soil of its signification, the black consciousness now reverts to it, investing it with liberating vitalities and mystifications of black essentialism, "the shameless... Field-Niggerism" (265), in narrator's terminology, in order to provide ontological legitimacy for the black experience. "This is all very wild and childish," the narrator explains, "but to hell with being ashamed of what you liked. No more of that for me" (265–66). The black body itself becomes an open wound of signification, where the question of shame powers its fundamental antagonisms on the streets of Harlem. Indeed, the battlefield that Harlem becomes at the end of the novel is over the disinscription of the black body that is able to reset the stage for possible pasts and alternate futures, disrupting the white narratives of historical progress.

The Unpresupposable Subject: "Man of Parts"

However, the narrator's repeated questioning of the self-consistency of black American experience foreshadows his emerging understanding that the legitimacy of black America sought in exclusionary structures of racial particularisms is yet another displacement of subjectivity that disables the multiplicity of subjective positions. Indeed, the internal difference that cuts across the closures of subject formation is already present as the "annoying" question that deflates the symbolism of his "birth" as a racial subject:

> They're my birthmark... I yam what I yam... What and how much had I lost by trying to do only what was expected of me instead of what I myself had wished to do? What a waste... But what of those things which you actually didn't like, not because you were not supposed to like them, not because to dislike them was considered a mark of refinement and education – but because you actually found them distasteful? The very idea annoyed me. How could you know?... I would have to weigh many things carefully ... simply

because I had never formed a personal attitude toward so much. I had accepted the accepted attitudes and it had made life seem simple...

(266–67)

Since racial visibility is "at once a *point* of identity," as Bhabha writes, and "at the same time a *problem* for the attempted closure within the discourse,"[48] the binarism of racial identification forces open a space of invisibility that gathers the unproductive excess which escapes hegemonic articulation altogether. Invisibility in the novel articulates the diasporization of racial difference, its slippage across the totalities that determine its politics. It anticipates what Hall refers to as "the politics of the end of the essential black subject."[49] For the narrator, who feels increasingly trapped in the process of subject formation where visibility is determined by the racial schemas of identification, this space becomes a metaphor for freedom and a space for ambivalence and disclosure of difference in subject formation.

Abandoning the Brotherhood and narrowly escaping from the nationalist clutch of Ras the Destroyer and his cohorts, the narrator inadvertently assumes invisibility through camouflage on the streets of Harlem, making others mistake him for one Mr. Rinehart, whose ambivalent phenomenology seems to resist oversimplified strategies of identification. As the signified repeatedly slips under the signifier in a series of displacements where the narrator is assumed to be "Rhine the runner and Rhine the gambler and Rhine the briber and Rhine the lover and Rinehart the Reverend" (*IM* 498), exposing the very movement of supplementarity and deferral of presence, the narrator's ontological stability is progressively attenuated: "What on earth was hiding behind the face of things? If dark glasses and a white hat could blot out my identity so quickly, who actually was who?" (493). Having no single signifier to represent him in the ossified schemas of racial difference, Rinehart's world of invisibility, as the narrator realizes, was one of "possibility," revealing the rhetorical structure of subjectivizing regimes:

It was too much for me. I removed my glasses and tucked the white hat ... away. Can it be, I thought, can it actually be? ... could he be all of them: Rine the runner and Rine the gambler and Rine the briber and Rine the lover and Rinehart the Reverend?... What is real anyway? But... [i]t was true as I was true. His world was possibility and he knew it... The world in which we lived was without boundaries. A vast seething, hot world of fluidity, and Rine the rascal was at home [in it]... It was unbelievable, but perhaps only the unbelievable could be believed. Perhaps the truth was always a lie.

(498)

Desperate to reclaim a sense of mastery and possession, the narrator quickly resorts to the strategies of renegrification of the world:

> Perhaps ... the whole thing should roll off me like drops of water rolling off Jack's glass eye. I should search out the proper political classification, label Rinehart and his situation and quickly forget it... I wanted to back away from it ... to consult someone who'd tell me it was only a brief, emotional illusion. I wanted the props put back beneath the world.
>
> (498, 500)

The fantasies of identity, propping the world back up, are provided on a regular basis in the Brotherhood by its "chief theoretician" (357) Brother Hambro, a white lawyer and an ideological advisor whose mind was "too narrowly logical" (500) to consider the legitimacy of what escapes it. For Brother Hambro, "scientific necessity" requires "the weak ... [to] sacrifice for the strong" (503). Due to new political alliances of the Brotherhood, the narrator's district with its disaffected members was to be renounced for the interests of the cause. Having no affective content that would split objectivity and make it alive, the decision is justified in good conscience by the perfunctory abstractions of teleological narratives:

> a part of the whole is sacrificed – and will continue to be until a new society is formed ... the aggressiveness of the Negroes ... [will] now have to slow ... down for their own good. It's a scientific necessity... They can't be allowed to upset the tempo of the master plan.
>
> (503, 504)

For the narrator, however, the living drama of the split subject is staged alongside the main drag of history, in its back alleys that open up dead ends and snags the hegemonic logics of the present cannot account for. "For him it was simple," as the narrator explains. "For *them* it was simple. But hell, I was *both*. Both sacrificer and victim. That was reality too, my reality. He didn't have to put the knife blade to his *own* throat" (506). Reality, for the narrator, emerges instead in the immanent state of contradictions contained in the techniques of power that determine the binarisms of his social existence but that remain only implicit in the expository narratives based on antagonisms that power the dialectic of progress. The narrator's refusal to abide by any determined assignations of identity brings this dialectic to a standstill, pointing towards alternative presents unseen in the binary articulations of his own. Indeed, as Foucault suggests,

> [m]aybe the target nowadays is not to discover what we are but to refuse what we are. We have to imagine and to build up what we

could be to get rid of this kind of political 'double bind,' which is the simultaneous individualization and totalization of modern power structures.[50]

Invisibility, in the novel, is a metaphor for disclosure of these contradictions and a waste product of the process of subjectivization that calls for a historical transformation of the subject. The invisible subject is in every sense an unpresupposable subject, a "singularity without identity," in Agamben's terms,[51] that cannot be thematized by the reductive typologies of the present, its "proper political classification[s]" (*IM* 498), but that emerges from within its contradictions. In "The Little Man at Chehaw Station," Ellison provides a graphic image of an unpresupposable subject that for him suggests "new possibilities of perfection."[52] Writing against "the ethnic sanctity"[53] and the inherited absolutisms of racial difference, Ellison is "reminded of a light-skinned, blue-eyed, Afro-American-featured individual who could have been taken for anything from a sun-tinged white Anglo-Saxon, an Egyptian, or a mixed-breed American Indian to a strayed member of certain tribes of Jews."[54] "This young man," he continues,

> appeared one sunny Sunday afternoon on New York's Riverside Drive near 151st Street, where he disrupted the visual peace of the promenading throng by racing up in a shiny new blue Volkswagen Beetle decked out with a gleaming Rolls Royce radiator. As the flow of strollers came to an abrupt halt, this man of parts emerged from his carriage... Clad in handsome black riding boots and fawn-colored riding breeches of English tailoring, he took the curb wielding – with an ultra-pukka-sahib haughtiness – a leather riding crop. A dashy dashiki ... flowed from his broad shoulders down to the arrogant, military flare of his breeches-tops, while ... a black Homburg hat, tilted at a jaunty angle, floated majestically on the crest of his huge Afro-coiffed head. As though all this were not enough to amaze, delight, or discombobulate his observers – or precipitate an international incident involving charges of a crass invasion of stylistic boundaries – he proceeded to unlimber an expensive Japanese single-lens reflex camera, position it atop the ornamental masonry balustrade which girds Riverside Park in that area, and activate its self-timer. Then, with a ballet leap across the walk, he assumed a position beside his car ... [and] began taking a series of self-portraits... Viewed from a rigid ethno-cultural perspective, neither his features, nor his car, nor his dress was of a whole. Yet he conducted himself with an obvious pride of person ... inviting all ... [to] wonder in response to himself as his own sign and symbol, his own work of art... And his essence lay, not in the somewhat comic clashing of styles, but in the mixture, the improvised form, the willful juxtaposition of modes.[55]

Ellison's subject, constituted as a "sign" by virtue of its opposites, in the "juxtaposition of [its] modes," represents the limit point of subjectivization that disrupts the individualizing strategies of identification and fixed systems of social organization. As a "man of parts," he is most visible, being the effractive figure "of visual peace," and yet, at the same time, most invisible, insofar as he resists identification within the dominant structures of visibility. What is revealed in this ambivalent figure of (in)visibility in Ellison's anecdote is the space of *non-relation* between the subjectivizing language of power and the subject that cannot be fully appropriated by it, and it is within this space of non-relation, which, for Ellison, is eminently American, that the possibilities of alternate futures reside:

> His Volks-Rolls Royce might well have been loaded with Marxist tracts and Molotov cocktails, but his clashing of styles nevertheless sounded an integrative ... compulsion to improvise upon the given. His garments were, literally and figuratively, of many colors and cultures, his racial identity interwoven of many strands. Whatever his politics, sources of income, hierarchal status, and such, he revealed his essential "Americanness" in his freewheeling assault upon traditional forms of the Western aesthetic... Culturally, he was an American joker. If his Afro and dashiki symbolized protest, his boots, camera, Volkswagen, and Homburg imposed certain qualifications upon that protest. In doing so they played irreverently upon the symbolism of status, property, and authority, and suggested new possibilities of perfection.[56]

In terms of the narrative, the disarticulation of the language of power that frees up alternate forms of enunciation is represented by the narrator's refusal to assume his own subjectivization within the constraining racial schemas that constitute his historical and social existence. His "hole in the ground," that is "*full* of light" to manifest his invisibility, to "confirm ... [his] reality [and] give birth to ... [his] form," (*IM* 6) is the space of non-relation and a laboratory of subject formation where new, unpresupposable identities not yet legible by the existing orders of history can emerge. It is only as invisible that the narrator's *own* form is reconstituted as visible. It "is incorrect to assume," as he explains, "that, because I'm invisible and live in a hole, I'm dead... I myself, after existing for some twenty years, did not become alive until I discovered my invisibility" (6, 7). For the narrator, to be riveted to fixed assignations determined by power relations and remain "unaware of one's form is to live a death" (7). The only way for agency and for true emancipatory politics to emerge is to multiply subjective positions. "Diversity is the word," the narrator declares in his Epilogue. "Let man keep his many parts and you'll have no tyrant states" (577). This resistance to subjectivizing processes is also where Foucault locates the political imperatives of our time. "The political, ethical, social, philosophical problem of our days," he writes, "is not to try to liberate the individual from the state and from the state's institutions but to liberate us ... from the type of individualization which is linked to the state ... [and] to promote new forms of subjectivity through the refusal of this kind of individuality which has been imposed on us for several centuries."[57]

Soliciting new economies of power relations, however, requires the exigency of deconstruction of the language of power in order to open up the space of non-relation, "a hole in the ground" that allows for definition of identities in "juxtaposition of modes."[58] In Foucault's terms, this space of non-relation could be seen as a heterotopic space, existing alongside history in history, an interrogative space accrued by the contradictions of history, and as a "simultaneously mythic and real contestation of the space in which we live," it can transform the relations of power by exposing the contingency of their definition.[59] For the narrator of Ellison's novel, this was a "thread of reality" (511), loosening the skein of its enduring illusions:

> I was both depressed and fascinated... My entire body started to itch, as though I had just been removed from a plaster cast and was unused to the new freedom of movement... [The fact that] you could actually make yourself anew ... was frightening, for now the world seemed to flow before my eyes. All boundaries down, freedom was not only the recognition of necessity, it was the recognition of possibility. And sitting there trembling I caught a brief glimpse of the possibilities posed by Rinehart's multiple personalities and turned away ... if Rinehart could use them in his work, no doubt I could use them in mine. It was too simple, and yet they had already opened up a new section of reality for me.
>
> (498–99)

The realization that his world is neither binary nor dialectic, that "men are different and that all life is divided" (576), that the foundations supporting it are fantasies of the white mythology and that its "beautiful absurdity" (559) throbs fiercely under our desperate attempts to put it "in a strait jacket" (576), is what compels the narrator underground. "[B]ecause up above there's an increasing passion to make men conform to a pattern" (576). Refusing the assignations of his historical existence and "its narrow borders" (576), he takes refuge in a hole alongside it in a space of non-relation where he will write his own narrative of liberation before resurfacing again. The world, indeed, may not be ready yet but in its fantasies of visible certainties, as the narrator tells us, "an invisible man has a socially responsible role to play" (581).

Notes

1 W. E. B. Du Bois, *The Souls of Black Folk* (New York: Dover Publications, 1994), 2.
2 Ibid.
3 Ibid.
4 Ralph Ellison, *Invisible Man* (London: Penguin Classics, 2001). Henceforth, *IM*; all citations in the main text.
5 Discussing the possibility of resistance to the normalizing procedures of power, Foucault considers subjectivization in terms of assuming the restricted notions of identity to which one is consigned by the individualizing strategies of power that "force the individual back on himself, and tie him to his own identity in a constraining way." It is a technique of power, Foucault further explains, that "applies itself to immediate everyday life [and] categorizes the individual, marks him by his own individuality, *attaches him to his own identity, imposes a law of truth on him that he must recognize and others have to recognize in him*. It is a form of power which makes individuals subjects." Michel Foucault, "The Subject and Power," in *Power: The Essential Works of Michel Foucault 1954–1984*, vol. 3 of *The Essential Works of Michel Foucault 1954–1984*, ed. James D. Faubion, 3rd ed. (London: Penguin, 2002), 330, 331, emphasis added.
6 For Du Bois, indeed, there are only two terms within which the persecuted black subject can be meaningfully articulated in racially determined social structure. The contradictory movement of subject formation is seen either in terms of "hypocritical compromise" or "radicalism:" "From the double life every American Negro must live … must arise a painful self-consciousness, an almost morbid sense of personality and a moral hesitancy … [that] tempt the mind to pretence or to revolt, to hypocrisy or to radicalism… The one type of Negro stands almost ready to curse God and die, and the other is too often found a traitor to right and a coward before force; the one is wedded to ideals remote, whimsical, perhaps impossible of realization; the other forgets that life is more than meat and the body more than raiment." Du Bois, *The Souls of Black Folk*, 122, 123.
7 Ralph Ellison, "The Little Man at Chehaw Station," in *The Collected Essays of Ralph Ellison: Revised and Updated*, ed. John Callahan, 2nd ed. (New York: Modern Library, 2003), 507.
8 Ibid.
9 Ibid., 517.
10 Foucault, "The Subject and Power," 336.
11 Ibid., 331, emphasis added.
12 Ibid., 331.
13 Aurelia Armstrong, "Beyond Resistance: A Response to Žižek's Critique of Foucault's Subject of Freedom," *Parrhesia: A Journal of Critical Philosophy*, no. 5 (2008): 20.
14 Foucault, "The Subject and Power," 342.
15 Ibid., 340.
16 Ibid., 342.
17 Ibid.
18 Ibid.
19 Ibid.
20 Jacques Rancière, "Politics, Identification, and Subjectivization," *October* 61 (1992): 60, emphasis added.
21 Ibid., 61.
22 Ibid., 61–62.

23 Ibid., 61.
24 Ibid., 62.
25 Ellison, "The Little Man at Chehaw Station," 507.
26 Rancière, "Politics, Identification, and Subjectivization," 62, emphasis added.
27 Du Bois, *The Souls of Black Folk*, 9.
28 Ellison, "The Little Man at Chehaw Station," 508.
29 "The Little Man at Chehaw Station" is an essay first published in *The American Scholar* in 1978 and later included in Ellison's collection *Going to the Territory* (1986). With the effects of the Civil Rights Movement still echoing through a racially torn and politically wounded America, the essay integrates Ellison's aesthetic concerns within the broader political reality of jealous cries for ethnic particularisms and for the prerogatives of blood that divest the American experience of its "wonder" and its "stubborn complexity." The problem of identity is condensed in America's "random assemblies of sensibilities," where "even the most homogeneous gatherings of people are mixed and pluralistic." For Ellison, however, this mystery of "Americanness" that resides in its ontological ambiguity, is worth keeping and "perhaps," as he continues, it "arises out of our persistent attempts to reduce ... [it] to an easily recognizable unity." Ibid., 502, 504.
30 Gerald Lyn Early, *Ralph Ellison: Invisible Man* (New York: Cavendish Square Publishing, 2009), 56.
31 For Bhabha, the moment of deconstruction that, in this case, I associate with the narrator's prophetic challenge to the discursive categories that articulate his social existence, is the moment of *proper* political intervention. "The language of critique," as Bhabha explains in "The Commitment to Theory," and that I see manifested in Ellison's writing, "is effective not because it keeps forever separate the terms of the master and the slave, the mercantilist and the Marxist, *but to the extent to which it overcomes the given grounds of opposition* and opens up a space of translation: a place of hybridity, figuratively speaking, where the construction of a political subject that is new, *neither the one nor the other*, properly alienates our political expectations, and changes, as it must, the very forms of our recognition of the moment of politics." Homi K. Bhabha, *The Location of Culture*, 2nd ed. (London: Routledge, 2004), 37, emphasis added.
32 Bhabha, *The Location of Culture*, 2004, 37.
33 Cf. Paul Gilroy's discussion of Richard Wright and his increasing critical investment in the differentiation of the black subject in *The Black Atlantic*. Paul Gilroy, *The Black Atlantic: Modernity and Double Consciousness* (Cambridge, MA: Harvard University Press, 1993), 153.
34 Du Bois, *The Souls of Black Folk*, 124.
35 Ibid.
36 Ibid.
37 Frantz Fanon, *Black Skin, White Masks*, trans. Richard Philcox (New York: Grove Press, 2008), 80.
38 Du Bois, *The Souls of Black Folk*, 108.
39 Ellison, "The Little Man at Chehaw Station," 509.
40 In his "Preface" to *The Wretched of the Earth*, Sartre argues, with Fanon, that the savagery of the oppressed, witnessed in the violent spasms of emancipation, is nothing but the oppressor's savagery turned against himself. The "boomerang ... flies right back at us, it strikes us, and we do not realize any more than we did the other times that it's we that have launched it." Frantz Fanon, *The Wretched of the Earth*, trans. Richard Philcox (New York: Grove

Press, 2004), liv. Hardt and Negri call this same moment "the boomerang of alterity" or the "inversion of the colonialist logic itself," which they, nevertheless, see as illusory, since it reappropriates the racial inheritances it is, at the same time, committed to abolishing. Cf. Michael Hardt and Antonio Negri, *Empire* (Cambridge, MA: Harvard University Press, 2001), 130, 131.
41 Fanon, *The Wretched of the Earth*, 148.
42 For Fanon, this desire is a direct effect of the social imperative to "'whiten or perish'" and is pathological since it creates a fantasy of identification, "hallucinatory lactification," that leverages black subjectivity against itself. Not internally determined, it has its origin in "the real source of conflict," which, for Fanon, is "the social structure" that "proclaims the superiority of one race over another" and makes "inferiority complex possible." Fanon, *Black Skin, White Masks*, 80.
43 In *The Souls of Black Folk*, Du Bois exposes the deep-lying flaws in the accommodationism of Washington's "Atlanta Compromise" that "counsels submission to civic inferiority" for the benefit of economic self-sufficiency. "In counselling patience and courtesy" in demands for civic and political equality, "Mr. Washington represents in Negro thought the old attitude of adjustment and submission," practically accepting "the alleged inferiority of the Negro races" that should focus "all their energies on industrial education, the accumulation of wealth, and the conciliation of the South." For Du Bois, Washington's "gospel of Work and Money" represents the "civic death" of black America, while it also surreptitiously legitimizes the continued persistence of racial discrimination. Du Bois, *The Souls of Black Folk*, 30–31, 32, 33.
44 In his essay, "Nietzsche, Genealogy, History," Foucault maintains that the body, far from being n(eu)atural, motivating foundationalist discourses and grand illusions of metaphysics, is radically historical, experienced *as mediated* through different stresses of its social history. For Foucault, it is the very articulation of history and the watershed of biopolitical disciplinary regimes. "The body," he writes, "is the inscribed surface of events (traced by language and dissolved by ideas), the locus of a dissociated self (adopting the illusion of a substantial unity), and a volume in perpetual disintegration. Genealogy, as an analysis of descent, is thus situated within the articulation of the body and history. Its task is to expose a body totally imprinted by history and the process of history's destruction of the body." Michel Foucault, "Nietzsche, Genealogy, History," in *The Foucault Reader*, ed. Paul Rabinow (New York: Pantheon, 1984), 83.
45 Bhabha, *The Location of Culture*, 2004, 104.
46 Upon his arrival in New York, the narrator resists the urge to confirm the fantasy of collective self-consistency assumed about the Black Belt by refusing to take "the special" of "pork chops and grits" recommended by the counterman, opting instead for "orange juice, toast and coffee." "You fooled me ... I would have sworn you were a pork chop man." Proud to differentiate himself from the racialized stereotype, the narrator considers this as "an act of discipline, a sign of change that was coming over [him]..." (*IM* 178).
47 For Stuart Hall, the boomerang of the repressed is crucial in the struggle to transform "the dominant regimes of representation" and the "discursive spaces" that author for black experience. It enables "the *contestation* of the marginality, the stereotypical quality, and the fetishized nature of images of blacks by the counterposition of a 'positive' black imagery." He considers "these strategies ... principally addressed to changing ... 'the relations of representation'" that "play a *constitutive*, and not merely a reflexive,

after-the-event, role." Stuart Hall, "New Ethnicities," in *Black British Cultural Studies: A Reader*, eds. Houston A. Baker Jr., et al. (Chicago, IL: University of Chicago Press, 1996), 164, 165.

48 Bhabha, *The Location of Culture*, 2004, 81.

49 Hall, "New Ethnicities," 166.

50 Foucault, "The Subject and Power," 336.

51 In *The Coming Community*, Agamben calls for a community that has lost its presuppositions and its operative concepts of belonging. Its subjects are no longer subjects but "whatever singularities" that have no assignable properties, "that form a community without affirming an identity, that ... cobelong without any representable condition of belonging." Whatever-being, he explains,

> has no identity, it is not determinate with respect to a concept ... rather it is determined only through its relation to an *idea*, that is, to the totality of its possibilities. Through this relation ... singularity borders all possibility and thus receives its ... [determination] not from its participation in a determinate concept or some actual property (being red, Italian, Communist), but *only by means of this bordering.*
>
> Giorgio Agamben, *The Coming Community*, trans. Michael Hardt (Minneapolis: University of Minnesota Press, 1993), 67, 86

52 Ellison, "The Little Man at Chehaw Station," 511.

53 Ibid., 509.

54 Ibid.

55 Ibid., 509–11.

56 Ibid., 511.

57 Foucault, "The Subject and Power," 336.

58 Ellison, "The Little Man at Chehaw Station," 511.

59 In "Of Other Spaces," Foucault is interested in sites "that have the curious property of being in relation with all the other sites, but in such a way as to suspect, neutralize, or invert the set of relations that they happen to designate, mirror, or reflect." In relation to utopias, these are "real places ... which are something like counter-sites," immanent to all political structures, and "a kind of effectively enacted utopia[s] in which the real sites ... are simultaneously represented, contested, and inverted... Because these places are absolutely different from all the sites that they reflect and speak about, I shall call them ... heterotopias." Michel Foucault, "Of Other Spaces," *Diacritics* 16, no. 1 (1986): 24.

8   The Body that Race Built

Shame, Trauma and Lack in Toni Morrison's *The Bluest Eye* and *God Help the Child*

Sheldon George

Toni Morrison's literary career begins in 1970 with what she has termed a "public exposure of a private confidence."[1] Her first novel, *The Bluest Eye*, fictionalizes a secret shared with Morrison in childhood, an African American classmate's disclosure of a desire for blue eyes. Morrison defines her classmate's disclosure as grounded in "racial self-loathing," describing it as the revelation of shameful "secrets" that, Morrison avows, were both "shared" by African Americans and "withheld from us by ourselves" (212). Through her publication of these secrets, Morrison sought to counter African Americans' "damaging internalization of assumptions of immutable inferiority" while challenging the "outside gaze" from which these assumptions originated (210). But, forty-five years after launching her career with *The Bluest Eye*, Morrison's task seems incomplete. In her 2015 publication, *God Help the Child*, Morrison returns to a similar story of shame and self-hatred with an adult protagonist whose mother taught her as a child to detest her blackness. However, unlike the characters in *The Bluest Eye*, some of whom are driven to insanity by their efforts to escape their racial identity, Morrison's new protagonist, Bride, learns as an adult to manipulate her blackness, redefining it as an exotic source of beauty. Morrison actively encourages readers to associate the two novels by characterizing Bride as having a "blue tint" in her eyes (6).[2] She acknowledges that images of blackness have, as Bride's mother, Sweetness, puts it, "changed a mite" and even the darkest of black people "are all over" the media now (176). But in returning to this topic of race and self-love, Morrison deliberately maps through her writing a psychological relation to shame that, despite shifting social conceptions of racial identity, persists across time for African Americans.

J. Brooks Bouson has shown how, through "stage[d] scenes of inter- and intra-racial violence and shaming in her novels," Morrison's early writings seek to "gain narrative mastery over and artistically repair" the psychological impact of the other's shaming gaze upon African Americans.[3] But what I am interested in exploring in this chapter is a recursiveness in Morrison's focus upon African Americans' psychological relation to the racialized body. I see at the core of this return a literary understanding of race that allows us to imbed shame within a broader psychoanalytic conception of a psychic lack that repeatedly afflicts all subjects but which, I argue, often impacts African Americans in distinctly pronounced ways. I approach a theory of shame and trauma by conjoining the work of traditional shame theorists with that of psychoanalyst Jacques Lacan to link trauma and shame to the psychic lack that Lacan famously positions at the center of subjectivity. Lacanian theory argues that when a subject is initiated into subjectivity through language, her newly formed consciousness splits away from the unconscious and those aspects of the psyche that escape language, thus producing in her a central void, a lack. This process of psychic splitting that founds identity is itself traumatic to the subject, and its trauma is significantly repeated, I argue, through racist acts that seek to ground the racialized subject's body and identity solidly upon lack. Each subject is driven by fantasies of wholeness, by a crucial desire to mask lack. However, such fantasies are actively challenged for African Americans by racist acts of shaming. Shame occurs in those moments when fantasies of wholeness are replaced by feelings of belittlement, insignificance and worthlessness, and the subject is forced to recognize the masks that hide lack. Taken to its extreme, shame pushes the subject toward a confrontation with trauma, a traumatic unveiling of lack that can shatter the self.

Both of Morrison's novels, *The Bluest Eye* and *God Help the Child*, comment upon the varied ways that African Americans attempt to reassert a fantasy of wholeness that can protect them from a confrontation with lack. An intertextual comparison reveals the lingering psychological impact upon African Americans of the shaming gaze that seeks this confrontation. *The Bluest Eye* envisions race as an externally imposed psychic image of the body that invades subjectivity to define the African American self as flawed and dirty. It thereby ties race to feelings of shame that urge one toward a desire for mimicry of iconic symbols of whiteness. What moves the novel's characters from shame to trauma is their inability to establish a psychic image of the self that both masks the lack pinned to the body and finds reinforcing support in the external world. Morrison has described this external world in America as a "racial house" built upon the "all-knowing law of the white father."[4] Her first novel presents American society as so actively hostile to racial blackness that it not only confronts African Americans with a perpetual sense of homelessness – experienced both environmentally and at the level of the body – but also drives the text's characters toward psychological breakdown.

Expanding upon the psychological implications of a long historical process of binding African American identity to shame and lack, *God Help the Child* insists that the bodily image of African Americans is produced ultimately by fantasy and discourse. Written decades after the Civil Rights movement and social efforts to resignify black as *beautiful*, the novel presents characters as accessing racial identity not through identification with an embodied other, or even primarily through a psychic self-image, but rather with the abstract linguistic signifiers of race. Characters embrace these signifiers as the support of psychic pleasures that seem to evade shame by supplying African Americans with a sense of pride, and even the masquerade of superiority. Acknowledging that African American social and political movements have significantly recuperated the still frequently shamed black body, the novel also reveals the paradoxical pleasures African Americans have learned to derive from the traumas of race. Read together, *God Help the Child* and *The Bluest Eye* thus trace a focus upon shame and the body that not only extends back into Morrison's own childhood but also shapes her production of her writing as a tool of psychological self-analysis for racialized audiences.

The Split between the Body and the Imago

One of the unique features of Toni Morrison's *The Bluest Eye* is its understanding that the black body can mediate a subject's relation to lack. The novel's young protagonist, Pecola Breedlove, an African American girl who wishes for blue eyes in an effort to escape her blackness, inhabits a body that "absorb[s]" all of the "waste which [is] dumped on her," allowing others to feel "wholesome after [they have] cleaned [them]selves on her" (205). Through this fantastical restructuring and cleansing of the self, made possible for others by Pecola's racial blackness, the novel presents race as capable of actualizing the illusory wholeness described by Jacques Lacan in his seminal work on the "mirror stage." This work allows us to conceptualize the subject's identity as grounded in a psychic image more reliant upon fantasy than upon the subject's embodied physicality. Morrison's novel roots the shame confronting African Americans and her literary characters in this discordance, explained by Lacanian theory, between the body and the psychic image.

Lacan presents in his theory of the mirror stage the notion of a split between the physical body and the "specular image or imaginary body" that constitutes the self as an ego.[5] He describes the ego as an imago or self-image that is formed through its differentiation from the reflected image of the mother with whom the child conflates himself until his acquisition of language allows for distinctions between "I" and "you," self and other. Before such distinctions, the child, limited in his motor capacity, begins to see himself as complete and agential through the "orthopedic" function of the mother who supports him in her arms in front of the mirror.[6] This fantasy of wholeness in the presence of the mother is what Lacan calls the Imaginary. But the child must leave the Imaginary to enter into the Symbolic, or the world of language, in which he will have to find a new means of supporting the fantasy of wholeness once facilitated by the mother, a fantasy that is made all the more necessary by the lack introduced by language itself as that which splits the psyche into its component parts, separating the conscious mind from the unconscious. In the end, the child emerges from the mirror stage with the sense of an independent self that is consistent and discrete only through the function of its identification with an other upon whom the psychic image of the body will be modeled; Lacan calls this other the ego ideal.

What Morrison's text realizes is that this ego ideal, upon which the psychic image of the body is modeled in order to sustain the fantasy of wholeness, is strongly bound to whiteness in pre-Civil Rights American society, finding its clearest manifestations in media celebrities who seem to embody the perfection whiteness promises. In drinking milk from a Shirley Temple cup, for example, Pecola dreams of consuming whiteness, of taking it in bodily and effecting a corporeal change that will move her closer to the perfected ideal that Shirley Temple manifests. At issue in Morrison's text is the body as the root of a self-identity that, for African Americans of this time period, is at odds with the ideal that agitates psychic fantasies. Lacan emphasizes that upon entrance into the Symbolic, it is only the child's body that finally grounds his sense of "mental … consistence" to ensure fantasies of wholeness.[7] The body is like a "bag" of "merely skin" that "holds things together," structuring and reinforcing an image of the self that is simultaneously physical and mental.[8] But in order to create this simultaneity, the physical body must be claimed psychically. Lacan explains that the body is inherently "foreign" to us, for ultimately "one 'has' a body, one 'is' not [one's own body] in any way"; but, he asserts, the "root of the imaginary" is the subject's belief that she "has a body to adore," first in blissful oneness with the mother and later in discrete coherence as a single, unified self.[9] This adoration is what allows for the narcissism of the ego, or the taking ownership of the foreign body as the self. The body, Lacan says, must serve as a "bandage," not only binding together the fragmented self but also making that self loveable and worthy of ownership, and this self as bandage must thus remain "clean." By demonstrating the significance of such cleanliness to self-love and psychic consistency, Morrison's text reveals the obstacles to fantasies of wholeness that emerge for African Americans whose bodies are sullied by the shameful images supplied to them by a racist Symbolic.

Lacanian theory not only implicates this Symbolic in the construction of a lovable self, but also designates the Symbolic as the "locus from which the" fundamental "question" of the subject's "existence" must "arise," the question of who or "what am I?"[10] Absent from Lacan's theory, however, is acknowledgement of the fact made abundantly clear by Morrison's work: that this essential question of one's subjective status is often answered in the Symbolic by notions of racial identity. Ignoring race, Lacan explicitly ties one's subjective understanding and narcissistic embrace of who or what one is to Symbolic ego ideals that psychically structure one's "form," producing for each subject an ego grounded specifically in two factors: the subject's sexed identity and her experience of herself as bound to "contingency" or a quiescence that may manifest lack.[11] But, as Gwen Bergner has argued, "race" must be seen as "a constitutive factor of identity," one that emerges through the acquisition of language in tandem with one's sexual and existential sense of self.[12]

In investigating how shame and racial identity map onto and inflect Lacanian notions of subjectivity, it is helpful here to recall the Du Boisian characterization of the African American psyche. Theorizing from his own position as an explicitly racialized subject, W.E.B. Du Bois argued that the discrimination afflicting black Americans can lead to a dualistic sense of self, a "contradiction of double aims" and an "unreconciled" identity that he calls "double consciousness."[13] Morrison's work suggests that this conflict over contending versions of black identity, the "twoness" that arises from always "measuring one's soul by the tape of a world that looks on in amused contempt," manifests as an effort to negotiate a lovable sense of self that can reinforce the fantasies of the Imaginary.[14] At issue is an effort to mediate through race a subjective sense of quiescence and contingency that, despite the designation Du Bois pins to this process, emerges in the form of struggles occurring at *both* the unconscious and conscious levels. As Kalpana Seshadri-Crooks argues, "racial difference" is "unconsciously assimilated by all raced subjects as a factor of language," because the racist Symbolic simultaneously assails subjects on both planes of the psyche.[15] Present in Morrison's novel is recognition that the contentious questions of identity that surface in double consciousness for African Americans are rooted in shameful images of the racial self that emerge from the Symbolic but penetrate the unconscious. And such images, the novel shows, may impede attempts to introject a fantasy ego ideal that refutes lack by affirming the Imaginary imago first constructed in the mirror as an undifferentiated, prelinguistic, sexless and raceless gestalt.

The Bluest Eye reveals this struggle between the Imaginary imago and Symbolic notions of race that penetrate into the unconscious by focusing upon characters for whom the shamed African American body remains foreign and unclaimed. Lacan explains that the two questions of subjectivity – Who am I as a sexual being, and what is the meaning and value of my existence? – become "knott[ed]" together in subjective relations to "love and procreation."[16] In *The Bluest Eye*, the inability to love the raced self dominates as the factor that knots together and contextualizes all questions of subjective identity. Pecola Breedlove struggles to take on characteristics of whiteness as she seeks an answer to the central question she articulates throughout the book: "How do you get somebody to love you?" (32). The black body itself becomes an impediment to love for Pecola, marking a lineage that binds her to a seemingly immutable condition of dejection. Since, as Lacan notes, a subject's image of self is "animated in each particular case by the whole ancestral history of real others," what determines Pecola's unworthiness of love is the fact that she is the child of a black family who has "accepted ... without question" the notion of their own detestable ugliness, taking this "ugliness in their hands" (39) and claiming it, "although it did not belong to them" (38).

Ultimately attempting to emerge into a lovable whiteness by casting off the abjected black body, Pecola nevertheless confronts the fact that her self-image must root itself narcissistically at the level of the psyche. In truth, Pecola struggles to displace existent psychic images of both the black body and the racialized self that have already been negatively cathected by the racist Symbolic to produce a conscious "conviction" that she is the child of "ugly people" (39).[17] Indeed, when confronted with her deepest feelings of shame over fighting-parents she wished would simply "kill" each other, Pecola is able to move closer to her dreams of whiteness by imagining the disappearance of her entire body, with the single exception of her eyes (43): "What was the point?" she wonders to herself; the eyes "were everything. Everything was there, in them. All those pictures, all of those faces" (45). Holding "the picture of [her parents] Cholly and Mrs. Breedlove," as well as her own image, the eyes are the orifices through which the psyche intersects with the Symbolic world of meaning (57). Lacan argues that the subject must "situate [her]self in the picture" that is painted by the meanings available in the external world; and this same picture, he elaborates, is taken in psychically: the external "picture is painted" in "the depths of [the subject's] eye," at the point where the eye functions to establish a correlation between external and internal portraitures of the self and its world.[18] Unable to unseat within her unconscious a preexistent image of her black-ugliness, Pecola dwells in a perpetual state of shame that emphasizes the discord between the self presented to her externally and the white imago she wishes to introject as support for her fantasies of wholeness.

It is exactly in such moments of stark disjunction, as one's subjective experiences force a reevaluation of one's lovable self-image, that shame is made manifest. Because shame involves an evaluation of the self from the "other's point of view," shame can be exhibited as a sort of "disembodied experience," an alienation in which the self discards full "body awareness" in favor of identification with the evaluating gaze of the other.[19] Shame fragments and splits the self, unraveling the wholeness ensured by the psychic image as a "bag" that wraps the self in a fantasy of consistency. Bound to heightened "self-consciousness" and "self-imaging in the eyes of the other," shame provides a bridge connecting the particular experience of Pecola to that of African Americans more broadly, tracking closely with the amplified awareness of white perceptions described by Du Bois.[20]

Du Bois' presentation of double consciousness as the "sense of always looking at one's self through the eyes of others" is taken to its extreme by Morrison's novel, driving inexorably Pecola's descent into insanity.[21] The novel presents Pecola as overcoming, only through madness, what Du Bois describes as the "contempt" and self "pity" that African Americans are urged to take on with the shame that both splits their identity – "an American, a Negro" – and allows them to "see [themselves only] through the revelations of the other."[22] Pecola dissolves this double consciousness by exacerbating its inherent split, fully identifying with the gaze of the Symbolic Other while severing all ties to a psychic image of herself as black, Negro (5). When the Symbolic's representation of this black self as dirty is traumatically affirmed by her father's incestuous act of rape, by his violent display of his feelings of "hatred mixed with tenderness" toward her, Pecola splits away from the damning pictures of the world by constituting a psychic reality in which the Other, the Symbolic itself, does not exist (163). Descending into insanity, she substitutes the Symbolic with an alter ego, a variant-self perceived only by her, who repudiates her blackness by seeing her blue eyes and reflecting back for Pecola an imago that defies the actual physicality of her body. Pecola's psychological trauma finally culminates in this radical splitting of the ego that actively shatters her psyche. Having thus severed her link to reality, she "spen[ds] her days ... walking up and down" with her hands "flailed" like "a bird in an eternal, grotesquely futile effort to fly," sustained only by the tenuous illusion of having achieved a fantastical whiteness (204).

The Body, Homelessness and Insanity

Morrison faults the racist American Symbolic for Pecola's insanity, showing that "the land of the entire country was hostile" to a vivifying black image of self (206). If Pecola must retreat into a shattered psyche to establish the imago she wishes for herself, it is because, Morrison suggests, African Americans are at home neither in the American Symbolic nor in their own physical bodies. Morrison has claimed that "the overweening, defining event of the modern world is the mass movement of raced populations, beginning with the largest forced transfer of people in the history of the world: slavery."[23] This mass uprooting is imagined by the text as generative of a perpetual, metaphysical state of homelessness. The text identifies this state through reference to African American fears of being "outdoors" with "no place to go," identifying this fear as "the real terror of life" (17). Being "put outdoors" without a home manifests "an irrevocable, physical fact, defining and contemplating [their] metaphysical condition"; homelessness, the text notes, marks "the end of something," serving as an obstruction to the fantasies by which African Americans establish a subjective, metaphysical relation to both their embodied and psychic existences. Recognizing this psychic experience of homelessness, this alienation from the body and the Symbolic, Morrison centers her work upon an effort both to "eclipse the racial gaze" of the other and to express African Americans' "yearnings for social space that is psychically and physically safe."[24]

In *The Bluest Eye*, Morrison expresses such yearnings through Pauline Breedlove, Pecola's mother. The text describes Pauline's experiences as structured by a longing for her ancestral southern home. But when Pauline's "dreams die" and her fantasies of wholeness are dismantled in the north, Pauline pins her life's failures to her physical body, depriving her body of polysemic and variegated associations that emerged in childhood (110). Significantly, the nail that injured Pauline's body, punching "clear through her foot during her second year of life," not only helped explain for Pauline many "otherwise incomprehensible" things, like why "she alone of all the children had no nickname," but it also, contrastingly, "saved Pauline Williams from total anonymity" (111), producing the slight "deformity" that singled her out as a special love-object for her future husband, Cholly (110). When Cholly first meets Pauline, "instead of ignoring her infirmity, pretending it was not there, he made it seem like something special and endearing" (116), attentively "tickling her broken foot and kissing her leg" to produce for her sensations and colors that she will retroactively associate with home (115). As Pauline later thinks of her home in the south, she thinks of June bugs that were "shooting everywhere" in a "streak of green" as she waited "down by the depot" to set off (112). The June bugs correspond to a particularly fluid relation to color and the body that Pauline loses in the city. Pauline explains that when she first met Cholly and he kissed her leg, "it was like all the bits of color from that time down home when all us chil'ren went berry picking after a funeral and I put some in the pocket of my Sunday dress, and they mashed up and stained my hips ... all of those colors [were already] in me ... [and] it was like them berries, that lemonade, them streaks of green the june bugs made, all come together" (115). The colors Pauline associates with home lack stable, hierarchal segregation, and when Cholly makes love to her, she feels "those bits of color floating up" into her body to form a "rainbow" inside, granting Pauline an embodied feeling of "power" and a certainty that, "I be strong, I be pretty, I be young" (130).

But Pauline cannot sustain this vivifying bodily sense of power and self-contentment when she moves to the city and confronts the shaming gaze of others. The "goading glances and private snickers" of the "few black women she met" in the city cause Pauline not only to "miss [her] people" back home but also to attempt to change her "country ways" (115). Pauline's dreams of self-control, the fantasy imago she wished to construct around a body that is strong, pretty and young, finally fall apart when, in the midst of sitting in a movie theatre with her face and hair made up like the movie stars she admires, she bites into a candy and pulls "a tooth right out of her mouth" (123). Here Pauline starts to imagine her body as not just damaged in this moment, but inherently flawed. Though she had actively sought to establish at the psychic level an imago that mirrors the white movie stars after whom she refigures her physical appearance through hairstyle and makeup, she comes to "build a case" for the failures in her life "out of her foot," reaching back into the past to construct her body and its physicality as permanently crippled (110). Whereas the child of the mirror stage secures her fantasy of power and control through identification with the orthopaedic image of another, Pauline's failure to mimic the other reinforces her sense of fragmentation and motor incapacity. Her acceptance of the impossibility of attaining whiteness, her reluctant embrace of a racialized black identity, brings with it a crippling sense of lack, for "after her education in the movies" Pauline was never able to "look at a face and not assign it some category in the scale of absolute beauty" (122). What Pauline assigns to herself and transmits to her daughter is the shamed conviction of a strict correlation between ugliness and her family's own embodied blackness.

Morrison connects such rigid correlations between color and beauty to a rejection of the black body that moves characters precipitously toward a state of insanity. This is the case explicitly with Pecola, but also with Soaphead Church, the character who fantastically grants Pecola her blue eyes. Soaphead is a paedophile driven by his neurotic pursuit for an abstract ideal of perfection that not even the movie stars so admired by Pecola and Pauline, and indeed not even God, can embody. It is an ideal that he associates with whiteness in his longing for a world of strict segregation and hierarchic order that reflects "the neatness of Dante" (173). As a "cinnamon-eyed West Indian with lightly browned skin" (167), Soaphead maintains a desire for the ideal that is fueled by the fact of his descent from a "British nobleman" who "introduced his white strain into the family in the 1800s." Soaphead's family aggressively sought to preserve the "blood of the noble group" and, like "a good Victorian Parody," learned to "separate [themselves] in body, mind and spirit from all that suggests Africa." Like Pecola, who aims at a synecdoche of whiteness in seeking after blue eyes, Soaphead's family mimic only "the most dramatic, and the most obvious, of [their] masters' characteristics" (177). They become "not royal but snobbish, not aristocratic but class-conscious." (177) Taking on "the worst" characteristics of whites, they value a hierarchy that defiles their own worth as racialized subjects, while simultaneously aspiring toward the immaculate, unblemished purity of whiteness (177). Soaphead's exposure to this class-conscious snobbishness helps to develop within him a "persistent nausea" that emerges from "the slightest contact with people," a nausea that gives him cause to "regard himself as discriminating, fastidious and full of nice scruples" (165). Rooted in a perverse disdain for the embodied other that extends naturally from but surpasses the racism of his family, Soaphead Church becomes what the text calls a "very clean old man" (167), an individual so obsessed with cleanliness and so repulsed by "all the natural excretions and protections the body was capable of" that he "settled on those humans whose bodies were least offensive – children" (166).

Fueled by racialized idealizations of purity that produce disdain for the body, Soaphead's fantasy life achieves final symmetry in a paedophilic love for "the light *white* laughter of little girls" (181, ital. added). His progression cautiously conveys how one may move naturally from racial thinking to pathology. Indeed, Soaphead's fantasy conception of race and purity roots him most broadly in what we must call a state of neurosis, defined most precisely as a condition in which the subject "substitutes" his own desires for the "demand of the father," or the representative of the Symbolic who ejects the child from a primal unity with the mother of the Imaginary.[25] It is the role of this representative to serve as the ego ideal that embodies a perfection the subject can attain in the Symbolic as substitute for the fantasy wholeness he loses in exiting the Imaginary. But the neurotic's problem is that the other with whom he identifies makes him feel his lack, his inherent distance from perfection and wholeness. This is precisely the case with Soaphead, who is found wanting by a father whose "controlled violence" drives him toward a "hatred of, and fascination with, any hint of disorder or decay" (169).

The race-based demands for purity and cleanliness that Soaphead "learned at the flat side of his father's belt" (170) lead to his dalliance with the priesthood (165); but, existing in a body with brown skin and cinnamon eyes that display his approximate relation to whiteness and, simultaneously, his insurmountable distance from it, Soaphead cannot cleanse himself sufficiently to be worthy of his faith. He desperately seeks after an absolute purity, and when he finds Velma, the woman who was to finally be the answer to his burning question – "where was the life to counter the encroaching nonlife" – he equates their "lovemaking with communion and the Holy Grail" (170). Velma recognizes that he is "suffering from and enjoying an invincible melancholy," and she leaves him "the way people leave a hotel" (177), refusing to build with him the home he longs for in a place "where [he can finally] *live*" (178). Unable to find a liveable divinity within or beyond the racist Symbolic, Soaphead indulges himself in his own fall from grace, lifting his eyes in "contemplation of [God's] Body and fall[ing] deeply into the contemplation" of the bodies of little girls (179).

In this fall, Soaphead displays the ways that shame may develop into an extreme example of neurosis, and even activate psychosis. In keeping with theories that define shame as involving a "whole self" image, an all-encompassing self-definition that emerges from failure, the subject of shame starts to move toward neurosis when his inability to meet the other's demands produces a sense of lack that causes him to feel "deep down" that he is "the most vain thing in existence, a Want-To-Be," a perfect failure.[26] What will finally root his neurosis, however, is not simply failure, but the fact that he aspires toward the "impossible," aiming at an ideal of perfection that is attainable by none.[27] Bowed in shame at his unworthiness before the unattainable, the neurotic eventually comes to deride not just himself but also the other upon whom the self is modeled, the ideal of perfection which had presented an apparent wholeness he thought he could attain. It is this sense of the imperfection of the other upon whom he has modeled himself that stirs Soaphead in angry resistance against both his father and God. And such rejection of the authority of the ideal father is precisely what *may* lead to psychosis.

Lacan defines psychosis as a "foreclosure of the signifier" of the Other, a rejection of the Symbolic and the meanings it establishes through the authority of the ego ideal that structures it.[28] He elaborates that this rejection can be directed at either "a real father" or "the One-Father" who stands as embodiment of an "ideal-reality," further specifying that this father is yet seen by the psychotic subject to "be at fault, to fall short, or even be fraudulent."[29] Accordingly, Soaphead slides toward psychotic foreclosure of the Symbolic by rejecting God on account of the "sloven and unforgivable error" he had made in "designing an imperfect universe" (173). For Lacan, psychosis is "a disturbance that occur[s] at the inmost juncture of the subject's sense of life" and self.[30] As Soaphead continues in his rebuke of God, we sense this disturbance as an existential query uniting in racial self-hatred the two questions addressed to the Symbolic by the subject; Soaphead not only questions the value of his encroaching nonlife but also accompanies his deep dependence upon Velma for personal and sexual identity with a proclivity toward "active homosexual[ity]" that is contradicted by his utter "disgust" for the thought of "caressing and being caressed by a man" (166). By resolving these conflicts of identity through a racial disdain that leads to complete rejection of the human body, Soaphead approaches a psychotic condition wherein he is bound to the prelinguistic reality of the Imaginary. Seeking after the gestalt, the illusory unity of the Imaginary, he is plagued by fantasies of "the fragmented body," the porous body that leaks and secretes, the differentiated body that, ironically, drives him back to and ultimately stabilizes his neurotic obsession with purity and cleanliness.[31]

Avoiding psychosis through his inability to fully discard the father and the ideals of whiteness and purity this father's Symbolic authority centers, Soaphead Church exists, finally, in a torturous, shame-driven state of neurosis and hatred for the father whose ideals secure his condition of lack. While choosing both to embrace and transgress this father's demand for order and cleanliness in seeking out little girls, Soaphead takes on an identity in the Symbolic only through his melancholic enjoyment of his own suffering. Within the Symbolic, he learns a name for himself, "misanthrope," a "label [that] provide[s] him with both comfort and courage," settling him in an adversarial relationship to the Symbolic while driving him, in direct rejection of the authority of the father, to give Pecola the blue eyes God did not (164). Here it is the neurotic, himself bordering upon madness, who catapults Pecola into a true psychosis, birthing from her desire for whiteness the delusions that sever a psychotic's link to reality. This desire only further escalates with her insanity, evolving into an obsessive quest for an impossible superlative: a search for the absolute bluest eyes that leaves her forever in unwinnable competition with others. Through Soaphead's stalled approach toward insanity and Pecola's complete psychic unraveling, the novel thus maps the structure of race along the very borders of neurosis and psychosis. It unveils the psychic dilemma race pushes all subjects toward, in which not even the most idealized other – not even God, and certainly not embodied white Americans – can achieve the perfection race leads one to madly pursue.

Fantasy, *Jouissance* and the Signifier

In her more recent novel, *God Help the Child*, Morrison returns to the topics of *The Bluest Eye*, except now with a focus upon a protagonist who believes she has achieved a perfected image of the self as *black*. Morrison's protagonist, Bride, seems to avert the shame that plagues *The Bluest Eye*'s characters by highlighting her racial blackness, "stressing it, glamorizing it" through wearing white clothes to accentuate her skin color (143). Working in the cosmetics industry, Bride successfully manipulates race as a source of pleasure by selling her "elegance to all those childhood ghosts" and the people who now "drool with [an] envy" that she experiences as not just "payback" but pure "glory" (57). But where shame can be defined as "a response to exposure" that confronts us with the "viewing other[s']" negative "opinion of ourselves," Bride's glorification of her body for her childhood ghosts yet traps her within the mechanisms of shame.[32] Though able to manipulate a changing fantasy relation to race in America, which the novel sets out to critically explore, Bride remains separated from a necessary self-awareness described in the text with the simple words "truth" and "clarity" (56).

In a 2008 interview with *Time*, Morrison emphasizes this historical shift in the fantasy relation of African Americans to race that has taken place since she wrote *The Bluest Eye*. When asked whether "young black girls are still dealing with the same self-acceptance issues" as Pecola Breedlove, Morrison responds, "No, not at all, not at all. They seem to me to be excessively confident in themselves ... they don't even know what I'm talking about." Morrison elaborates: "I find young African American women much more complete. They seem to have a confidence, almost a feeling of superiority, in some ways, that I recognize, that they take for granted." It is precisely this taken-for-granted confidence and superiority, which has emerged in opposition to the shame imposed upon blackness, that Morrison puts to task in *God Help the Child*. Morrison has stated that she wrote *The Bluest Eye* after the "reclamation of racial beauty in the sixties stirred" in her questions about why this beauty needed "wide public articulation to exist."[33] Now, decades later,

Morrison shows that public display and acceptance of black beauty can yet mask the shame associated with race. She uses the new novel to caution African Americans against a fundamental misrecognition of the self that can emerge with the glorification of racial identity.

While *The Bluest Eye* presents most specifically the glorification of whiteness as bound more to an impossible fantasy than to the body, *God Help the Child*, along with much of Morrison's later prose writings, couples conceptualizations of race in relation to images of the body with a presentation of blackness in particular as grounded primarily upon racial signifiers. Morrison has argued that because blacks have historically been viewed through stereotypes that are often self-contradictory – seen as, for example, "either submissive children, violent ones, or both at once" –the "fundamental characteristics of blacks" in American society are "folded into" a "general miasmas" of "incoherence" and "racial irrationality."[34] *God Help the Child* suggests that, removed from any relation to actual African Americans, blackness produces subjective identification with abstract signifiers of race that act as what Morrison calls "metaphorical shortcuts": "racially informed and determined chains" of meaning in relation to which the subject positions herself.[35]

Booker, Bride's lover, communicates the contemporary understanding that "scientifically there is no such thing as race". He observes that if race is "just color," we must see the use of "race as a choice" (143). This choice is motivated in the text by certain pleasures derived from racial identity. Suggesting the ways that blackness in contemporary America is reduced to a signifier that is often productive of this pleasure, minor characters like Jerri, Bride's fashion advisor, recognize that "Black sells," and is indeed "the hottest commodity in the civilized world" (36) – so hot that Bride's white best friend, Brooklyn, can "add [to herself] an allure she wouldn't otherwise have" simply by twisting her "blond hair into dreadlocks" (44). Dislodged from any single defined meaning, racial blackness is embraced in the text for its capacity to produce *both* pleasure and pain. Thus expanding *The Bluest Eye*'s revelations of race's relation to shame, the text situates race within a broader domain of fantasies through which characters compensate for lack.

Morrison has noted the psychoanalytic insight that "the subject of the dream is the dreamer," adding that this dreamer achieves through her fantastical psychic productions an "extraordinary meditation on the self."[36] *God Help the Child* shows its characters constructing through the fantasy of race a self-reflexive meditation that operates upon lack through the signature dream processes of condensation and displacement. Lacan's work reveals that these dream processes, identified by Freud, express themselves in fantasy and everyday life through the linguistic mechanisms of metonymy and metaphor. Arguing that what Freud discovered in displacement was really the "transfer of signification that metonymy displays," the shifting of associative meaning from object to object, Lacan simultaneously identifies condensation with "the super-imposed structure of signifiers" at play in metaphor, the substitution of one signifier for another that replaces it.[37] Metonymy is characterized by continual movement, a sliding from object to object in an effort to "find" that which produces *jouissance*.[38] Where *jouissance* ultimately signifies the simultaneous pleasure and pain of an unbearable bliss that threatens to shatter the psyche, the very bliss achieved by Pecola, it is associated in the fantasies of the subject with the impossible, pleasure-filled whole-ness of the Imaginary. Ultimately, the subject securely positioned within the Symbolic only ever experiences a euphoric *jouissance* at the level of fantasy, and only does so through the function of metaphor, by which a found object, such as racial identity, can substitute itself for what is lost, perilously filling the place of a lack that should never be filled.

We see metonymy at work in Bride. Lacan argues that the subject's desire, rooted in lack, is ever "caught in the rails of metonymy, eternally extending toward the *desire for something else*," for the ever-distant and ever-changing object that will fill this lack.[39] Throughout the text, Bride's actions are fueled by a desire to be touched, a desire attributable to her parental relations. Not only is Bride abandoned by her father, but her mother is repulsed by her deep black skin and refuses all physi-cal contact with her. Understandably, Bride metonymically displaces her desire to be touched by her parents onto Booker when they first meet. She immediately falls for Booker when he approaches her from behind, embracing her around the waist as they dance at a concert; and when their relationship dissolves and he leaves her, what she realizes she had valued most was that there was "no place on [her] body his lips did not turn into bolts of lightning" (37). Through Bride, the text outlines a relationship to the body that is strikingly similar to that unveiled in *The Bluest Eye*. Though Bride, unlike Pecola and Pauline, is able to say with conviction, "I'm young... I'm successful and pretty. Really pretty... I have what I have worked for," Bride remains dependent on a fantasy of beauty that is grounded in an other's vision of her body (53). In Book-er's presence Bride feels "relief"; she feels "curried, safe and owned" (56). Reliant upon Booker to curry, groom and clean a bodily image *she* may then own psychically, Bride naturally becomes "miserable" when Booker leaves (53). Without the metonymic placeholder that not only promises her fulfillment but also supports her fantasies, Bride's psychic imago begins to atrophy, as she is transformed in her own mind into the "scared little black girl" she used to be, becoming once again "flat-chested and without underarm or pubic hair" (142).

If Pecola's plight reveals the dangers of escaping the life of a scared little black girl through fantasies of whiteness, Bride's struggles reveal the dangers of attempting to do so through embrace of racial blackness. There is something peculiarly unhealthy about Bride's relationship to her black body. After Booker eventually leaves her without explanation, Bride can tolerate her loneliness only by herself currying her body, using his shaving brush and the "dull edge" of his razor to compulsively "carve dark chocolate lanes through swirls of white lather" on her face. The text suggests the meaning of this act by inviting readers to make pertinent metonymic associations of their own. Two paragraphs after its description of Bride's actions, the text divulges that her "neighbors and their daughters" had always said of Bride, "She's sort of pretty under all that black" (35). Through metonymic transferal of meaning across its paragraphs, the text conveys that the process of blanketing herself in a whiteness that accentuates and glorifies her blackness leaves Bride balanced upon a razor's-edge performance of race that not only threatens her with self-injury but is also performed for the evaluating gaze of an other. Here race is not a choice, as Booker suggests, but a psychic compulsion. The text shows Bride as having been shamed by the other, infected with the same sense of herself as worthless and dirty that dominates Pecola's self-image. The first other of psychoanalysis is of courses the mother, and it is indeed Sweetness who will not touch the black skin that Bride's slight rotation of the razor would lacerate with a transformation of pleasure into pain. But beyond focusing merely upon the mother's gaze as the source of Bride's troubled body-image, the text presents an understanding of the black body in relation to *jouissance*, suggesting that it is this connection to a pleasure capable of transforming into pain that articulates Bride's trauma.

Bride's psychological conflicts emerge from the ways that whites historically have enjoyed the black body. The text traces a pathological relation to pleasure and touching that starts with whites' control over blacks, a relation calculated to bring whites pleasure through their rejection and derision of African Americans. Similar to Bride, who recalls, "distaste was all over [Sweetness'] face when I was little and she had to bathe me" (31), Sweetness recalls her own mother's stories of how there "were two Bibles" when her mother got married, explaining that her parents "had to put their hands on the one reserved for Negroes". But, in spite of this separation, Sweetness continues, whites insisted her mother "scrub their backs while they sat in the tub and God knows what other intimate things they made her do" (4). The result of this cleaning and pleasuring of the white body that coincides with scorn for the black other is Sweetness finding that she can only "hold on to a little dignity" and secure some semblance of pleasure in her own self-image by separating herself from blackness and the child who embodies it: forcing her daughter to call her "'Sweetness' instead of 'Mother' or 'Mama'" (6). Effecting a traumatic relation to the black body, here transmitted inter-generationally, Sweetness' actions cause Bride to associate the innately pleasurable touch of a mother with pain, until, eventually for Bride, pleasure comes to be achieved *only* through pain. As Bride reveals, her childhood longing was so intense that she "used to pray [her mother] would slap [her] face or spank [her] just to feel her [mother's] touch" (31).

Sweetness's rejection creates a void in Bride, an absent sense of self-worth that has no clear association for Bride because it extends into a history that, as a child, she does not understand. But through the signifiers of race, Bride embraces a newly contextualizing identity. When she is eight years old, she testifies against and helps to wrongfully convict her teacher of child molestation. As an adult, she recognizes that in pointing out this teacher in court she was really pointing her finger at Mr. Leigh, her landlord, whom she witnessed raping a young boy. She had been only six years old, and when he chased her away calling her a "nigger" and a "cunt," she didn't know what the words meant, but "the hate and revulsion in them," she says, "didn't need definition" (56). Finally achieving an all-consuming self-definition through the racial signifier that here remains enigmatic for her, Bride reveals that such "name-calling" convinced her "not being a 'nigger girl' was all [she] needed to win" (57).

This self-definition achieved by Bride signals the function of metaphor, localizing in the word "nigger" all the feelings of revulsion and hate with which Bride had been acquainted in her life. Lacan states that when metaphor is achieved, "everything radiates out from and is organized around [its] signifier."[40] Situated "at the precise point at which meaning is produced in nonmeaning," metaphor emerges when a single signifier so "dominates" meaning that it seems to "stick perfectly to the signified," to the "amorphous mass of thoughts" that may lay within the subject as an unexpressed "image" or "feeling."[41] Through this dominance of race as metaphor, Bride brings an end to the "incessant sliding" of amorphous thoughts and feelings that defy her understanding, concentrating in the word "nigger" a meaning that touches equally upon Bride's own constitutive lack as a subject, the pleasures of her grandmother's employer, and the self-scorn of her mother.[42]

The shame that descends from her grandmother's white employer's *jouissance* becomes a particularly defining component of Bride's identity, against which she thus produces a newly invented glamorous self. But Bride develops a limited sense of this self, coming to see the world only through her race and the pain it has caused her. Tellingly, when the woman she wrongfully accused is released from jail and Bride seeks to make amends, Bride allows the woman to beat her so badly that she needs plastic surgery, passively taking the beating without even seeking to "protect" herself (32). Bride notes chapters later that the beating was "like Sweetness's slap without the pleasure of being touched" (79). Nonetheless, she keenly recalls the woman's touch, feeling hours after the incident the woman's "hard fingers clenching [her] hair" and the woman's "foot on [her] behind" (32). Bride's obsession with a touch, even one that brings pain, displays the ways that limiting her identity to the metaphor of race produces in her a psychic relation to pain that remains determinative of her interactions with the external world. Focused upon race, Bride acquires a self-centred concern with the pleasure and pain her body may grant her that impairs her capacity for relationship. She remains emotionally stunted, able only to enjoy Booker for the "sexual choreography" (134) of their "lovemaking" while refusing to "know" him as "somebody thinking things" (61). Instead of truly loving him, she uses Booker to reinforce her self-image as a "shield that protect[s] her from any overly intense feeling, be it rage, embarrassment or love" (79).

Jouissance and the Ancestor

Similarly to Bride, Booker is harmed by the vicissitudes of *jouissance*. Allowing the novel to imbed its discussion of shame and race within analysis of broader subjective efforts to mask lack, Booker experiences the *jouissance* of others as a source of identification. Specifically, this is structured around the death of his brother, Adam, who was murdered by a paedophile. Booker is unable to get past this loss because he has always seen his brother as a lost part of himself. Before Adam, Booker had a twin "who did not survive birth," and whose loss he had already collapsed with his own lack, designating this twin eventually as the absence he has always "felt [as a] warm void walking by his side" (115). In time, the "shape of the void fade[s]" and is metonymically "transferred" into "a kind of inner companion" that is supplemented by Adam. Through this collapsing of borders between self and other, Booker's brothers come to stand for the lack that is intimate to each subject. In Adam's loss, Booker makes present this internal absence that he will then be able to mourn, deploying Adam's loss as the metaphor through which he reaches the point where he can bring meaning to the nonmeaning of his own psychic lack. As Booker eventually recognizes, he holds on to Adam's death not because he misses Adam, but "rather," because he "miss[es] the emotion that [Adam's] dying produced" (161).

The text reinforces this case: that it is not to Adam that Booker is attached, but rather to *jouissance*. Booker tattoos Adam's name on his left shoulder, a gesture initially in keeping with Booker's desire to memorialize his brother's death. Booker last saw his brother riding off on his skateboard, gliding like a "spot of gold moving down a shadowy tunnel toward the mouth of a living sun" (115). In order to mark that "final glow of yellow tunnelling down the street, Booker place[s] a single yellow rose on [his brother's] coffin" (116), later "reenacting the gesture" by having "a small rose tattooed on his left shoulder" (120). Booker seeks through these acts not just to record the passing of a light that has always been internal to himself, but also to "freeze and individualize his feelings," "separate them" out from the "sorrow" of the rest of his family (120). But in devising this means of individualizing sorrow, Booker also actively emulates his brother's murderer, metaphorically replacing his love of Adam with the paedophile's brutal hatred, by entering into psychic and physical spaces he associates with the killer.

After the murderer is caught, "what Booker wanted was not the man's death" but "his life" (120). As the paedophile used Adam for his own pathological pleasures, so too does Booker gain access to the *jouissance* of his own lack by bringing back his dead brother to "run" his "life" (156), turning his own "brain into a cadaver and [his] heart's blood formaldehyde" to prolong their mutual suffering (157). Through Adam, he accesses a "feeling so strong it define[s]" him, "leaving" behind a "thrilling" "absence" for Booker to "live" in (161). Dwelling in this absence itself, creating a home out of it, Booker contemplates how to signify "pain and despair without end," asking himself, "wasn't there a tribe in Africa that latches the dead body to the back of the one who had murdered it?" (120). Booker finally eternalizes his own unending despair, coming to wallow in the presence of his own lack, by metaphorically placing himself in the position of the murderer. As he sits to tattoo the rose through which *he* will be the one to carry his brother on his shoulder for the rest of his life, Booker thinks, "Was this the same chair the predator sat in, the same needle used on his paste-white skin?"

Lacan argues that what occurs in metaphor is not "the juxtaposition" of "two equally actualized" signifiers, images or feelings, but rather the phenomenon of one feeling being "replaced" or at least occluded by "the other."[43] Through tattooing his brother's light to himself, Booker accesses a feeling of sorrow that transfers from the paedophile's *jouissance* to redefine Booker's love as abuse. This *jouissance*, which already collapses love of children with wanton disregard for their lives, binds Booker to what he calls the "casual evil" of the abuser (135). When Bride tells Booker that his aunt, Queen, who had failed to come to her own daughter's aid when her daughter accused Queen's husband of child abuse, nonetheless loved her daughter because she kept pictures of her all over her walls, Booker retorts: "well the motherfucker who murdered my brother had all his victims' photos in his fucking den" (169). The act of memorializing the lost slides into an image of self-centered cruelty in the text. Thus, when Booker finally arrives at the moment in which he says something with the truth and clarity longed for by the novel, it takes the form of an apology: "I apologize [Adam] for enslaving you in order to chain myself to an illusion of control... No slaveowner could have done better" (161).

Equating his love of his brother to the tyranny of the slave master, Booker's words frame the text's desire to force its readers to reconceptualize the losses to which we cling, shining new light upon the departed whom we enslave to the *jouissance* we arrive at through fantasies such as race. Indeed, the text ultimately calls into question the very fantasy of race itself, conceptualizing race as one of the ways through which characters "cling to a sad little story of hurt and sorrow – some long-ago sorrow and pain" (158). Whereas the core sorrow of African Americans is slavery, the text suggests that, through the persistent fantasy of race,

African Americans often fatally reanimate and haul on their own backs the dead slaves of American history, resurrecting them as ancestors who return only in the form of a metaphor of pain which defines and structures African Americans' own relation to *jouissance*. The book's title, *God Help the Child*, suggests its deep contemplation of a traumatic *jouissance* that has descended from these slaves as racial ancestors. But, in a time when, as Booker suggests, race is more readily acknowledged as truly not existing, the use of race relies less directly upon actual dead slaves than upon metonymic and metaphoric processes that give meaning to the abstraction of blackness. Precisely by identifying in Bride the abstraction of a "blackness [that] thrilled him" (133), a *jouissance*-filled blackness that enables him fantastically to transform Bride into a statue carved for his own pleasure – a "midnight Galatea" with "obsidian-midnight skin" – Booker comes finally to "see" in Bride's "eyes" the "starlight" he longs to recover (133). Though the text appears to shift away from a direct focus upon race with Booker's story, contemplating more abstractly the vicissitudes of *jouissance*, it finally shows how race in American society has been historically transformed, most specifically through the slave ancestor, into mechanisms of *jouissance*, into the means of African Americans' access to an unbearable pleasure.

This understanding of race and the ancestor interestingly complicates and expands Morrison's conception of home and the ego ideal as it is presented in both *The Bluest Eye* and Morrison's early prose writings. In a 1984 essay titled "Rootedness: The Ancestor as Foundation," Morrison argues for the importance of evaluating "Black literature on what the writer does with the presence of an ancestor."[44] Looking at the work of African American authors whom she helped champion in her capacity as editor for Random House, Morrison idealistically describes ancestors in black literature as "timeless people whose relationship to the characters are benevolent, instructive and protective," and who provide "a certain kind of wisdom" (343). Morrison links the sense of homelessness that invades the African American psyche to the "absence of an ancestor," an ancestor whose presence would have "determined the success or happiness of the character" (343). Declaring as early as 1980 that "the ancestor is not only wise," but also "values racial connection, racial memory over individual fulfillment," Morrison asserts that "the devastation of the protagonist [in black literature] never takes place unless he succeeds in ignoring or annihilating the ancestor."[45] However, in *God Help the Child*, it is the ancestral presence, Booker's aunt Queen, who prevents Booker from working through the loss and lack that devastate him.

Not only did Queen direct Booker to "mourn" his brother "for as long as he need[s] to," but she did so because she too had suffered a loss and does not have the full wisdom to note and overcome its effects (147). Though her daughter is still alive, she effectively lost this daughter when she failed to protect her from molestation; her love continues through the memorializing pictures on her wall that mirror both Booker's tattoo and the photos kept by Adam's murderer. Booker reveals that, Queen, the ancestor, "keeps everything," and it is this very act of holding on to the past that initially misleads him into believing "heartbreak should burn like a star" (163). Booker eventually comes to recognize however, that the stars that streak their light toward us "died thousands of years ago and we're just now getting their light"; thus reconceptualizing his relation to the irretrievable luminescence he associated with Adam, Booker finally acknowledges a need to let the objects of the past "explode, disappear" (163). When Queen is killed in a house fire, she comes to represent the passing of the ancestor who binds us to the pain of this past. Seeming to serve as substitute for the white ego ideal that so dominates *The Bluest Eye*, she is an ancestor the characters actively mourn and embrace, as Booker and Bride come together to cleanse her scorched body, bathing "her one section at a time" (166). But in the end, they must let go of her, and of the past they have clung to. Where the ancestor represents a celebration of "racial memory over individual fulfillment," Booker and Bride must first embrace, but then move on from the ancestor to achieve the individual fulfillment their relation to the past has impaired.[46]

Conclusion

Reflecting on what initially destroyed his relationship with Bride, Booker concludes that it was, "Lies. Silence. Just not saying what was true or why" (155). Extrapolating beyond the text, the idea of recovery through the breaking of a silence is precisely what roots Morrison's own literary career. As a child, when confronted by her friend's disclosure of her desire for blue eyes, Morrison responded with silent congeniality, later divulging that, "the sorrow in her voice seemed to call for sympathy, and I faked it for her, but, astonished by the desecration she proposed, I 'got mad' at her instead."[47] Initially silencing her anger at an image of her friend with "very blue eyes in a very black skin" that "violently repelled" her because it was, Morrison admits, "doing [harm] to *my* concept of the beautiful," Morrison years later would write *The Bluest Eye* in embrace of a "struggle" for "writing that was indisputably black," eventually returning decades after to directly problematize this very blackness in *God Help the Child*.[48] Where it is the signifier – language itself – that inscribes the body with meaning, Morrison turns to novel writing in order first to recuperate the sullied, shamed image of the black body which she confronted in her friend's desire; later, she unveils the fantasies and pleasures that bind the black body and psyche to trauma and past sorrows. Embracing the novel form in an effort to challenge the myths that have defined blackness, Morrison views literature not only as mythopoetic in its capacity to counter the discourses of race, but also as a source of deeper psychic and personal awareness, a tool capable of telling "people something they didn't know" about themselves.[49]

Acknowledging that "the narrative into which life seems to cast itself surfaces most forcefully in certain kinds of psychoanalysis," Morrison embraces an artistry that mirrors the work of the analyst, dialoguing with her reader to highlight "what the conflicts are, what the problems are."[50] Just as "the analyst cures through dialogue," Morrison's writing rejects her earlier silence by opening up a literary exchange that seeks to "transfer … the problem of fathoming" shame to the readers who remain "implicated" in the desires unveiled in her texts.[51] In analysis, dialogue between patient and analyst allows for a "mapping of the subject" in relation to the fantasies that force the patient's desires off track.[52] In this process, the purpose of the analyst's dialogue is not to define authoritatively the proper objects of the patient's desires, but rather to once again agitate desire, shifting it metonymically onto an individualized path that no longer stagnates the patient in a torturous relation to his obsession. Morrison's artistry seeks after this same fluid relation to desire and meaning, attempting to free the African American subject from Imaginary ideals bound to whiteness, and from structures of *jouissance* bound to the racialized signifier and the ancestor.

Indeed, arguing that "the text … cannot be the authority" but instead "should be a map" that helps to "clarify" not "solve social problems," Morrison seeks "active participation" from her reader.[53] Her writing positions readers as both analysts, assembling the discourses of characters who present as patients of a pathological desire, and also patients themselves, placing their desires side by side with those of the characters in order to map their own relation to a character's pathology. Morrison dedicates *God Help the Child* simply to "You," her reader. While Bride echoes the post-Civil Rights achievements of African Americans in using race to create a positive image that is indisputably black, Morrison's most recent novel works together with her first to help readers design a self that extends beyond race. In Morrison's return to an embattled image of blackness shamed by the gaze of a racist American Symbolic, Morrison grants readers the novels themselves – a gift for "You" – as the means of remaking the self-identities race has built for each of us.

Notes

1 Toni Morrison, "Afterword," in *The Bluest Eye* (New York: Plume, 1993), 212.
2 Toni Morrison, *God Help the Child* (New York: Alfred A. Knopf, 2015).
3 J. Brooks Bouson, *Quiet as It's kept: Shame Trauma and Race in the Novels of Toni Morrison* (New York: SUNY Press, 2000), 18.
4 Toni Morrison, "Home," in *The House that Race Built*, ed. Wahneema Lubiano (New York: Pantheon Books, 1997), 4.
5 Jacques Lacan, "Le Sinthome," trans. Luke Thurston (*Ornicar*, 6–11, 1976–1977), 16.
6 Jacques Lacan, "The Mirror Stage as Formative of the *I* Function as Revealed in Psychoanalytic Experience," in *Écrits: The First Complete Edition in English*, trans. Bruce Fink (New York: Norton, 2006), 78.
7 Lacan, "Sinthome," 19.
8 Ibid., 18.

9 Ibid., 60, 19.
10 Jacques Lacan, "On a Question Prior to Any Possible Treatment of Psycho-sis," in *Ècrits: The First Complete Edition in English*, trans. Bruce Fink (New York: Norton, 2006), 459.
11 Lacan, "Question," 459.
12 Gwen Bergner, *Taboo Subject: Race, Sex and Psychoanalysis* (Minneapolis: University of Minnesota Press, 2005), xxxi.
13 W.E.B. Du Bois, *The Souls of Black Folk* (New York: Penguin, 1989), 11.
14 Du Bois, *Souls of Black Folk*, 11.
15 Kalpana Seshadri-Crooks, *Desiring Whiteness: A Lacanian Analysis of Race* (New York: Routledge Press, 2000), 25.
16 Lacan, "Question," 461.
17 For a useful reading of race as psychically cathected, see Farhad Dalal, *Race, Colour and the Process of Racialization* (New York: Routledge, 2002).
18 Jacques Lacan, *The Seminar of Jacques Lacan, Book XI: The Four Fun-damental Concepts of Psycho-Analysis*, trans. Alan Sheridan (New York: Norton, 1998), 96.
19 Helen Block Lewis, *The Role of Shame in Symptom Formation* (New Jersey, NJ: Lawrence Erlbaum Associates, 1987), 17.
20 Lewis, *The Role of Shame*, 15.
21 Du Bois, *Souls of Black Folk*, 5.
22 Ibid.
23 Morrison, "Home," 10.
24 Ibid.
25 Jacques Lacan, *On the Names-of-the-Father*, trans. Bruce Fink (Boston, MA: Polity Press, 2013), 77.
26 Andrew P. Morrison, *Shame: The Underside of Narcissism* (New Jersey, NJ: The Analytic Press, 1989), 12; Jacques Lacan, "The Subversion of the Sub-ject and the Dialectic of Desire in the Freudian Unconscious," in *Ècrits: The First Complete Edition in English*, trans. Bruce Fink (New York: Norton, 2006), 700.
27 Jacques Lacan, "Desire and the Interpretation of Desire in *Hamlet*," in "Lit-erature and Psychoanalysis: The Question of Reading Otherwise," Special Issue, *Yale French Studies*, 55/56 (1977): 36.
28 Lacan, "Question," 465.
29 Ibid., 481, 482.
30 Ibid., 466.
31 Ibid., 448.
32 Donald L. Nathanson, M.D., *The Many Faces of Shame* (New York: The Guilford Press, 1987), 5.
33 Morrison, "Afterword," 210.
34 Toni Morrison, *Birth of a Nation'hood* (New York: Pantheon Books, 1997), xi, x, ix, xviii.
35 Toni Morrison, *Playing in the Dark: Whiteness and the Literary Imagina-tion* (New York: Random House, 1992), xi.
36 Morrison, *Playing*, 17.
37 Jacques Lacan, "The Instance of the Letter in the Unconscious," in *Ècrits: The First Complete Edition in English*, trans. Bruce Fink (New York: Norton, 2006), 425.
38 Lacan, "Instance," 425.
39 Ibid., 431.
40 Jacques Lacan, *The Seminar of Jacques Lacan Book III: The Psychoses*, trans. Russell Grigg (New York: Norton, 1997), 268.
41 Lacan, *The Psychoses*, 423, 267, 265, 264, 261.

42 Lacan, "Instance," 419.
43 Ibid., 422.
44 Toni Morrison, "Rootedness: The Ancestor as Foundation," in *Black Women Writers (1950–1980): A Critical Evaluation*, ed. Mari Evans (New York: Doubleday, 1984), 343.
45 Toni Morrison, "City Limits, Village Values: Concepts of the Neighborhood in Black Fiction," in *Literature and the Urban Experience*, ed. Michael C. Jaye and Ann Chalmers Watts (New Jersey, NJ: Rutgers, 1981), 43.
46 Morrison, "City Limits," 43.
47 Morrison, "Afterword," 209.
48 Ibid., 209, 211.
49 Morrison, "Rootedness," 340.
50 Morrison, *Playing*, v; "Rootedness," 341.
51 "Aggressiveness," 86; Morrison, "Afterword," 214.
52 Lacan, *Four Fundamental Concepts*, 273.
53 Toni Morrison, "Memory, Creation and Writing," *Thought* 59 no. 235 (1984): 389, 387.

9 "The Lyric a Form / of Shame Management?"

John Goodby

I

I've often wondered about shame, in all its various allotropes and guises, and about its connection with my poetry. This is because it looms larger in my experience, I think, than for many people. As a child I was cripplingly shy, embarrassable and highly susceptible to tears – I could find myself blushing furiously and my eyes watering at nothing more than having to walk past someone in the street, humiliated by a sense of vulnerability to their gaze and their physical closeness. That hypersensitivity extended to the more usual sources of shame. As a rank conformist at school, I largely avoided punishment, but when it did happen, in an era of corporal punishment, it would reduce me to a quivering, pink-faced wreck. I could easily have believed back then, with Edmund Talbot in William Golding's *Rites of Passage*, that it is possible "to die of shame." This intensity of response was matched by the variety of forms shame could take, at my parents asking about a film ("Lord Jim") my friend's parents had taken me to (it had a brief topless episode, which I hadn't even noticed), or in sympathy at my Mum's mortification when a shop refused her check, or at Enid Blyton's toe-curling use of the word "dear" ("her dear red shoes"). In each case, a powerful, involuntary physical response – flush, trembling, blushing, tears – would accompany the emotion.

This involuntary, physical aspect may account for the link between shame and poetry, and its often sexual form. When, at seventeen, I read the episode in Joyce's *A Portrait of the Artist*, in which Stephen Dedalus is confounded by the sight of the word "foetus," I sympathized, as so many do. Stephen's shame results from his sudden knowledge that the sexual fantasies he believed to be private have some purchase in the outer world, even though that world is still ostensibly the one of his childhood. Desire, lust, is a source of shame, then; but shame can also give an edge to the pleasure, as Stephen also goes on to discover, and the similarities between poetry – rhythmic, arational, bodily language – and the commonest source of adolescent shame, masturbation, can be traced readily enough (it's no coincidence that they so often enter our lives at the same time, or that poets deemed to be "visceral" – John Keats, Algernon Charles Swinburne, Dylan Thomas – are also dubbed masturbatory).

Still, just as you eventually have to learn sexual relationships with others, so you must also learn to distance yourself from your emotions if you want to improve on those dire, early scribblings. The only difference in my case was that the first efforts at poetry and partnership also coincided with the effort to suppress my extreme shyness, and perhaps led me to overdo it. Not much makes me well up or brings a lump to my throat these days – it's usually something trivial, like a cheesy movie or poem, an account of personal struggle against the odds – although, ever since I can remember, I've found it hard to cry at the one time when it's most allowed, most *necessary*, namely, at the death of someone close. Even when I could blub at the drop of a hat I couldn't do that, and now I seem to do so only unbecomingly, while remaining relatively dry eyed at grievous loss. Perhaps I can only cry when it is unbecoming, embarrassing, shaming? Whatever it is, the drawn-out grief of bereavement only kicks in in the wake of a failed love relationship.

One result, in writing terms, is that quite a lot of my recent poetry is about erotic mourning, centered on shaming but practically imaginary scenarios of transgression from my permanent relationship. Generically, this mode has a predecessor in a subspecies of elegy in Latin poetry – there are examples by Gallus, Catullus and Ovid – but it's fairly rare. Of course, while it contains an element of confession, it seems to me that my main reason for this subject matter is because it allows in fantasy a renunciation of responsibility, a bypassing of the fixed structures – established relationship, the ego – that impede linguistic self-discovery. The pretexts may be shameful but they lead to pleasurably transgressive traffickings with the libido of the linguistic unconscious. In any case, as Denise Riley has noted, beyond the shame potential lurking in any assumption of authorial superiority, the self-reflexivity of poetry is dogged by an innate "linguistic guilt," the writer's sense that there is no coherent center or meaning in language, and that its workings are arbitrary (or "involuntary") – in which case, I may as well be hung for a sheep as for a lamb. Nor is that arbitrariness necessarily malign; writing may well be like herding cats, but the slippage and crumbling of language which comes from trying to control it releases the *jouissance* of poetry, and – if only for a short time – releases the self from its iron bonds.

II

A few years back, I published *Illennium* (2010), a collection of 72 cut-up sonnets which broaches some of these subjects. It takes as its model Ted Berrigan's *The Sonnets* (1964), and follows his use of chance and aleatory procedures, derived from Duchamp and John Cage, for collaging scraps of through-written poems, diaries, descriptions of paintings, articles, letters, translations, and sundry other cultural stuffs. Riddled and reinforced by leitmotifs – evocative lines and phrases wrenched from their original contexts, which both focus and disperse affect – Berrigan's sequence interweaves the most ethereal and mundane materials in a way that seems to accord with a never quite grasped dream logic, but which also enacts the compulsive repetition of specific painful details concerning "the trajectory of a single attachment within a tangled set of friendships." *Illennium*, too, arose from such a "tangled set of friendships," and one in particular which flared briefly in 1998. Never exactly a "relationship," it ended soon after it (almost) began, but left me grieving for months. Nothing like closure, let alone reconciliation, was available, and normal confessional poetic strategies were no use at dealing with the horrible residue. What I gradually came to see – over several years, in fact – was that *The Sonnets'* fractured facturings of surreal whimsy and seriousness might allow both for the open, cathartic display of the facts of the shameful case, and for a calming dispersal of the lyric self. And because shame was so central to what I wanted to (un)say, I decided to try to find out more about it.

I discovered that shame, long-neglected by sociology and psychoanalysis, was being rediscovered and reexplored. One essay belonging to this rediscovery that struck me in particular was "Shame as the Master Emotion of Everyday Life," by Suzanne M. Retziger and Thomas J. Scheff, which I discovered while trawling the web.[1] This described a history of the neglect, especially by psychologists ("it seems to be shaming to talk about shame"), which it countered by theorizing shame as a hitherto unacknowledged "core emotion," overlooked for so long because its ineluctably collective aspect threatened late capitalist myths of individualism and self-autonomy. This, in turn, meant that shame was constantly misrecognized in personal relationships too, leading to vicious cycles of shame, anger at being made to feel shame, shame at that anger, and so on. It confirmed, in other words, what the fallout from the friendship and my life-history seemed to teach me, that dilute shame was so pervasive in everyday life that it was like water to a fish, shaping all our thoughts and deeds in some way or other, the counterpart, in affective terms, of ideology – an unacknowledged legislator. More, the essay yielded a vocabulary that fitted many of the *mises-en-scènes* of my poem: "facework" [saving face], "feeling traps," "the shame / anger spiral." It also distinguished usefully between resentment (anger directed outwards) and guilt (directed towards the self), and, crucially, treated shame as a process. The essay's claims were ultimately too sweeping, but its appeal and appositeness couldn't be gainsaid, and I applied it with gleeful opportunism to *Illennium*.

In doing so, I became what Retziger and Scheff called a "shame worker," though not a systematic one, constellating their ideas and taxonomies as a matrix within which the narrative of friendship – its intellectual and sexual undertones, its codes and terms of endearment, its sociohistorical contexts, its humor, cajolery, and recriminations – might cohere in the mind of the reader. In a line I took as an epigraph for the book ("Shame knowledge may allow researchers to make visible what is usually invisible, the actual state of any relationship where dialogue is available"), my emphasis was on the "may," any totalizing "explanation" resisted. The tonal range tended to extremes, with heavy sociological formulae jostling with flippancy and downright prattishness, romantic idealism with abasement, abstractions with named figures and places, news items and social activities such as concert-going, drinking, and watching television ("The Fast Show" is a key text, and the snippets of collaged text flash up with the speed of TV trailers). Sonnet XXV, for example, splices together a nickname ("Peach" > "Peach Melba" > "Melba"), sexual innuendo ("How close to come without coming"), news item (the Bill Clinton/Monica Lewinsky affair: "'it depends on what the meaning of "is" is'"), the words of one of the principals (*I know this is as hopeless ... as usual*"), the death of Ted Hughes ("Lie thou, Ted, now"), and a local reference ("The Antelope" is a pub in Mumbles, Swansea):

> From feathers flagrant sweet thick ankles fingers not slender
> Wetly ache & throe   be Melba to me
> scalp rash & wrathful skies
> How close to come without coming   Humpty asks
> The straightforward face   "Are you and she
> yet it is   needs no con firming
> so vividly hidden demurral would be tautologous
> "(not so secret!)"   Wetly ache & throe
> *I know this is as hopeless and impractical*
> *as usual*   The face
> glows jonquil
> This is   married men Lie thou, Ted, now
> and "it depends on what the meaning of the word 'is' is"
> My dream: to fetishise a hairy escapade
> next door to The Antelope   only dreaming the day?

Baleful erotic melancholy, guilt, shame, and embarrassment ("ache & throe," "rash & wrathful skies") are writ large, but are partly contained within a framework of more disparate material that relativizes, without extinguishing, their anguished, doomy tone. The form inscribes the couple's idealistic refusal of conventional notions concerning shame and a resultant renunciation of deviousness ("no con"), but the refusal itself is opaque and evasive, its verbal materials "vividly hidden" in plain sight. In this sense, like *Illennium* as a whole, Sonnet XXV invokes several senses of "shameless" – brazen heartlessness, sheer unembarrassability, refusal of prudish censure, mere naivety – all at once.

Certain authors noted for dealing with shyness, shame, embarrassment, and their cognates are particularly important as intertextual conscripts. Keats' "blushful"-ness and engorgings (and Christopher Ricks' critical analysis of them) feature, as do Jules Laforgue, Arthur Rimbaud, Malcolm Lowry, Dafydd ap Gwilym. Some are made embarrassing against their intentions, as in Sonnet XXIII: a cut up of an Enid Blyton Famous Five story produces the line "'She's just crazy on Dick,' said Joan ... How *could* Dick stand up for that awful girl," one of several double entendres so blatant they're almost single. Tennyson gets "tin memoriam," Keats' "Ode on a Grecian Urn" contributes "O attic ape! Fair altitude!" and the opening scene of *Antony and Cleopatra* is maimed in "There's buggery in the love that can be reckoned." Shakespeare's sonnets, *the* canonical sequence (Sonnet 129's self-disgusted "expense of spirit," but also the idealizing urges of, say, Sonnet 57) are ever-present, and an episode of broadcast secrecy from *As You Like It*, in which Rosalind's suitors nail their anonymous poems to trees in the Forest of Arden, makes an appearance:

> Nigel harping on about Parker's *Angela's Ashes*
> shot through a green-tinged filtrum
> but creased, you colour puce, vermeil, poppy,
> coral, stammel, madder, cochineal
> annealed, vermilion, magenta – its hot flushes
> Hang there, my verse, in witness
> of my violet gums   Such a nut is Rosalind
> for happiness   slaughtered
> Tongues I'll hang on every tree
> The fair, the chaste   unexpressive she. "My secret
> love (not that secret really!)" Truly con
> sensual   blindfoldingly sweet
> So? can't help wanting you here with me now,
> dreaming of the day   Or at every sentence end.

By this point in the sequence, there are accusations of forgetting "what shame meant," of giving off signals of shame (blushing) while acting in a way which signals the loss of the compassion, of humanity, even, which gives rise to shame. Blushing may now be anger, a face "madder & madder" at the evidence of its misbehavior, playing on the rose "madder" tint of a blush. The "straightforward" is anagrammatically becoming "straightfroward," the "Peach" is being "impeached." Later on, the shame is lost in brazenness, bringing in the brass of Shakespeare's Sonnet 65 – "Since neither brass, nor stone, nor earth nor boundless sea / But sad mortality o'ersways their power" – though "brass" has dropped an "s" and we have "Dad morality" via some perfervid slippage. What was a delectable, semi-licit situation, teetering deliciously on abandonment to shame, has become the courting of occasions for humiliation; with the speaking subject in meltdown, the "ill" of *Illennium* is pathologically highlighted.

Language mimics this disintegration. Pun, the most shameful trope, and the one viewed as least compatible with literary dignity by the style police, is to the fore, and often in the most groaningly embarrassing ways: a chapter in a study of Irish poetry is titled "From Eire to Modernity," a distant friend is "So Nia & yet so far," an emotional immolation that occurs on a sofa is a "settee-suttee." These can be within and across other languages; my knowledge of these is embarrassingly small, but at one point, for example, we're told that "all men songe." "Mensonge" is French for "lie," and the speaker of the sequence is a true liar, but the split gives "men" who "songe," that is "dream," which may qualify the harshness of "mensonge" in the direction of delusion, although not too much, I hope. While the gendering of shame discourses is noted, for example – "'We are ashamed to seem evasive in the presence / of a straightforward man, gross in the eyes / of a refined woman'" – the sexism of this dealing out of attributes by Retzinger and Scheff is meant to be noticed, as is the narrator's own sexism, apparent in a pun like "thongs for the mammary." There's other wordplay too, usually of the echolaliac, verging on puerile variety: "softened as so often," "you reck recklessly," "a slave is no salve."

It isn't for me to say whether any of this adds up to a serious lyric response to a shameful episode, or to shame more generally – Laurie Duggan, a poet I admire greatly, complimented me on *Illennium*'s willingness to be flippant, which might sound rather double-edged, but I see as getting the point. This is "the lyric [as] a form of shame management," and it may be that all lyric is that to some degree. Certainly, a poem on the subject has to incorporate that knowledge. The lyric *ékstasis* is continually and irritatingly cast in a transcendental, quasi-theological mode even now, especially in mainstream poetry, and the use of shame theory to expose this sham shame is a legitimate way past it. It's serious enough if you take it seriously: the theory is paraphrased in *Illennium* as "Guilt / pertains simply to one's deeds or actions, shame / is ontological, of self," and it doesn't get much heavier than that. Which recalls the gay US poet John Weiners, who, when asked how he wrote his poetry, answered, "I just write down the most embarrassing thing I can think of." This stands as the epigraph to the final poem in *Illennium*, and it sounds like a joke (it is), but it's a scarier practice than most poets who make a premium of their honesty usually achieve. Here, to finish this section, is Sonnet X VII, which begins with an anagram, and continues with a spoof student essay question, the title of an M.A. dissertation on R.S. Thomas, and works through references to a dead friend, a line from another poem in *Illennium* (it samples Keats' "I am sure of nothing but the holiness of the heart's affections" via Edwin Morgan's "Message Clear"), an un-outed neglected Irish modernist, shame theory, Enid Blyton, and a

statement about sincerity on poetry and the sincerity of this poem which
is as ambiguous as I can make it:

XXIV

Ken Livingstone = King votes Lenin, or
"'Fanny Price is the theme of, not
a character in, *Mansfield Park*.' Discuss."
I'll discuss 'Keeping the Short Boundaries Holy'
poetry meetings with Vic at The Viv or Viv at The Vic
The straightfroward face blutacked to the blinds
        an   i   t   s   he h a t   e   s
blutacked to the office blinds, all clunky
& Roman: LIX CVIII VIV
MacGreevy's use of painterly imagery
deflects both from the reality he sees and the emotions
he experiences Forget 'maybe'
'Red Tower isn't a place. Red Tower is a man.'
if I ever write a poem that raw I'll be amazed

III

I want to finish by claiming, briefly, that shame can also be usefully
applied to some of the contexts of writing poetry and of canon-
making; if it's (almost) the "master emotion" of everyday life, why not
of everyday poetry life too? So here's another shaming confession, to
begin; I should have written more poetry than I have, and I am embarrassed that I've produced far more criticism than poems, in acts of
writing which have eschewed real risk. In fact, I've probably used the
professional requirement to write criticism as an excuse to avoid writing poetry. To complicate this further, the poetry I *do* write is divided
between what are (mis)called "mainstream" and "alternative" kinds,
corresponding to the rather apartheid-like split in British poetry culture. Thus, my early poems appeared in Faber's *Poetry Introduction
8*, in 1993, but after a conversion to linguistically innovative poetry
around 2000, *Illennium* (hence its title) became the first fruits of a
very different writing.

And yet, despite this, from time to time I found myself returning,
red-cheeked, to write well-crafted, carefully disheveled mainstream poems, cynically produced to enter in poetry competitions. The idea was to
expose – to my own satisfaction, at least – the all-too-imitable, prepro-
grammed nature of the poetry culture that revolves around these events,
and which rules in *Poetry Review* and over London poetry publishers'
lists and poetry festivals, and that so shamelessly, ignores the riches of
modernist-derived poetry in Britain that one is embarrassed on behalf of
the otherwise intelligent and sensitive people responsible for it. In 2006,

I managed to win first prize, £5,000, in the Cardiff Poetry Competition, with "The Uncles," a fairly schmaltzy piece I'd hacked out in about forty minutes (easily the best rate of pay I'm ever likely to receive). In 2008 and 2009 I won another competition and made third in another, with equally faked-up pieces.

So what did it prove? Not much. What is "fake," what "sincere," in poetry anyway? Competitions which elicit the same trite lyrics continue to proliferate. There has been some sign of rapprochement between the mainstream and self-styled avant-garde, but not that much. The best poets ignore the biases and go on writing, relying on the sifting effects of time and taste. Perhaps the point is that the shamelessness I exposed has deep historical roots, beyond the movement with which it is associated, and that it may persist for many decades yet. If this is so, it may be my criticism will do most to redeem my own shame at not writing enough poems. The reason for this is that my critical work is a reappraisal of Dylan Thomas, the classic case of a poet who embarrasses the poetic and critical powers and a perfect instance of what I'd call canonical shame. Most poets and critics of Thomas forget Yeats' injunction not to confuse the conscious artist with "the bundle of accident and incoherence who sits down to breakfast," and read Thomas' poetry through the myth of the man. Too busy moralizing from the person, usually in default left-Leavisite mode, they miss its acute intelligence, beauty and daring, and the deep paradox of one of the most obscure poets in the language ("Altarwise by owl-light") being the author of "Poetry Please" favorite lyrics ("Fern Hill"). Above all, they miss understanding his work as a response to modernism which turned subaltern marginality – precisely what the metropolis saw as shameful weakness – into a hybrid, mongrel strength.

As a result, since the 1970s, Thomas has been written out of standard narratives of British poetry, dismissed as a colorful dead-end at best, a self-indulgent windbag at worst. The tradition of the empiricist, well-made lyric of Hardy, Auden, Larkin, and their successors is widely regarded, even now, in academia, as "*the* English tradition" (the definite article is Donald Davies'). And yet, like the proverbial elephant in the drawing room, Thomas is too big to be completely ignored, so from time to time officially sanctioned big hitters are wheeled out to maintain the line that he was an adolescent poet only, regressive and all the rest of it. Each conveniently ignores Thomas' writing of the body, his poetry of married love, war, nuclear-threatened pastoral and, above all, a method of always working "from words" rather than "towards" them which acknowledges linguistic guilt and opens poetry up to the liberating energies of the linguistic unconscious. The detractors thus reflect the embarrassment of a poetry culture which can't grasp how the author of "Fern Hill" also wrote the experimental "Altarwise by owl-light," and those who are truly interested in shame and the act of writing could do worse than start by comparing the poetic practices of the Patersons, Farleys, and Duffys with those of Thomas; if they do so, I believe, they will assuredly arrive at a better sense of the true complexity of the interaction between canonical and creative shame in British poetry of the last half century.

The point is not just that Thomas is a closet modernist, of course, but that the range of his poetry is an embarrassment to the divisions which poetic neo-modernists and neo-traditionalists alike have erected around their fiefdoms. However, I am embrarrassingly naïve enough to feel that the linguistic energy and invention of Thomas and his rather neglected successors is particularly timely because it cannot help but resist the language of instrumental reason, of HiEdBiz, corporations, and politicians, and that it does so more successfully than that of quirkily ironic, identity-discovering fare, however ostensibly radical. The medium is the message where poetry is concerned, and not in some merely decorative, surface sense. So it is that, in order to overcome my shame at not writing more poetry, I tell myself that by helping to shake up Audenary accounts of mid-century poetry I contribute to poetry of the present, albeit indirectly, and that in exposing a (bad) canonical shame I've helped free up a (positive) creative variety. It's a simplistic credo, but however much we might blush to admit it, shame is essential to poetry because risk and exposure, however involuntary, are at the heart of its sweet mortifications. Poetry, in this sense, is the news that stays news because it offers the most complete, perhaps the only alternative – bodily, mindful, shameful, shameless – to the powers that would "name and shame" us from above; because it alone can do so from below.

Note

1 T.J Scheff and S.M. Retzinger, "Shame as the Master Emotion of Everyday Life," *Journal of Mundane Behavior* 1.3 (2000): 303–324.

10 Vulnerability and Vulgarity
The Uses of Shame in the Work of Dodie Bellamy

Kaye Mitchell

In *Carnal Appetites* (2000), Elspeth Probyn addresses "questions of appetite, of excess, of fear, shame and disgust," arguing that "by bringing the dynamics of shame and disgust into prominence we are forced to envision a more visceral and powerful corporeal politics."[1] The relationship that she proceeds to posit between disgust and shame is, in my opinion, too schematic, and her definition of both too narrow,[2] but in Probyn's recognition of "the way in which disgust and shame may illumine the body's capacities for reaching out and spilling across domains that we would like to keep separate, or hidden from view," she offers a useful starting point for reading the work of Dodie Bellamy.[3] As a novelist, poet and essayist emerging from the alternative literary scene in San Francisco, associated since the 1980s with the "New Narrative" movement, Bellamy has produced a body of work that thwarts genre boundaries and, in her own words, "[champions] the vulnerable, the fractured, the disenfranchised, the fucked-up."[4] Probyn's "spilling out" arguably expresses both the content and the form of much of Bellamy's work: from its confessional and sexually explicit elements, to its use of appropriation from apparently culturally discrete sources such as canonical poetry, high theory, pop culture and pornography. Bellamy pursues this "unguarded embrace of cultural artifacts," while eschewing what she calls "the mainstream avant-garde's condescension towards pop culture – using it as a source of parody that the author remains intellectually and morally superior to." Instead, she refuses that distance, that superiority, claiming that "a more honest and interesting approach to pop culture is to delight in its tackiness but at the same time admit you're profoundly moved by it."[5] The "profound" and the "tacky" are thereby positioned as not mutually exclusive; "unguarded," meanwhile, expresses remarkably precisely both the method (scattershot) and the feeling (vulnerable, unprotected) of this "embrace of cultural artifacts."

Significantly, Bellamy also connects this (fascination with) "lowness" to femaleness, asserting that "[a]ggressively female experience and the female body are still denigrated by the avant-garde, and thus, to write from the position of one's femaleness is still to commit oneself to low culture."[6] In this chapter, I want to argue that such modes and methods allow Bellamy to tread a line between vulnerability and vulgarity, in a manner that exemplifies the double-functioning of shame, particularly for the writer who "write[s] from the position of [her] femaleness": that is to say, shame functions both as constitutive and as critical of femininity; it invokes and involves both a desire for spectacle and a desire for self-concealment. As Silvan Tomkins writes, "In shame I wish to continue to look and to be looked at, but I also do not wish to do so."[7] Bellamy's work, I suggest, is not simply or straightforwardly *shameless*, because it demonstrates a keen awareness of, and commitment to, a certain "low culture" of female embodiment and a degraded "feminine" culture of the mainstream and the "tacky"; its relationship to shame is not, therefore, one of redemption or overcoming, but rather something more immersive, complex and complicitous, which potentially produces more dissonant effects both formally and politically.

Such an understanding of shame – and its relationship to femininity – both builds on and complicates that posited by Sandra Bartky in *Femininity and Domination* (1990), where she argues that "It is in the act of being shamed and in the feeling ashamed that there is disclosed to women who they are and how they are faring within the domains they inhabit."[8] Bartky asserts that shame is "gender-related" in the sense that "women are more prone to experience" shame than men, and because "the feeling itself has a different meaning in relation to their total psychic situation and general social location than has a similar emotion when experienced by men."[9] Shame, then, experienced as or through "a pervasive sense of personal inadequacy' and as or through 'the shame of embodiment," reveals "the 'generalized condition of dishonour' which is women's lot in sexist society."[10] For women, feelings of shame "are profoundly disclosive of [their] 'Being-in-the-world.'"[11] The simultaneously structural and personal nature of shame for women is certainly something that Bellamy's work explores and exemplifies; however, the question that inaugurates this chapter is what is altered in this experience of shame – and disclosure of self – when the "act of being shamed" is instead an act of self-shaming, an embrace of a shamed position or an apparently shameless appropriation of material that may itself be shameful; all of these practices are found in Bellamy's work and/or form part of her writing philosophy. What forms of self-disclosure-through-shame are thereby made possible? What relationships are instantiated between shame and femininity, shame and writing in the "exultation in lowness" that is Bellamy's writing?[12] To what extent might we read this phrase – "exultation in lowness" – as a distinctly gendered expression of what, for Giorgio Agamben, forms part of the definitive experience of shame (and, indeed, of "the fundamental sentiment of being a *subject*"): "to be *subjected* and to be *sovereign*"?[13] Arguably, gendered embodiment, for

Bellamy, is indissociable from her writing practice, and is the locus of her experiences of both subjection and sovereignty.

The apparently shameless and transgressive elements of Bellamy's writing have been frequently noted. Bellamy's work might be read as "transgressive" in the sense discussed by Peter Stallybrass and Allon White in *The Politics and Poetics of Transgression*, because of the extent to which it allows the "low" or "base" to trouble the "high" or "exalted," thereby challenging the most fundamental "mechanisms of ordering and sense-making" in Western cultures, and producing, in turn, a deliberate disorder at the level of the page.[14] However, while Stallybrass and White identify, usefully, "a striking ambivalence to the representations of the lower strata (of the body, of literature, of society, of place) in which they are both reviled and desired," an ambivalence that includes both "repugnance" and "fascination," Bellamy illuminates the gendered nature of the hierarchies of high and low culture and emphasizes the inextricability of repugnance and fascination in the particular case of the simultaneously shameful and desired female body.[15]

In a recent reading of Bellamy's work, Christopher Breu positions it as part of "a 'minor' practice of postmodern writing that engages with the obscene, abjected and disavowed materials of late-capitalist existence," a "counter-tradition" which "is often called the 'literature of transgression' and is associated with writers such as William Burroughs, Thomas Pynchon, J.G. Ballard, Samuel Delany, and Kathy Acker."[16] He contrasts this "late-capitalist literature of materiality" with more "immaterial" metafictional practices.[17] Breu reads Bellamy's work as "[articulating] an explicitly feminist and queer politics of materiality and embodiment, one that affirms rather than recoils from those aspects of our existence marked as abject, disruptive, and all-too material" and as "[juxtaposing] the theoretical and the intimate, the abstract and (representations of) the brutely material in order to produce a discomfort that is simultaneously stylistic and affective."[18] The "brutely material" carries with it the shameful taint of the debased and coarse – again, what is refused are the distancing gestures and self-consciousness of intellectualism or of any position of moral superiority – and the "discomfort" produced exemplifies the transmissibility of shame, its highly contagious nature.[19] In confirmation of this point, Bellamy has claimed that she "often [writes] about material I feel resistance to, material that makes me uncomfortable, because that creates a charge for me, a sort of erotics of disclosure";[20] if this "erotics of disclosure" implies a (shameful?) pleasure on the part of both writer and reader, the persistence of discomfort and the admission of vulnerability make this a much more ambivalent experience than the *affirmation* of the abject that Breu finds in Bellamy's work. That action of affirmation is also troubled, I suggest, by Bellamy's undermining and/or disorientation of the authority of the speaking "I" in much of her work – most notably in those works employing cut-up.

Cunt-Ups (2001)

In *La seconde main ou le travail de la citation* (1979) (*The Second Hand or the* Work *of Citation*), Antoine Compagnon praises the brilliance and potential of the practice of citation:

> Blessed citation! Among all the words in our vocabulary, it has the privilege of simultaneously representing two operations, one of removal, the other of graft, as well as the object of these operations – the object removed and the object grafted on, as if the word remained the same in these two different states. Is there known elsewhere, in whatever other field of human activity, a similar reconciliation, in one and the same word, of the incompatible fundamentals which are disjunction and conjunction, mutilation and wholeness, the less and the more, export and import, decoupage and collage? The dialectic of citation is all-powerful: one of the vigorous mechanisms of displacement, it is even stronger than surgery.[21]

In *Cunt-Ups* (2001), that "dialectic" is complicated, its possible synthesis disrupted, by Bellamy's practice of splicing together apparently incompatible materials (semantically, aesthetically, generically and politically incompatible), in a manner that emphasizes disjunction, even while exploring the seamless conjunction and transmutation of bodies and body parts; there is no "reconciliation" here, but rather a tireless process of juxtaposition and discordance which emphasizes the jarring joy and shame of desire. As Jennifer Cooke explains the method of *Cunt-Ups*:

> The source texts ... were a mixture of Bellamy's own writing and some work by unnamed others; these were then subjected to the cutting technique that Burroughs specified by slicing each page into four. Each cut-up includes a mixture of these different squares which were then taped together, typed up, and "reworked."[22]

Bellamy had initial misgivings about cut-up:

> It seemed to me that only someone who had no access to an intuitive sense of reality would need to cut the text and tape it back together to get to this non-linear place. It seemed, in my reductive view of things, a very male thing to do a cut-up.

But decided to "[use] pornographic material for my cut-ups and [rename] the form 'cunt-ups,'" claiming that "It's a joke, but it's also a feminist reclaiming of the cut-up."[23] In *Cunt-Ups*, Bellamy uses the cut-up method "to enact the interconnectedness between body and thing, to create a frenzy of desire that subverts any stable abstraction of the lover's body as object,"[24] which is here revealed in all its "brute" – sometimes titillating, sometimes disgusting – materiality. She takes the material from her "lovers' pornographic rantings," from "the language of critical theory or abstraction," and from the confessions of serial killers such as Jeffrey Dahmer.[25] In this way, irreconcilable discourses and registers are compelled to coexist – indeed, to conjoin; boundaries between the proper and the improper, between high and low, are irremediably transgressed.

The pornographic element is to the fore, with the text's ceaseless repetition of "cunt," "cock," "asshole," etc. – a peppering of obscenity that is, by turns, comical, discomfiting, embarrassing and titillating. Whether or not *Cunt-Ups* is, as Bellamy claims, an attempt to "[take] back" the "male form" of pornographic language and "[subvert] it to my own ends,"[26] its jarring obscenities force us to consider language as a tool of both violence and arousal (sometimes simultaneously), while raising questions about what, precisely, constitutes the obscene, the unspeakable or the shameful. This sexualized language makes the text also, on Cooke's reading, a "failure" – though this is not presented as a criticism. As Cooke explains:

> Our words for sex are crude and *Cunt-Ups*, as its title suggests, knows this well. As a sensory experience, sex is hard to capture in language... In this respect, *Cunt-Ups* necessarily fails and that is part of the point. As the text says itself, "No language will ever fit, no language will give light to the mysteries of my overwhelming need to tell you that I want" (p. 55) ["Cunt-Up #17"]. Sex, then, would be a limit case for representation, a threshold where language falters or is impoverished. At the same time, language can reach out and make you react, turning you on.[27]

Elspeth Probyn has claimed that "a form of shame always attends the writer. Primarily it is the shame of not being equal to the interest [in Tomkins's sense] of one's subject";[28] in the quite different context of postcolonial writing, Timothy Bewes has written of "a certain inadequacy of all forms with respect to representing experience."[29] In the writing of sex, that shame "of not being equal to" is magnified, and the writing carries with it various additional varieties of possible shame: at the "crude" (in all senses: unrefined, rudimentary, imprecise, coarse) nature of sexual language; at the 'failure' truly to capture the "sensory experience" of sex; at the impossibility, for Bellamy, of expressing her "overwhelming need"; at the social and/or moral impropriety of the utterance of carnal desire itself (particularly by a woman writer); at the (un)artistic taint of the pornographic within the literary (the "low" sullying the "high"); at the unpredictability of arousal, when language "[reaches] out and [makes] you react." Desire emerges here as voracious, all-consuming: the one who desires is consumed by this desire, unable to think of anything else (desire is thus simultaneously agency and passivity, liberation and constraint);

but the desire itself is also a desire to consume, to ingest/incorporate the body of the other. The second half of "Cunt-Up #4" repeats the phrase "I want" eleven times: "I want to milk your come... I want to split you in half ... I want to take your skin off," etc;[30] while "Cunt-Up #13" declares, "It's like my cunt starts in the middle of my chest. It's like there's a heart that's fibrillating, sucking in my breath."[31] The final "Cunt-Up" ends, appropriately, with the subclause: "my wanting."[32]

The presentation of violence and obscenity in *Cunt-Ups* is complicated further by the fact that it is nearly impossible to discern, at each point, who is doing what to whom; there are no stable subjects (or even subject positions) here, and thus no easy attributions of victimhood or tyranny; any sense of shame is, consequently, scattered, unattributed (though not thereby absent). Instead, organs are interchangeable, free-floating, and bodies refuse to cohere into "male" or "female"; shifting pronouns disrupt the ownership of bodies and actions. There is at work, instead, a diffuse agency, such that it is hard to tell who is active and who passive: "I contact either myself or you, I recall being involved at this time when I moved our hand across my body."[33] Cut-up and collage – or what Bellamy refers to elsewhere as "procedural practices and appropriation" – thus become "tools to break open and challenge the ego-driven narrative."[34] The dispersal of ego facilitates, in turn, a dispersal of both desire and shame – again, their *dispersal* rather than their *disappearance*. In the graphic prose poems of *Cunt-Ups*, desire becomes flexible and free-floating, and bodies are endlessly changeable and permeable, penetrated and penetrating:

> My thoughts flutter down your purple neck and that gives me a hard-on. Your hips hugged against my belly, be inert, be happy, I just want to feel you with both feet overhead, all my fight waits to fuck your swollen pink and white spaces, to jostle you around gently until you turn blue. I kiss your finger and touch the head of your cock, you're wild now, invisible.[35]

The aggression here – "fight," "fuck" – is intermingled with tenderness; even spaces are materialized ("your swollen pink and white spaces"), lack becoming flesh. Yet the "purple neck" and "swollen pink" evoke bruising as well as arousal, and the text repeatedly returns to imagery of dismemberment: lovers becoming killers and their victims, and vice versa; the body taken apart by desire, endlessly penetrated and invaded by the other.

> All these parts coalescing into a heart, we had sex and used sleeping pills, rose, and your cock in the center fucking, strangled me and then dismembered my body for the first time.[36]

In "Cunt-Up #4" she writes, simply: "I'm getting quicker at cutting up the body I was born with," suggesting the critical compartmentalization

of the female body, its brutal objectification, as well as more literal vio-
lences enacted upon it.[37] All organs become sexual here and every part
of the body is open to the lover's touch – but also to violation: "your
cock pokes up, divining my guts, my heart, my lungs, the undersides,
I have no right to my organs, their incorrect shapes and desire."[38] This
is a radical, uninhibited, unconstrained intimacy, a merging of bodies,
but one that threatens a dissolution of self, and always carries the risk of
injury: "I'm going to kiss you and when you fall asleep I'll stab you like a
knife."[39] The surface "vulgarity," then, conceals a radical vulnerability,
a sense of self-as-wound.

The dismemberment at the level of theme is also, of course, enacted by
the text itself as a product of dis- and re-memberment, and Bellamy's practice of cut-up produces a kind of obscenity by juxtaposition.[40] As David
Banash argues, "cut-ups do conceptual, aesthetic, and quite literal violence to ideas of writing";[41] here that "violence to ideas of writing" is used
to explore – without reflective, redemptive, explanatory or moralizing
commentary – the violence that bodies do to each other, the pleasures
and pains of embodiment, the violence of language and the discomforts of
obscenity; the text is "perverted" – in various senses. As Bellamy has commented, on her practice of collage, "I often change such stolen passages to
the first person, I absorb and pervert them, make them *me*";[42] this absorp-
tion, however, does not quite amount to anything as settled and authorita-
tive as ownership. Edward Robinson, in his history of cut-up, asserts that:

> [i]ntegral to the nature of breaking down the control system were
> the random and collaborative aspects of the approach to the [cut-up]
> experiments. The random factor meant that not only was the control
> language held over the writer being broken down, but also the con-
> trol the writer has over the words is diminished.[43]

This surrendering of "control," this refusal of the claim to full authorship (and full authority), might suggest that cut-up – and other forms
of appropriation – has limited appeal for women authors still trying to
find a voice, to claim a right to speak or write, and to establish their
authority, and yet, for Bellamy (and for crucial female forebears such
as Kathy Acker),[44] it represents a deliberate violation of the sanctity of
the male-authored text and a protest against a feeling of imprisonment
within a patriarchal symbolic order. And yet, again, despite the "aggressive" sexual explicitness of *Cunt-Ups*, the blending and contortion of
bodies and sentences models also a kind of vulnerability – physical, emotional, sensual, artistic – to the other; bodies and texts are intertwined,
inextricable, interpenetrating in a continual fluctuation of the sovereign
and the subjected, the shameless and the shameful.

Such dangerous fluidity is evident also in the way that the text runs
over with bodily fluids that might be the product of sex or violence, or

both, and which demonstrate a kind of exultation in abjection; these are leaky bodies that overspill their boundaries – as female bodies have stereotypically been held to do;[45] here, that unboundedness of bodies is gleefully ungendered. Cooke finds in *Cunt-Ups* "tenderness," "hard sex," "desire" and "love," as well as a lot about writing; but she also notes that:

> there's a lot in *Cunt-Ups* which is disgusting… Disgust is contextual and sex is particularly good as a litmus test of this: what I might find disgusting with someone else, with my lover I find erotically charged, beautiful and exciting. Disgust, like lust, is a bodily affect, one that *Cunt-Ups* deliberately courts.[46]

What are the effects, for the reader, of the text's courting of the disgusting? Perhaps the point is that, in the absence of clear subject positions, it is impossible to locate affects such as shame or disgust, or rather, any shame is taken on, worked through, by the reader. We feel addressed by, implicated in, the text – "Typing these words I was dragging your cunt behind me, you know it, you've wet everything we've touched, ripe like fallen fruit, like the earth," Bellamy writes, in "Cunt-Up #19"[47] – and for one critic of the later *Cunt Norton* (2013),[48] "we feel guilty, like children caught touching each others' privates. To me, it's like Bellamy is my mother and my mother is watching me masturbate. She transforms me into one of her victims and accomplices."[49]

Bellamy's text raises questions, then, about what we might find personally disgusting or socially shameful, presenting embodiment and desire as experiences that oscillate unexpectedly (as her text does) between pleasure and shame; the depictions of bodies in *Cunt-Ups* refuse aestheticization, abstraction or transcendence, preferring instead the carnal and animal. This is politically risky, given the cultural associations of female flesh with meat and the apparent shamefulness of such rapacious sexual appetites; indeed, Bellamy has elsewhere written about being a "bad experimental feminist," due to her commitment to "[addressing] raw emotion" in her work, in a way that is "embarrassingly nonfragmented and direct," and because "I was always eager to fuck."[50] If *Cunt-Ups* appears to privilege sex over emotion, Bellamy is nevertheless insistent that the cut-up technique is *not* a means of presenting "heightened emotion" that is "displayed but not owned," boasting instead that "in my writing I favour a direct assault of over-the-top emotion, hysteria even"; the use of "assault" hints at how excessive emotion becomes a weapon directed triumphantly outwards, while "hysteria" unashamedly claims a conventionally feminized condition of disruptive, bodily feeling.[51] *Cunt-Ups*, accordingly, includes some moments of unexpected, uncanny lyricism and feeling:

> You don't know how infinite the course of my humiliations for you, singing actually – torch songs of nullity of being/being outside my

kind of love, the kind of love the top of the wall carved a hole in. The rock. They opened the door, and tied me down, a runnel of water/a returned letter.[52]

Here, intimations of suffering and torture meet romantic cliché ("torch songs") and a shifting self/body transformed by desire. Yet despite describing *Cunt-Ups* as "a very romantic book" in which she is "collapsing romance and porn,"[53] Bellamy makes it clear that love involves a confession of unappeasable need and a reduction of self to "nullity" or object status that is ineluctably humiliating:

> You can't see me because I'm still a thing. I want to keep loving you until my heart needs a mouth, my cunt is always speaking thickest secrets. I want to kiss you too, I want love and longing, and your praises.[54]

the buddhist (2011)

In Bellamy's 2011 publication, *the buddhist*, it is "love and longing" rather than sexual desire that is foregrounded, but the text nevertheless deploys the twin approaches of vulnerability and vulgarity as part of its exploration of the more shameful aspects of embodiment and literary expression. *the buddhist* gathers together a short, autobiographical story of the same title and a series of blog posts from Bellamy's "Belladodie" blog. Together, these pieces chart the demise and aftermath of Bellamy's relationship with a man identified only as "the buddhist." The book combines elements of confessional memoir with much self-reflexive musing on the writing of that story, alongside commentary on Bellamy's day-to-day life and involvement in the experimental poetry scene. In the course of the entries she refers to the blog as "my project of dailiness, endurance, embarrassment," and the narrative, correspondingly, holds in tension revelation and boredom, spontaneity and mundanity.[55] "As I continued the blog," she tells an interviewer, "I came to view it as performance art."[56]

In *the buddhist*, Bellamy allows "emotional excesses to bleed around my words" (the bodily metaphor again apparent), but she also explains that "I've tried to use my babbling about loss and betrayal as an opportunity to refine and promote a political/aesthetic position."[57] So "babbling" is validated as a kind of theorizing and the personal and subjective are put in the service of the political and collective, exemplifying Bellamy's claim that "an in-your-face owning of one's vulnerability and fucked-upness to the point of embarrassing and offending tight-asses is a powerful feminist strategy."[58] This claim is perhaps borne out by a recent interview with Judith Butler, in which she asserts that "gender assignment finds us, from the start, vulnerable to its effects," and she figures vulnerability not as a form of "pure passivity" or as an absence of will, but rather as "the condition of responsiveness" that might lead to quite productive or positive challenges to "the terms by which we are addressed."[59] On Butler's reckoning, we are "vulnerable" in the sense that we are *subject to* the "enormous discursive practice" of gender, and vulnerable because we require these "forms of enabling address" – what she elsewhere refers to as *recognition*. In the case of the kind of disappointed/unreciprocated love narrated by *the buddhist*, that need for recognition – and therefore that vulnerability – is particularly pronounced, that "condition of responsiveness" particularly heightened. Recall Butler's claim, in *Undoing Gender* (2004), that we "are undone by each other. And if we're not, we're missing something. If this seems so clearly the case with grief, it is only because it was already the case with desire. One does not always stay intact."[60] Bellamy's refusal to "stay intact" is evident in her "owning" of her "vulnerability and fucked-upness," but also in the deliberately fragmentary nature of her text. For Butler, a rejection or denial of vulnerability is linked to "fantasies of sovereignty" (at the state level but also at a personal level); in texts such as *Excitable Speech* (1997) and *Precarious Life* (2005), she "endorses an engagement that is anchored in and arises from acknowledgment (not disavowal) of human interdependence and incompletion," an acknowledgment of our vulnerability, our susceptibility to injury at the hands of the Other.[61]

In its candid acknowledgment of vulnerability in a manner which yet attempts to deploy that vulnerability as a feminist strategy of shaming, *the buddhist* can be read alongside formally very different texts such as Chris Kraus's *I Love Dick* (1997), Marie Calloway's *what purpose did i serve in your life* (2013), or the artist Sophie Calle's project/installation, *Take Care of Yourself* (2009).[62] These works explore and document (rather than "confessing") experiences of romantic injury and vulnerability, shame and self-abasement. Anna Watkins Fisher has discussed Kraus and Calle as practicing a kind of parasitism, and she asks "how parasitism might articulate itself as an experimental art practice as well as a performance model for contemporary feminist politics"; both Kraus and Calle, she argues "[perform] the figure of the parasite as a figure of overidentification," insisting on "loving men who reject them."[63] Bellamy arguably does something similar in *the buddhist*, finding a renewal of self and renaissance of creativity in the apparent shame of her rejection:

> Over and over I'm finding that after the lover leaves, from a reader's perspective, that's when things get really exciting, for that's when a woman can finally settle into herself. It's as if the absent lover creates an opening to surprising depths of humanness.[64]

Furthermore, like Kraus – who cites the crucial influence of the feminist body artist Hannah Wilke upon *I Love Dick* – Bellamy declares that "what I'm doing here resonates with the history of feminist performance art,"[65] referencing the work of Carolee Schneemann, whose "Interior Scroll" (the paper slowly pulled from her vagina during a 1975 performance) riffs:

> I met a happy man, / a structuralist filmmaker … he said we are fond of you / you are charming / but don't ask us / to look at your films /… we cannot look at / *the personal clutter* / *the persistence of feelings* / *the hand-touch sensibility.*[66]

In *the buddhist*, Bellamy marshals her "personal clutter" and gives her "feelings" full sway, but the "personal" is transformed via her "noisy corporeality" and the deliberate "vulgarity" of her writing.[67] She thereby inserts her work into a tradition of feminist avant-gardism which extends through poetry, prose and conceptual art, taking in Kathy Acker's "aggro assertion of female subjectivity – aggro deconstruction of female subjectivity – aggro fuck you to received notions of female subjectivity,"[68] and Sylvia Plath's "exultation in lowness":

> [Plath's] "high" poetry may be formally brilliant, but its content embarrasses. Her domestic squabbles, her depression, her female rages. From her I learned to grope around in the dark muck of femaleness, to embrace the terrors and embarrassments that emerged.[69]

We might note here how the "dark muck of femaleness" is bound up with "embarrassment": the shame of the (merely) personal ("domestic squabbles"), the shame of excessive emotion ("depression," "female rages") and, it is implied, the more primal shame of the female body itself ("the dark muck").

In connecting these experiences to the structural conditions of gendered vulnerability by situating their work in relation to a tradition of feminine and feminist self-exposure, artists such as Kraus, Calle and Bellamy touch on a "primary vulnerability" with very particular social and cultural consequences for women. Such a primary vulnerability also works against a kind of sovereignty at the level of the self and of the text – hence the foregrounding of a shame that both produces and undoes the self, hence the texts' formal and other incoherencies (the text itself is "undone"), hence the disruption of any kind of stable narratorial "I" – while exploring qualities of "interdependence and incompletion." That vulnerability is, however, in Bellamy's work, always in tension with what she describes as the "feral." Asked about the graphic sexual content of her work, Bellamy avers that: "all I ever wanted was to be feral, feral for me equals writing – my problem has always been how to enact the feral in a bourgeois world I wasn't raised to navigate."[70] To be "feral" means for Bellamy the embracing of pornographic imagery, a blurring of genres, a *shameless* mixing of high (poetic) and low (pornographic) content, but it also indicates a variety of sexual insatiability or voraciousness:

> My cunt flesh belches and fissures, torques itself inside out – this is the carnage of abandoned love – sex is dangerous, the buddhist told me over and over again – my cunt drools and spews, its juices glistening like a perfect orange on a rainy afternoon, my cunt shrieks never enough never enough never enough.[71]

Her unbounded body – emitting its "belches" and "juices" and "shrieks" – becomes, here, the locus of a vengeful, violent and limitless desire, obstinately insistent and inappropriate in its needs, its protests.[72] (This "carnage" has its detrimental effects, however: the passage hints at the bacterial infection with which Bellamy has just been diagnosed, so her "cunt flesh" expresses here both desire and disease.)

The opening "story" of *the buddhist*, by contrast, begins with a much tamer description of Bellamy having rather painful contorted sex with the eponymous subject of her narrative. There is little sense of shame in the scene or its narration and Bellamy combines an awareness of the potential absurdity of the situation with a sense of its transformative beauty and power: "Upside-down, legs dangling above me, I'm like an orchid hanging from the branch of a banyan tree in a botanical garden in Florida, an extraterrestrial white flower with a flushed pink core glowing in the generic hotel room light."[73] In this description, the natural and fecund (orchids, banyan trees, botanical gardens) wilt somewhat in the glare of the ersatz and kitsch (the "generic hotel room light"), yet the "flushed pink core" of Bellamy's desire dominates. Nevertheless, a friend asks her, "are you really going to get naked with him – at your age?" recommending something that she calls a "post-menopausal sex burqa," and Bellamy herself subsequently brands this opening story "a piece so obscene it makes my soul blush," despite the fact that it is less candid than other episodes in *the buddhist* and considerably less sexually explicit than much of her other writing.[74] The question of what is appropriate for a woman of her "age" resurfaces at several points in the narrative, with Bellamy noting that "Middle aged women are such easy prey, like they're supposed to walk around with eyes averted, hanging their heads in shame at their wreckage."[75] This Bellamy defiantly refuses to do, instead expressing the contradictory desire:

> To embrace the fucked-up, to move towards a maturity and strength that can include and express weakness and embarrassing content of all sorts without shame, to allow myself the full resonance of being a female subject … living in a fucked up nation, in a fucked up world, in the 21st century.[76]

To be "fucked up" – and to confess this – is, here, no barrier to "maturity and strength," while Bellamy implies that the foregrounding of "weakness" and "embarrassing content ... without shame" expresses the experience of "being a female subject ... in the 21st century." Vulnerability, weakness, and embarrassment are thus reworked as positions of strength and possibility, while Bellamy's intensely personal, acutely emotional experiences speak to the structural inequalities facing women in respect to their bodies and desires. When Bellamy asserts that "To deny behaviors and experiences gendered as weak or 'feminine' is not feminist or queer, it's heteronormative to the hilt. Like Kathy Acker, I long to quiver and terrify in the same gasp," her juxtaposition of quiver/terrify similarly posits a model of female agency that combines vulnerability and confrontation, or, more radically, stages vulnerability *as* confrontation.[77]

Despite elsewhere describing her work as "a user-friendly experimentalism, with lots of narrative candy and humor [sic], a sort of avant-garde lite,"[78] Bellamy nevertheless declares that "It was a long hard road for me to feel okay about the sort of straightforwardness I perform in *the buddhist.*"[79] It is certainly narratively much more accessible than *Cunt-Ups* and *The Letters of Mina Harker* (1998); what is carried over from these earlier works, however, is Bellamy's belief that "conceptual practices don't remove the self – they're Rorschach blobs into the self" and that "the conceptual – especially in the work of women – [cannot] be separated from the body."[80] The leaky, recalcitrant, uncontrollable, borderless, desiring/demanding feminine body (in Bellamy's presentation of it) is here mirrored by the mutating, disorienting syntax of the text, by its mix of the erudite and the vernacular, by its abrupt, discomfiting shifts between desire and disgust. Of course, the centrality of the body to women's conceptual art and writing has proven to be a contentious source of debate, as I have discussed elsewhere,[81] with Jennifer Ashton bemoaning the fact that "the new women's poetry understands 'innovation' as a direct extension and production of women's bodies," on the one hand, and Jennifer Scappettone retorting that for "women vanguardists," "the return to the body – which involves no unmediated return to a body proper – is a provocative feature of poetry riotously opposing a culture that continues to cast women as certain kinds – peculiarities – of subjects."[82] In Bellamy's case, the graphic, uncompromising communication of desiring, imperfect, voluptuous female carnality constitutes precisely both a stylistic and a political provocation; it forms part of her project of staging both vulnerability and vulgarity as offence and thus reworks feminine debasement as an experimental feminist strategy. As she explains in an essay entitled "Body Language":

> I'm particularly intrigued by writing that addresses the body – illness, ingestion, desire, display, sexual passion, subtle eroticism. The

writers I most admire celebrate vulgarity and emotion... Writing can
and should offer an emotional engagement with materiality. That
engagement can be highly mediated or direct, but that engagement
begins a politics, a morality of writing.[83]

In *the buddhist*, what is embarrassing – even shameful – is not the candid, occasionally vulgar, language, or the engagement with the "brutely
material" (to hark back to Breu's description), but rather the owning of
desire and the speaking of emotion (the investing/imbuing of materiality *with* emotion), betraying an "interest" (in the Tomkins sense of the
term) that refuses to be cowed. In one episode, Bellamy takes an Ambien
and "brainstorms" in her journal, offering us disconnected fragments of
thoughts and feelings:

> As an antidote to my urge to privilege bookish mode over bloggish
> mode, here are my journal rants, typed up, as unedited as possible...
> Notion of embarrassment – pushing towards discomfort... I love the
> idea of giving the impression of the unmediated in writing – to type
> in all caps WHY WON'T YOU FUCKING LOVE ME.[84]

The "notion of embarrassment – pushing towards discomfort" is notably unattributed – whose embarrassment, whose discomfort is at stake,
here? If Bellamy is content to pour out her own minor humiliations in an
"unmediated" way (or rather: in a way that gives "the *impression* of the
unmediated"), she also uses this as part of her attempt to "[seduce] the
reader into profound discomfort."[85] The narrative's metamorphosis from
blog to book also allows Bellamy to reflect upon what constitutes "real
writing" ("bookish mode," as distinct from "bloggish mode") and to see
the gender bias in this: while male poets may be able to present their
"letters and journals" as part of their "writing practice," she wonders:

> Would these guys consider a woman blogging about her heartbreak as
> part of a serious writing practice? I doubt it. Is my refusing to consider
> this blog Real Writing an internalized misogyny? My posts are too
> slight, too femmy, too sloppy (I'm a compulsive reviser), too easy.[86]

Yet she subsequently concludes that "the difference [between blog and
book] isn't about value – one form isn't more valuable than the other –
the difference is about labor and intensity,"[87] and the very form of the
blog – its open-endedness, its participation in collectivity as her readers
respond and empathize, its unfiltered, immediate quality, its multiple
false endings (repeatedly she says, "it's time to wind up the buddhist
vein," before going on to write yet more about him)[88] – these qualities
allow Bellamy the kind of emotional working-through that the end of
the relationship with the buddhist requires. Eventually she must let go,
declaring: "I can no longer hang on to the buddhist – the book, the

person, or the blog. May I be wiped clean of all griping, abandonment, desire, melancholy, and rage."[89]

For Bellamy, the writing of *the buddhist* allows her to fashion her personal narrative as, simultaneously, emotional catharsis and social commentary:

> Writing about the buddhist here has been public display, of course, but it's been a public display of trying to figure something out, I'm not sure what it is – something about desire, obviously, and the trajectory of mourning – but also about boundaries, about secret/public, about embodiment and meaning, and the frailty of the ego, about the embarrassment and shame of being left or rejected, about pushing myself into ever uncomfortable spaces in writing.[90]

Shame – the "shame of being left or rejected" – is not only the subject matter here; it is also both stimulus for and consequence of the "public display" of the text; "public display" indicates, in particular, the functioning of shame as spectacle, as a particular way of *being seen*. Shame speaks both to this testing of "boundaries" and to this engagement with the contradictions, the combined pleasures and terrors, of "embodiment" and selfhood ("the frailty of the ego"); finally, shame also becomes a *mode* of writing here, a narratorial policy of "pushing [oneself] into ever uncomfortable spaces." Importantly, Bellamy herself is not untouched by this – by the shame of what and how she writes – finding herself sometimes "unexpectedly mortified" when giving a reading.[91] As she explains, in "Low Culture":

> I'm working towards a writing that subverts sexual bragging... A female body who has sex writing about sex – no way can I stand in front of an audience reading this stuff and maintain the abstraction the "author"' A BODY some writers glory in this but I feel miserable and invaded – as if the audience has x-ray vision and can see down to the frayed elastic on my panties. But, really, it is I who have invaded my own privacy.[92]

Writing, then, does not release Bellamy from shame; there is nothing triumphalist, consolatory or straightforwardly redemptive in her take on the debasements of the feminine. Bellamy refuses to disavow the uncomfortable visibility of the "female body who has sex writing about sex"; she refuses to separate body and text or to take refuge in "the abstraction the 'author.'" I began this chapter with Probyn's claims that "bringing the dynamics of shame and disgust into prominence" could facilitate "a more visceral and powerful corporeal politics" and a more productive awareness of "the body's capacities for reaching out and spilling across domains that we would like to keep separate, or hidden from view."[93] As I hope I have shown, Bellamy keeps little-to-nothing "hidden from view," and the dynamics of shame and disgust form the larger part of her subject matter and mode of expression. In forcefully confronting her readers with her own particular vulnerability – in allowing that vulnerability to spill out of the text, shamefully, inappropriately, vulgarly even – she emphasizes our own "primary vulnerability," our own, necessary, "interdependence and incompletion," as Butler phrases it, thereby figuring writing as affective community. And in choosing to "[invade her] own privacy," she acknowledges the formative, ineliminable role of shame in both the public and private construction of femininity, and in the act of writing.

Notes

1 Elspeth Probyn, *Carnal Appetites: foodsexidentities* (London: Routledge, 2000), pp. 3, 9.
2 Probyn claims that:

> The moment of disgust that is produced by the encoding of bodies is geared to generating shame in the reader. From shame at one's feelings of disgust, these images sow the seeds of a more visceral accounting of difference, a bodily reaction to bodies.
>
> (Carnal Appetites, p. 129)

But she is really looking here at a very particular kind of disgust – at the body of the other – in a way that fails to take account of the broader experience and remit of disgust, e.g. its protective and/or hygienic function, its connection to dirt and disorder. She also assumes that we will feel shame at our disgust – when in fact it is more likely that we will feel (moral) superiority of some kind. In fact, it seems to me that what she is talking about is not really disgust, and that the self-disgust she touches on (the chapter opens with her averring that: "Like many, I spent much of my childhood feeling disgusting," *Carnal Appetites*, p. 127) is really shame (at bodily/personal imperfection) rather than disgust.
    Probyn quotes Tomkins' view on disgust, that it has "evolved to protect the human being from coming too close" (Silvan Tomkins, *Affect, Imagery, Consciousness Vol. III* (New York: Springer, 1991), p. 15), and suggests that: "Shame, on the other hand, is in part generated by the recognition of having been too close, where proximity to the other has been terminated." (*Carnal Appetites*, p. 133) Again, this is rather too neat an opposition – what Tomkins calls "interest" is not quite the same as "proximity." She suggests that "if taste is socially and historically constructed, then so too must extreme distaste and disgust" [sic], but it doesn't follow that if taste is socially constructed, disgust must be too; arguably there are varieties of disgust that are social and varieties that are biological. When she asks: "why does disgust feel simultaneously so primal and so social?" the answer is simply: because it is both! Or perhaps: because there are different varieties of disgust. Her attempts to present disgust and shame as "distinct yet doubled" are interesting, but tend to result in reductive definitions of each in order to show them as "doubled" (*Carnal Appetites*, p. 133).
3 Probyn, *Carnal Appetites*, p. 134.
4 www.belladodie.com/about/ [accessed 12 July 2016].
5 Dodie Bellamy, "Low Culture," in Mary Burger, Robert Glück, Camille Roy and Gail Scott (eds.), *Biting the Error: Writers Explore Narrative* (Toronto: Coach House Books, 2000), pp. 226–37 (235, 234).

6 Dodie Bellamy, *Academonia* (San Francisco: Krupskaya Books, 2006), p. 126.

7 Silvan Tomkins, "Shame-Humiliation and Contempt-Disgust," in Eve Kosofsky Sedgwick and Adam Frank (eds.), *Shame and Its Sisters* (Durham: Duke University Press, 1995), pp. 133–78 (137).

8 Sandra Bartky, *Femininity and Domination* (London: Routledge, 1990), p. 93.

9 Bartky, p. 84.

10 Bartky, p. 85. As Bartky explains in a footnote, Husseen Abdilahi Bulhan, in *Frantz Fanon and the Psychology of Oppression* (New York: Plenum Press, 1985), "characterizes a 'generalized condition of dishonor' as a status in which one's person lacks integrity, worth and autonomy and in which one is subject to violations of space, time, energy, mobility, bonding and identity." (133, fn6).

11 Bartky, p. 95.

12 Bellamy, *Academonia*, p. 126.

13 Giorgio Agamben, *Remnants of Auschwitz*, trans. by Daniel Heller-Roazen, (New York: Zone Books, 2002), p. 107. My emphasis in second quotation.

14 Peter Stallybrass and Allon White, *The Politics and Poetics of Transgression* (Ithaca: Cornell University Press, 1986), p. 3.

15 Stallybrass and White, pp. 4–5.

16 Christopher Breu, "Disinterring the real: Dodie Bellamy's *The Letters of Mina Harker* and the late-capitalist literature of materiality," *Textual Practice* 26:2 (2012): 263–91 (266).

17 Breu, p. 267.

18 Breu, pp. 268, 271.

19 Eve Kosofsky Sedgwick describes shame as "both peculiarly contagious and peculiarly individuating." See "Queer Performativity: Henry James's *The Art of the Novel*," *GLQ* 1:1 (1993): 1–16 (5).

20 Sarah Todd, "An Interview with Dodie Bellamy," *Girls Like Giants*, 17 April 2012. Accessible at: https://girlslikegiants.wordpress.com/2012/04/17/an-interview-with-dodie-bellamy/ [accessed 12 July 2016].

21 Quoted in, and translated by, Marjorie Perloff, in *Unoriginal Genius: Poetry by Other Means in the New Century* (Chicago: University of Chicago Press, 2010), pp. 3–4.

22 Jennifer Cooke, "*Cunt-Ups* by Dodie Bellamy" [review], *Hix Eros Poetry Review* 5 (2014): 8–10 (8).

23 Sara Wintz, "From Cut-Up to *Cunt Up*: Dodie Bellamy in Conversation," Harriet Poetry Blog at the Poetry Foundation, November 2013. Accessible at: www.poetryfoundation.org/harriet/2013/11/from-cut-up-to-cunt-up-dodie-bellamy-in-conversation/ [accessed 8 December 2016].

24 Dodie Bellamy, "Statement," in Caroline Bergvall, Laynie Browne, Teresa Carmody and Vanessa Place (eds.), *I'll Drown My Book: Conceptual Writing by Women* (Los Angeles: Les Figues Press, 2012), pp. 338–39 (339).

25 Bellamy, *Academonia*, p. 75.

26 Bellamy, "Low Culture," p. 232.

27 Cooke, pp. 9–10.

28 Elspeth Probyn, *Blush: Faces of Shame* (Minneapolis: University of Minnesota Press, 2005), xvii.

29 Timothy Bewes, "The Call to Intimacy and the Shame Effect," *Differences: A Journal of Feminist Cultural Studies* 22:1 (2011): 1–16 (5).

30 Dodie Bellamy, *Cunt-Ups* [2001] in *Tender Omnibus* (New York: Tender Buttons Press, 2016), [Cunt-Up #4].

31 Bellamy, Cunt-Up #13.

32 Bellamy, Cunt-Up #21.

33 Bellamy, Cunt-Up #9.

34 Bellamy, "Statement," in Bergvall et al., p. 338.

35 Bellamy, Cunt-Up #20.

36 Bellamy, Cunt-Up #3.
37 Bellamy, Cunt-Up #4.
38 Bellamy, Cunt-Up #4.
39 Bellamy, Cunt-Up #13.
40 NB this is perhaps even more strikingly the case in Bellamy's later *Cunt Norton* (2013), in which canonical poetry by the likes of Shakespeare, Tennyson, Yeats, and others, taken from the culturally revered *Norton Anthology of Poetry*, is spliced with Bellamy's pornographic narrative; the masculine canon (Emily Dickinson is the only female poet to be "cunted" here) is thus violated by Bellamy's crude language and irreverent, penetrative desire. As Ariana Reyes comments, in her Foreword to *Cunt Norton*: "Shakespeare is commended to his or their proper androgyny [...]. In this book, Ginsberg is better and gayer than Ginsberg. [...] To take the bracing, medicinal Burroughsian cut as far as Dodie Bellamy takes it, such that it both cuts and makes to pour forth, means to render each cut into true congress: to cunt means to mark the spot where rupture and fusion become indivisible." (unpaginated).
41 David Banash, "The History and Practice of Cut-Ups," *American Book Review* 32:6 (2011): 10–11 (10).
42 Bellamy, "Low Culture," p. 232.
43 Edward S. Robinson, *Shift Linguals: Cut-Up Narratives from William S. Burroughs to the Present* (Amsterdam: Rodopi, 2011), p. 43.
44 In early works such as *The Burning Bombing of America* (1972) and *Rip-Off Red, Girl Detective* (1973), Acker makes use of Burroughs-style cut-up, incorporating passages from other works. Her work then shifts, according to Edward S. Robinson's reading, "from syntactic cut-ups toward outright plagiarism and a method that could be more accurately described as cut and paste than cut-up," e.g. in *The Childlike Life of the Black Tarantula by the Black Tarantula* (1973) and *The Adult Life of Toulouse Lautrec by Henri Toulouse Lautrec* (1975). In these works, "Acker intercut larger sections of narrative from different sources. Where she overtly plagiarized from her source texts, by simply copying sections of them out, she sought to 'represent' the texts, and address the question, 'if I repeated the same text, would it be the same text?'" Robinson, p. 154.
45 See, for example: Susan Bordo, *Unbearable Weight* [1993] (Berkeley: University of California Press, 2004); Avril Horner and Angela Keane (eds.), *Body Matters: Feminism, Textuality, Corporeality* (Manchester: Manchester University Press, 2000); Janet Price and Margrit Shildrik (eds.), *Feminist Theory and the Body: A Reader* (New York: Routledge, 1999).
46 Cooke, p. 10.
47 Bellamy, Cunt-Up #19.
48 Dodie Bellamy, *Cunt Norton* (Los Angeles: Les Figues Press, 2013).
49 Andrew Ketcham, "Cunt Norton" [Book review], *New Orleans Review*. Accessible at www.neworleansreview.org/cunt-norton/ [accessed 7 December 2016].
50 Dodie Bellamy, *the buddhist* (Berkeley: Allone Co. Editions, 2011), p. 42.
51 Bellamy, *Academonia*, pp. 74–75.
52 Bellamy, Cunt-Up #1.
53 Bellamy, "Low Culture," p. 232.
54 Bellamy, Cunt-Up #5.
55 Dodie Bellamy, *the buddhist* (San Francisco: Allone Co. Editions, 2011), p. 84.
56 Sarah T., "An Interview with Dodie Bellamy."
57 Bellamy, *the buddhist*, pp. 37, 49.
58 Bellamy, *the buddhist*, pp. 34–35, 42.
59 Sara Ahmed, "Interview with Judith Butler," *Sexualities* 19:4 (2016): 482–92 (485).

60 Judith Butler, *Undoing Gender* (London: Routledge, 2004), p. 30.

61 George Shulman, "On Vulnerability as Judith Butler's Language of Politics: From 'Excitable Speech' to 'Precarious Life,'" *Women's Studies Quarterly* 39:1/2 (2011): 227–35 (232).

62 For more information on Calle's exhibition, see: www.paulacoopergallery. com/exhibitions/sophie-calle-take-care-of-yourself/press-release [accessed 8 January 2017].

63 Anna Watkins Fisher, "Manic Impositions: The Parasitical Art of Chris Kraus and Sophie Calle," *WSQ: Women's Studies Quarterly* 40:1–2 (2012): 223–35 (223, 224).

64 Sarah T., "Interview with Dodie Bellamy."

65 Bellamy, *the buddhist*, p. 89.

66 Quoted in Amelia Jones, *Body Art / Performing the Subject* (Minneapolis: University of Minnesota Press, 1998), p. 3.

67 Bellamy, *Academonia*, p. 115.

68 Bellamy, *the buddhist*, p. 89.

69 Bellamy, *Academonia*, p. 126.

70 Bellamy, *the buddhist*, p. 143.

71 Bellamy, *the buddhist*, p. 144.

72 cf how Susan Bordo, in *Unbearable Weight*, reads "images of unwanted bulges and erupting stomachs" as "a metaphor for anxiety about internal processes out of control – uncontained desire, unrestrained hunger, uncontrolled impulse." (189).

73 Bellamy, *the buddhist*, p. 13.

74 Bellamy, *the buddhist*, pp. 12, 34.

75 Bellamy, *the buddhist*, p. 29.

76 Bellamy, *the buddhist*, p. 35.

77 Bellamy, *the buddhist*, pp. 34–35.

78 Bellamy, *Academonia*, p. 51.

79 Sarah T., "An Interview with Dodie Bellamy."

80 Bellamy, "Statement," in Bergvall et al., p. 338.

81 Kaye Mitchell, "Introduction: The Gender Politics of Experiment," *Contemporary Women's Writing* 9:1 (2015): 1–15.

82 Jennifer Ashton, "Our Bodies, Our Poems," *American Literary History* 19:1 (2007): 211–31 (214); Jennifer Scappettone, "Bachelorettes, Even: Strategic Embodiment in Contemporary Experimentalism by Women," *Modern Philology* 105:1 (2007): 178–4 (180, 181).

83 Bellamy, *Academonia*, pp. 81–82.

84 Bellamy, *the buddhist*, pp. 85–86.

85 Bellamy, *the buddhist*, p. 44.

86 Bellamy, *the buddhist*, p. 73.

87 Bellamy, *the buddhist*, p. 111.

88 Bellamy, *the buddhist*, p. 108.

89 Bellamy, *the buddhist*, p. 130.

90 Bellamy, *the buddhist*, p. 70.

91 Christopher Higgs, "Colonized on Every Level: An Interview with Dodie Bellamy," *The Paris Review*, July 29, 2014. At: www.theparisreview.org/ blog/2014/07/29/colonized-on-every-level-an-interview-with-dodie-bellamy/ [accessed 12 July 2016]. The choice of "mortified" is an interesting one on Bellamy's part; "mortification" can mean both "great embarrassment and shame," and "the action of subduing one's bodily desires" (i.e. "mortification of the flesh") – something that Bellamy notably refuses to do.

92 Dodie Bellamy, "Low Culture," p. 226.

93 Probyn, *Carnal Appetites*, pp. 9, 134.

11 Writing Shame and Disgust in Susan Gubar's *Memoir of a Debulked Woman*

J. Brooks Bouson

Susan Gubar, a scholar whose work is foundational to feminist literary studies, records her experiences as an ovarian cancer patient in her 2012 book *Memoir of a Debulked Woman*.[1] "Enduring ovarian cancer mires patients in treatments more patently hideous than the symptoms originally produced by the disease," writes Gubar, who was sixty-three and approaching retirement when she was diagnosed with advanced ovarian cancer in November of 2008 (3). Aware of the gendered legacy of what Jane Schultz calls a "double silencing" – the "silence surrounding cancer testimony abetted by women's hesitation to relate intimate details about their bodies" (73) – Gubar refuses to resort to euphemism as she writes about her illness, and, instead, chooses to describe, in agonizing detail, her plunge into the horrific world of the bodily abject. Offering testimony about her humiliating experiences as an ovarian cancer patient, and dealing with shameful body matters, she frames her experiences as an ovarian cancer sufferer as an authorial struggle against reticence.

Gubar's *Memoir of a Debulked Woman*, in Jane Schultz's terms, "forces readers into the nether regions of discourse" by giving voice to "what has often been exiled to the realm of the unmentionable" (75). This is evident in responses to Gubar's work. Since publication, commentators have described it variously as a book that is "brutally honest," "difficult to read" and "not for the queasy";[2,3,4] as a "searing" first-person account that is "grueling in its detailed depiction of bodily afflictions";[5] and as a "no-holds-barred" memoir that "will make you flinch in places you didn't know you had".[6] Gubar's writing is certainly frank and expository, and it openly risks shaming and disgusting her readers. In fact, I would like to suggest in this chapter that Gubar is determined to put shame and disgust to work politically in two ways: first, by addressing important questions about the current medical treatments available to women suffering from ovarian cancer, and second, by scrutinizing the range and cultural appropriateness of the emotional and writerly responses to such gendered illnesses.[7]

A Debulked Woman

"Debulking – the surgical removal of a part of a malignant growth that cannot be totally excised – remains the standard initial response to advanced ovarian cancer," explains Gubar, who recalls that when she was first diagnosed she was totally unprepared for the "horrific ordeals" she would undergo as a cancer patient (4, 3). Left in a "stunned state" by the rapidity of her surgery, Gubar decided to record her experiences in "an effort to catalog the physical and mental states" she was passing through "with the hope of then comprehending their significance" as she became subjected to what she calls "the ruthless instruments, technologies, and formulas of the medical machine" (77, 218). Like the "wounded storyteller" described by Arthur Frank in his well-known analysis of illness narratives, Gubar is pointedly aware of the necessity of reclaiming her story and language from the medical machine.[8] "Ill people still surrender their bodies to medicine, but increasingly they try to hold onto their own stories," writes Frank. "Refusing narrative surrender becomes one specific activity of reflexive monitoring, and thus an exercise of responsibility" (16). The wounded storyteller gives voice "to an experience that medicine cannot describe," and, in so doing, seeks to "reclaim" the experience of suffering and "turn that suffering into testimony" (18). As Gubar in the role of the wounded storyteller overcomes her inhibitions and makes the private public by writing about her experiences as a cancer patient, she makes use of her considerable gifts as a literary writer by combining autobiographical writing with critical, literary, and theoretical reflections. Indeed, Gubar's love of the "quirky unpredictability and stylistic panache" she sometimes finds in the personal writings of feminist scholars[9] emerges again and again in her memoir, especially as she writes about shameful or viscerally disgusting matters.[10] A complex autopathographical performance, Gubar's memoir conveys at one and the same time the rupture in Gubar's life caused by her cancer and her attempt as a memoirist and scholar to narratively repair her identity and reclaim her subjectivity from the "medical machine" that has taken over her life. Over and over, Gubar admits that feelings of shame and disgust impede her writing. Crucially, however, it is these same feelings which impel her to complex writerly displays. She intertwines passages of poetry, quotations from other cancer memoirs, scholarly digressions on the female body, as well as cultural, literary and medical accounts of cancer into her narrative alongside repeated descriptions of her suffering and mutilated body.

Even as Gubar draws on heuristic and literary devices to give narrative meaning to her wounded body and traumatized psyche in *Memoir of a Debulked Woman*, she is mindful of Susan Sontag's well-known injunctions against metaphoric thinking in *Illness as Metaphor*.[11] "The most truthful way of regarding illness – and the healthiest way of being ill – is one most purified of, most resistant to, metaphoric thinking," as

Sontag insists (3). Commenting on how the controlling metaphors used to describe cancer draw on military language, Sontag writes:

> There is the "fight" or "crusade" against cancer; cancer is the "killer" disease; people who have cancer are "cancer victims." Ostensibly, the illness is the culprit. But it is also the cancer patient who is made culpable. Widely believed psychological theories of disease assign to the luckless ill the ultimate responsibility for both falling ill and for getting well. And conventions of treating cancer as no mere disease but a demonic enemy make cancer not just a lethal disease but a shameful one.
>
> (57)

In the view of G. Thomas Couser, Sontag has shown us that "the prevailing tropes of cancer add insult to the injury inherent in the disease, imposing a heavy penalty on the ill" (44).[12] Despite this, "much of the discourse that Sontag condemned continues to plague us"; indeed, it is "difficult for individuals, no matter how powerful of intellect," to change cancer discourse, which is "anonymously created and communally perpetuated" (45). But in the view of Martha Stoddard Holmes, "our task, after Sontag, is to rethink metaphor as a site of self-direction rather than one of interpellation by medical discourse".[13] For Holmes, Sontag's argument against metaphors is "dangerous ... as a stopping place":

> A desire to retire certain metaphors is all too easily translated into a "metaphors are bad" or "good metaphor / bad metaphor" policy, and once we start scrutinizing "negative images," it's all too easy to slip into a ban on all images, all representation, because of the inherent potential that our figures will do harm. And, of course, stopping metaphors is like ceasing to eat or to breathe.
>
> ("After Sontag" 265)

Gubar puts it in gentler terms. "Despite Susan Sontag's admonition against illness metaphors, images insist on creeping back," the metaphors for cancer used by other writers (67).

> A cankerworm, eel, embryo, or cockroach; a wilding twin, bully, emperor, beast, assassin, or demon, cancer strengthens itself at the expense of the weakened and unsuspecting human being whom it attacks and within whom it lodges to gain in strength.
>
> (69)

Gubar quotes knowledgeably from a variety of sources as she examines how other writers have described cancer. These include Reynolds Price, who refers to the cancer in his spinal cord as a "lethal eel" and a "lethal twin"; Anne Sexton, who refers to her mother's ovarian cancer as an "embryo/ of evil"; Liz Tilberis, who describes her own ovarian cancer as "a cockroach, defying an arsenal of poisons"; Siddhartha Mukherjee, who calls cancer the "emperor" of disease; and Katherine Russell Rich, who says that cancer makes the body "into its own assailant – its own assassin" (see pages 66–69). As Gubar becomes well-read in cancer memoirs and an expert in the metaphorics of disease, she is careful to contest generic conventions that require her to resort to euphemistic speech when referring to her own sick body. And yet in her harrowing account of her surgery and post-surgical complications, "debulking" remains as the organizing metaphor. As she develops the point in an interview: "Massive amounts of tissue are taken out of your body. Various chunks are taken out of your life. I lost my professional life... Your emotions, your spirit get *debulked*" (italics mine).[14] For Gubar, this metaphor is *real*.

Post-Operative Bodies and Squeamish Language

Reflecting on the general absence of public narratives of ovarian cancer, which has been described as a "silent" or "whispering" disease, Martha Stoddard Holmes remarks that the "'whisper' metaphor" inadvertently calls attention to the shame attached to ovarian cancer since "we whisper about things that are shameful".[15] While Gubar's book is hardly a whisper, neither can it avoid the shame which accompanies bodily abjection. "Rubbing a reader's nose in repugnant body disorders strikes me as a revolting and perverse act," Gubar states at the outset.

> The thought of people I know and people I don't know acquiring intimate information about the most private aspects of my being twists me into knots. I worry, will these people, the known and the unknown, be embarrassed of or for me since at many moments I am ashamed of myself?
>
> (xii)

When Gubar remarks that her decision to write about her shame "twists" her "into knots," she points to the embodiness of shame, the way that shame is "not only a *self*-conscious emotion" but is also "*body*-conscious".[16] Gubar is also aware that writing shame, as Elspeth Probyn has commented, can take a "toll" not only "on the body that writes" but also on "the bodies that read or listen" (140).[17]

Expressing concern for her readers, Gubar worries that people reading her memoir will find it a "yucky downer," and she is aware that some readers may want to turn away in shame or recoil in disgust as they read the "graphic and sometimes gross physical incidents" she includes, material "that not everyone will want to read, but that cannot be excised from reflections on the current treatment of ovarian cancer" (23, 31). Yet despite her at times "almost pathological unwillingness" to describe her bodily condition to others, Gubar overcomes her "reticence or self-censorship" through writing, determined not to resort to what she calls the "squeamish euphemisms" often used to "glamorize the fight against cancer and thus bracket or inhibit efforts to deal with suffering and degradation, deterioration and death" (31, 32). It is through this determination not to self-censor that Gubar's writing attains its political form as a protest, not against a disease, but against a disease's cultural reception and the invasive healthcare protocols which have become its naturally accepted corollary.

> Have you ever heard of a debulked woman? Have you ever seen one? I am one such living, breathing, debulked woman, though no one ever explained to me how such a being comes about, what such a condition means, or how it would feel, so I'm still finding my own debulked ways of being in a decidedly bulky world.
>
> (58)

Gubar remarks that she finds the word "debulked" an "ugly adjective" to describe her postoperative condition: "Think of debulking as evisceration or vivisection or disemboweling, but performed on a live human being" she writes, describing the standard surgery for ovarian cancer, which entails the removal of the ovaries, uterus and fallopian tubes as well as cancerous tissue in the abdominal cavity (59–60). In her postoperative figuration of her debulking, Gubar states that she has been "hollowed at the hub," and when her legs and ankles swell after the surgery, she sees herself as a grotesque spectacle: "an eviscerated trunk borne along by ballooning extremities" (71, 72). "The sick or dysfunctional body trumps not only mind and heart but also volition or will," she avers. "I no longer 'have' or 'relate to' a body. This injured body rules me" (74).

When the "taxidermied" Gubar looks in the mirror, she sees "a pale crone's visage" (76, 75). Enduring a succession of visitors after her surgery as a "surrealistic cancer salon" takes place in her living room, Gubar feels as if she is on display: "'You look great!' accompanies an air kiss hollowed out by bodies withdrawing so as not to hurt me in a tight clasp or so as not to be contaminated by the evil that lurks within me" (82). The social hollowing here is mimetic as the eviscerated body of the patient finds replication in the empty words of the interlocutor: social grace becomes an avoidance measure, social tact an insult to the already violated body. Told after her surgery that she has papillary serous stage III ovarian cancer and that cancerous tissue remains lodged on her bladder, Gubar learns that patients like her have an 80 percent – 85 percent chance of recurrence: without chemotherapy, such patients are likely to survive for a few months, while with chemotherapy they may live an

additional three to five years. Undergoing what she calls "gutting, drain-
ing, bagging, and poisoning," Gubar, after the removal of her uterus,
ovaries, fallopian tubes, appendix, omentum and parts of her colon, endures chemotherapy, even though she is convinced that it will "simply
forestall the inevitable" (33, 102).

As Gubar recounts, sometimes in mortifying detail, her shameful
and disgusting bodily afflictions, she is mindful of the shame and disgust long associated with the female body in Western culture. Because
women are "cast in the role of the body," the negative term in the mind/
body binary, writes Susan Bordo, they come to feel uneasy with their
femaleness, and "shame" and self-loathing over their "degraded" corporeality.[18] Women are also associated with what Julia Kristeva famously
called 'the abject': bodily substances and waste products – such as tears,
saliva, feces, urine, vomit and mucus.[19] The abject is defiling and disgusting, but since it is part of the self and body, it cannot be totally
expelled or rejected. Representing the horror of physical embodiment,
the abject produces a visceral reaction: "Loathing an item of food, a
piece of filth, waste, or dung. The spasms and vomiting protect me. The
repugnance, the retching that thrusts me to the side and turns me away
from defilement, sewage, and muck" (2). In cognate terms, Elizabeth
Grosz calls attention to the bodily shaming of women in our culture as
she describes the "volatile" and unclean female body, which is variously
represented "as a leaking, uncontrollable, seeping liquid; as formless
flow; as viscosity, entrapping, secreting".[20]

Echoing Kristeva and Grosz in her account of the cancerous body with
its loss of control, Gubar offers her own intimate reflections on the abject
and volatile in Western culture when she experiences what other women
writers of cancer memoirs euphemistically call "plumbing problems" (122).

> I have looked through the works of women writers, especially of
> so-called illness narratives and cancer memoirs, but cannot come up
> with anyone who goes beyond vague mentions of 'plumbing prob-
> lems' ... though almost all accounts of chemotherapy mention diar-
> rhea and constipation.
>
> (122)

Reflecting on the vague and uncommunicative – and shame-protective –
speech of other cancer memoirists, Gubar comments:

> "Is this reticence a reaction against the age-old identification of
> women with waste that dates back to the time of the church father
> Tertullian, who defined woman as a 'temple built over a sewer'?. . .
> Possibly because of monthly menstruation or vaginal discharge or
> lactation, the female body in the West has recurrently been imagined
> as a seeping, secreting viscosity".
>
> (122–23)

Perhaps this "ancient connection between females and filth explains why women rarely bring up the topic," she declares (123).

And yet Gubar admits her own squeamishness, specifically around bowel issues: "Despite my inbred reticence, I forge ahead with this writing by keeping in mind a purported comment of Roland Barthes: 'when written ... shit does not smell.' But why am I resorting to academic quoting of academic quoting here?" (123). She finds herself caught in a double bind. Barthes is leading her towards what she wants to say: that *real* shit does smell. Yet, at the same time, the Barthes' citation covers over what she wants to express: academic discourse is too clean, even when it is suspicious of its own procedures of hygiene. Does what Gubar calls her "mini-cultural history" (124) on the long-held association of women with waste and bodily processes serve to parenthesize the squalid body itself? "This long-winded digression is, after all, easier to sustain," she confesses, than writing about her bowel issues (123). If, as some theorists speculate, disgust has until recent times been "shunned as a subject of serious inquiry ... in part because its unsociable stink threatens to transfer to those who study it",[21] then it is fair to say that Gubar embraces "unsociable stink," both as she experiences it and as she represents it – admitting all the while both an embarrassment for the stink of defecation and a concern lest that stink be elided by academic discourse. In sum, Gubar's determination to make the private public by speaking about disgusting body matters is risky business.

As Colin McGinn comments of disgust, because it belongs in "the area of human experience most protected by taboo and hedged with euphemism," it is difficult to talk about. Because the "realm of the disgusting is by its nature repellent" and because dwelling on the topic "can lead quickly to the emotion itself," the act of breaking silence on disgusting phenomena "can elicit alarm" (3).[22] Yet Gubar feels that it is necessary to write through experiences of illness, making them into a matter of public interest, even at the risk of disgusting her readers.[23] Rather than resorting to the "squeamish euphemisms" (32) used by other cancer memoirists, Gubar takes her readers into the realm of the disgusting by describing what happens to her when she is shopping in a supermarket. When she suddenly feels waves of cramps, she cannot "bear the thought of soiling" herself in public:

> The vulnerability of the ill in public places comes home to me. I do not belong in this normal space. I am disabled, deficient... The cancer or the chemo takes the upper hand. I am merely its battered envelope, a conveyance of crap...
>
> (121)

As Gubar develops this account, the shame of defecation and the shame of writing about it occupy the same threshold between the private and public spheres, doubling movements which are literal as well as meta-phorical and linguistic. A rushed trip to the public restroom brings "massive explosions," Gubar writing that "the stink and filth of shit spills out to splash me with self-loathing, a numb sense of my own stained, sullied being" (124, 125). Sara Ahmed has noted how the speech act "That's disgusting!" is "performative," for it "can work as a form of vomiting, as an attempt to expel something whose proximity is felt to be threatening and contaminating," and thus to "designate something as disgusting is also to create a distance from the thing" (93, 94).[24] Accordingly, when Gubar speaks and writes about her body disgust and describes feeling a loss of bodily control, she uses alliterative speech to channel her bodily experiences. "Explosive, my body has become an excremental and execrable traitor... If our bodies are indeed ourselves, my self shames me with its interminable or un-voidable waste" (126–27). Repeated "s" sounds or the harsher "ex" sound evoke and emphasize the bodily experience she is describing as the *s*tink of *s*hit *s*pills and *s*plashes her with a *s*elf-loathing for her *s*tained and *s*ullied being and her *ex*plosive body becomes an *ex*cremental and *ex*ecrable traitor. Indeed, as we (the readers) mouth, or spit out, these words, we perform in our speech the kind of spitting out behavior that, as Ahmed notes, is provoked by an aversive disgust response. Beyond squeamishness and sentiment then, the expulsive physicality of language creates a bodily intimacy between the reader and the written text in Gubar's memoir.

Over the course of her treatment, Gubar endures medical procedure after medical procedure because of the complications she suffers from her debulking. Ending up with a leak from a hole in her sutured colon, she develops an abscess that must be drained through a long tube inserted into her right buttock and then through two larger drains. After that, she must undergo an ileostomy, a procedure in which a loop of the small intestine is brought up through the skin of her abdomen. "Presumably, I am too well educated to be ashamed by a physiological phenomenon beyond my control, but all the social mores surrounding evacuation and excretion conspire to make the ileostomy unspeakable and unspeakably anxiety-provoking" (155). From the stoma – the rust-red knob of intestine pulled outside the body – comes a mass of brown liquid that collects in a pouch which she then empties into the toilet. "I am perpetually dirty, defecating incessantly from my belly" (153), Gubar says of this further bodily humiliation. Deliberately she mires her readers in the disgusting as she describes her damaged, mutilated body and the "liquefied crap" that intermittently erupts from the stoma (152).

> I cannot help but think that the stoma seems and feels like an anti-phallus. Moist and concentrically circled, it looks like the thick last joint of a fat finger or the tip of a circumscribed boy's penis. When it is doing its peristaltic spasms (to eject waste), this small spigot

bears a resemblance to the head of a one-eyed snake or slug trying to worm its way out of my stomach.

(155–56)

The term "anti-phallus," which is suggestive of an inverted symbolic relation to desire, marks a living fascination with what is most repellent – the disgusting protuberance which belongs yet does not belong to the mutilated body. As Katie Jones observes,

> the fact that we sometimes choose to imagine disgusting things at all, to the extent of lingering on the particular details that make them disgusting [reveals] an element of attraction that can draw our attention towards the object of our disgust even as we are repelled.
>
> (11–12)

In her determination to tell the truth about her body, Gubar seems aware of, and intent on satisfying, the morbid curiosity of her readers, while equally conveying her own fascinated horror and visceral disgust at the sight of her mutilations.

When Gubar reads a scholarly book about cancer literature that draws on postmodern and feminist theories of the body to argue that women writing about cancer can employ the "trope of leakiness" in order to "reclaim their medicalized bodies," she finds the author's theory-laden (and shame and disgust avoiding) argument not only "offensive" but also "silly":

> I hooted at the idea that bodily 'leaks can be reconceptualized as a transgressive form of fluid embodiment' ... More revolting than revolutionary, my encounters with 'fluid embodiment' involved being drained and bagged in ways that would make me gag for months afterward.
>
> (129)[25]

Describing the "capacity" of disgust to "take hold" of our bodies, Rachel Herz comments that disgust is "literally a gut emotion," and thus many of the ways we describe the things that disgust us – "sickening," "nauseating," "it makes me want to vomit" – refer to digestion (197).[26] When Gubar describes how her contact with bodily fluids and waste products makes her "gag," she reveals the viscerality of disgust and the powerful way it can "hijack" the mind (see Herz 38) and take hold of the physical body. Again and again, she impresses us with her linguistic play and verbal inventiveness as she writes about "foul matters" (155), yet she also repeatedly brings readers back to the disgusting and shameful reality of her wounded body in order to heighten the visceral impact of her memoir. Gubar is clearly aware that her account of her mutilated and leaky body may provoke disgust in her readers. But she repeatedly returns to the physically awful and viscerally disgusting in her account as she offers a pointed political and feminist critique of the horrific medical treatments she must undergo as an ovarian cancer patient.

Entering a "barely sentient level of existence" as the side effects of her chemotherapy accumulate, Gubar describes what she calls the "posthumous existence" of chemo-time (175, 166). The Keatsian reference is apt, suggesting as it does the attempt to write beyond idealism and towards the precarity of the body; to write through the humiliation of dying – to momentarily survive one's own death – by openly exhibiting it in its most shameful aspect. Although she experiences a "rush of returning vitality" after the chemotherapy ends, she is aware that she is "healthy-but-only-for-a-while" (209, 215).

> In a remission of advanced ovarian cancer, it is impossible to consider the body purified or cleansed since it often harbors cancerous cells that will return… A better term for my condition might be dormancy, for the cancer is not gone but dormant, and therefore being in remission does not make me a cancer survivor.
>
> (215)

While cancer stories often present the cancer patient as a heroic individual doing battle with the invader disease and follow the classic cancer plot trajectory of "crisis, rescue, and recovery" (Stacey 7),[27] Gubar's memoir offers no final sense of triumph over disease.[28] "The life I have left to lose remains a shadowy semblance of my existence before cancer," Gubar realizes (228). By finishing her memoir two years and one month after her diagnosis, Gubar achieves the "happiest ending" she can imagine, and her hope is that her book will "do some good work in the world" (263, xiii).

Living on

In their feminist analysis of the recent history of women's illness narratives, Sayantani DasGupta and Marsha Hurst write that contemporary women's illness narratives speak "what was once unspoken, making public what was once private" (1).[29] Because until recent times the experience of illness was considered "the sole purview of the medical practitioner," the story of women's illnesses "is the story of the personal made public or, if you will, made political" (1, 5). Just as post-1960s feminism has helped spur a women's health movement and health-care activism, so it has also given women suffering from cancer, a disease that in certain forms has been viewed as a stigmatizing illness, both "the motivation and confidence" to write about their experiences as cancer patients. Accordingly, the number of works by women detailing their experiences with cancer "has increased exponentially since the early 1990s" (De-Shazer 5, 1). Yet while there has been a "proliferation of breast cancer accounts," there remains a "paucity" of memoirs about ovarian cancer,[30] which is something that Gubar set out specifically to help remedy in *Memoir of a Debulked Woman.*

Taking "an activist's stance" (xiii) she not only reclaims her experiences, but she also refuses symbolically coded optimism. Instead, she does battle with her reticence through writing. Gubar clearly believes that her writing is politically important and that by recording her experiences she can help others. Yet beyond this point of principle, she seems compelled by illness to write of the shameful body in terms which resist the seductions of a redemptive narrative, or fully therapeutic remedy, but rather which return consistently to the indignity of living with, and the prospect of dying from, ovarian cancer. Gubar's frequent admissions that she is both ashamed and disgusted add a sense of emotional vulnerability to this testimony, at once challenging the reader with the abjection of the cancer sufferer and using the *debulked* body to frame pointed questions about the current treatment of ovarian cancer patients and the broader cultural reception of the disease.

Since the publication of *Memoir of a Debulked Woman,* up to the time of writing this chapter in 2016, Gubar has continued with her task of writing about her experiences in a series of *New York Times* blogs. Enrolled in a targeted-therapy clinical trial of an experimental drug in 2012, Gubar passed her five-year survival prognosis in November 2013 and she describes her response to her "cancer-versary" in a November 2014 blog. The "shocking impact of a cancer diagnosis needs to be remembered," she writes, for "it marks a disruptive discontinuity in consciousness," and its anniversary "commemorates an end and a beginning – in this case a traumatic beginning." Aware that her "death sentence has not been commuted but temporarily stayed," she finds herself enjoying her "gravy days." "I am a lucky woman, reveling in the unearned bounty of more time and a thicker earthly existence than I had ever expected".[31]

Yet Gubar also reflects in a later piece on what it is like living in the "cancer closet." "While coping with cancer, I often feel like an impersonator of my former self," writes Gubar.[32]

> I am a sick person trying to appear healthy. While the contest between destructive cells and aggressive therapies persists, it seems strategic to pretend to be normal. All sorts of props – a wig, make-up, hats, billowing pants and shirts – provide a semblance of what I used to look like" ("In and Out of the Closet").

Thus while Gubar has been very public in her discussion of her illness, she nevertheless finds herself hiding her shameful cancer identity in her daily life and trying to pass as normal. In this way, shame is there, always necessary, always to be confronted again.

Notes

1 Gubar, Susan. *Memoir of a Debulked Woman: Enduring Ovarian Cancer.* New York: W. W. Norton, 2012.
2 Kirkus Reviews. *Memoir of a Debulked Woman* (review). (9 April 2012). Available online at www.kirkusreviews.com/book-reviews/susan-gubar/memoirdebulked-woman/ [accessed 11 February 2017].
3 Geffner, Mira. *Memoir of a Debulked Woman* (review). (16 January 2014). *Bay Area Cancer Connections.* Available online at http://bcconnections.org/ovarian-cancer/susan-gubar/ [accessed 11 February 2017].
4 Rogers, Deborah, and Karen Shook. "Silent Killer's Eloquent Victim." *Times Higher Education Supplement* (30 August 2012): 42. Available online at www.timeshighereducation.co.uk/books/memoir-of-a-debulked-woman-enduring-ovariann-cancer/420982.article.
5 Bladek, Marta. "Memoir of a Debulked Woman: Enduring Ovarian Cancer (review)." *Medical Humanities* 39.2 (2013): 142–43.
6 Mintz, Susannah. "Memoir of a Debulked Woman: Enduring Ovarian Cancer (review)." *Literature and Medicine* 30.2 (Fall 2012): 370–77.
7 Remarking on the ways in which the second-wave feminist movement "put shame to work politically," Janice Irvine writes that "feminists helped transform the broader emotional culture and, in the process, helped push shame out of the closet in their attempts to either heal it or convert it to anger" (74). Feminists also put shame to work in the 1980s: "Identifying and confronting shame was pivotal to feminist abortion rights and anti-violence politics, particularly in the child sexual abuse movement of the 1980s," and the act of "putting shame into the public conversation on sexual abuse was part therapy and part politics" (74).[33] In a similar way, when Gubar puts shame into the public conversation about ovarian cancer, her act of writing is "part therapy" and "part politics."
8 Frank, Arthur. *The Wounded Storyteller: Body, Illness, and Ethics.* Chicago, IL: University of Chicago Press, 1995.
9 Gubar, Susan. "Introduction." *True Confessions: Feminist Professors Tell Stories Out of School.* Ed. Susan Gubar. New York: W.W. Norton, 2011. ix–xviii.
10 In the introduction to her 2011 edited collection *True Confessions: Feminist Professors Tell Stories Out of School*, Gubar recalls that, when she solicited essays for the collection from leading feminist scholars, she wanted to capture in the personal accounts of her writers "the quirky unpredictability and stylistic panache" that she missed in much of the "rigorous scholarship" she perused to "keep up in the field" (xi). She was also fascinated, as a literary scholar, with examples of feminist criticism that paid regard to the "aesthetic pleasures" that had attracted her to the study of literature in the first place (xv). In *Memoir of a Debulked Woman*, Gubar offers an example of this hybrid style.
11 Sontag, Susan. *Illness as Metaphor.* 1977, 1978. New York: Random House–Vintage, 1979.
12 Couser, G. Thomas. *Recovering Bodies: Illness, Disability, and Life Writing.* Madison: University of Wisconsin Press, 1997.
13 Holmes, Martha Stoddard. "After Sontag: Reclaiming Metaphor." *Genre: Forms of Discourse and Culture* 44.3 (Fall 2011): 263–76.

14 Szabo, Liz. "Professor Writes about Painful Effects of Ovarian Cancer." *USA Today* (20 May 2012). Available online at http://usatoday30.usatoday.com/news/health/story/2012–05–20/Susan-Gubar-ovarian-cancer/55092236/1 [accessed 11 February 2017].

15 Holmes, Martha Stoddard. "Pink Ribbons and Public Private Parts: On Not Imagining Ovarian Cancer." *Literature and Medicine* 25.2 (Fall 2006): 475–501.

16 Nurka, Camille. "Feminine Shame/Masculine Disgrace: A Literary Excursion through Gender and Embodied Emotion." *Cultural Studies Review* 18.3 (December 2012): 310–33.

17 Probyn, Elspeth. *Blush: Faces of Shame*. Minneapolis: University of Minnesota Press, 2005.

18 Bordo, Susan. *Unbearable Weight: Feminism, Western Culture, and the Body*. Berkeley: University of California Press, 1993.

19 Kristeva, Julia. *Powers of Horror: An Essay on Abjection*. Trans. Leon Roudiez. New York: Columbia University Press, 1982.

20 Grosz, Elizabeth. *Volatile Bodies: Toward a Corporeal Feminism*. Bloomington: Indiana University Press, 1994.

21 Miller, Susan. *Disgust: The Gatekeeper Emotion*. Hillsdale, NJ: The Analytic Press, 2004.

22 McGinn, Colin. *The Meaning of Disgust*. Oxford and New York: Oxford University Press, 2011.

23 An aversive reaction, disgust centers around "the urge to pull away from, get rid of, and generally avoid that which is causing the feeling," writes Rachel Herz (29). Thus, disgust is described as "a viscerally felt rejection" (Jones 11)[34] of objects or substances that elicit disgust. As Carolyn Korsmeyer explains:

> Numerous studies have demonstrated that peoples across the globe ... respond to the same categories of elicitors. The objects that arouse disgust include bodily waste products: excrement, pus, menstrual blood. ... Infections and mutilations are included, along with the gore that they can produce, for the organs and fluids that properly function hidden away in our interiors become disgusting when loosed from the envelope of the skin. (754)[35]

While the "elicitors for disgust are fundamentally sensory," notes Korsmeyer, disgust is such a "powerful" emotion that "even an imagined scene brings on recoil; hence its force when deployed by artists" (755).

24 Ahmed, Sara. *The Cultural Politics of Emotion*. New York: Routledge, 2004.

25 DeShazer, Mary K. *Fractured Borders: Reading Women's Cancer Literature*. Ann Arbor: University of Michigan Press, 2005.

26 Herz, Rachel. *That's Disgusting: Unraveling the Mysteries of Repulsion*. New York: W.W. Norton, 2012.

27 Stacey, Jackie. *Teratologies: A Cultural Study of Cancer*. New York and London: Routledge, 1997.

28 In the view of Kathlyn Conway, illness narratives disseminate "the cultural story of triumph" (17).[36] In our culture, "we hide suffering" and insist that those who are ill and disabled

> rise above their suffering, battle their disease, and believe that everything will be fine in the end.... By subscribing so insistently to the narrative of triumph, we participate in a hysterical denial, as if by chanting 'triumph' we can ward off mortality. (18)

The standard and oft-repeated story of "self-improvement by breast cancer," writes Judy Segal, contains these components: "I found a lump; I was scared; I stayed positive and I fought; I recovered; now I am a better person; in some ways, cancer is the best thing that ever happened to me." To Segal, this story is not only "unwaveringly self-righteous" but by insisting on the necessity of a positive attitude, it is "coercive" (311).[37] Kirsten Gardner argues in a similar vein that the dominant cancer narratives of early detection then cure and a return to normalcy, which are used in the contemporary pink ribbon breast cancer campaign,

> celebrate survival and awareness, but rarely address the bleaker realities of cancer. Pink symbolizes breast cancer without telling us much about it. Where do women encounter narratives about caregivers who hold the shoulders of patients vomiting violently after a round of chemo? Or about bathing the breast cancer patient who is too weak to wash herself? (335)[38]

While disruptive cancer texts have challenged this detection-and-cure storyline, "early detection has remained a powerful and pervasive trope," one that "unifies women around a simple, straightforward, and hopeful message of triumph over breast cancer" (345).

29 DasGupta, Sayantani, and Marsha Hurst. "The Gendered Nature of Illness." *Stories of Illness and Healing: Women Write Their Bodies.* Ed. Sayantani DasGupta and Marsha Hurst. Kent, OH: Kent State University Press, 2007. 1–7.

30 Schultz, Jane. "Valid/Invalid: Women's Cancer Narratives and the Phenomenology of Bodily Alteration." *Tulsa Studies in Women's Literature* 32.2/33.1 (Fall 2013 / Spring 2014): 71–87.

31 Gubar, Susan. "Living with Cancer: Gravy Days." *New York Times blog* (20 November 2014). Available online at http://well.blogs.nytimes.com/2014/11/20/living-withcancer-gravy-days/ [accessed 11 January 2017].

32 Gubar, Susan. "Living with Cancer: In and Out of the Closet." *New York Times blog* (16 April 2015). Available online at http://well.blogs.nytimes.com/2015/04/16/living-with-cancer-in-and-out-of-the-closet/.

33 Irvine, Janice. "Shame Comes Out of the Closet." *Sexuality Research & Social Policy* 6.1 (March 2009): 70–79.

34 Jones, Katie. *Representing Repulsion: The Aesthetics of Disgust in Contemporary Women's Writing in French and German.* New York: Peter Lang, 2013.

35 Korsmeyer, Carolyn. "Disgust and Aesthetics." *Philosophy Compass* 7.11 (2012): 753–61.

36 Conway, Kathlyn. *Illness and the Limits of Expression.* Ann Arbor: University of Michigan Press, 2007. Reprinted under the title *Beyond Words: Illness and the Limits of Expression.* Albuquerque: University of New Mexico Press, 2013.

37 Segal, Judy. "Cancer Experience and Its Narration: An Accidental Study." *Literature and Medicine* 30.2 (Fall 2012): 292–318.

38 Gardner, Kirsten. "Disruption and Cancer Narratives: From Awareness to Advocacy." *Literature and Medicine* 28.2 (Fall 2009): 333–50.

12 On Writing-Up
Shame and Clinical Writing

Oliver Sacks and Julie Walsh

...it still strikes me myself as strange that the case histories I write should read like short stories and that, as one might say, they lack the serious stamp of science. I must console myself with the reflection that the nature of the subject is evidently responsible for this, rather than any preference of my own.

—Sigmund Freud, 1895[1]

I have no "literary" aspirations whatever, and if I write "Clinical Tales" it is because I am *forced* to; because they do not seem to me a gratuitous or arbitrary compound of two forms, but an elemental form which is indispensable for medical understanding, practice, and communication.

—Oliver Sacks, 1986[2]

I have always been intrigued by the logic of writing *down* notes (clinical or otherwise) in order then to write them *up*. What is it exactly that happens between these stages of writing? Can we really say that the first is a simple act of recording or documenting, while the second is a more elaborate process of reconstruction? The "write up" perhaps brings to mind the more ambiguous notion of the "stitch up" with its connotations of fabrication and willful misrepresentation. Similarly, the figurative use of the verb "to doctor" – as in *to doctor the evidence* – might remind us of the multiple powers that reside in the personage of the physician who may be writing up and/or stitching up your case. It would seem that the capacity to disguise or dissemble is somehow integral to the project of clinical writing. But so too must the idea of the "stitch up" imply the physician's care, his work of suturing a wound, or attending to the frayed nerves of a patient. Finding its high point in the clinical narrative or case history, the ameliorative power of storytelling can also be read as a desire to assuage the patient's suffering; to give form to the fractured or dislocated elements of experience. And what of the pleasures of spinning a yarn?

From his first book, *Migraine*,[3] to one of his last, *Hallucinations*,[4] Oliver Sacks finessed the art of the "clinical tale." With it he conveyed the many ways in which the fabric of one's personal identity can become unstitched by a range of neuropathological phenomena. As a medical practitioner and a writer, Sacks held that the greatest endeavor of medicine was to help an individual construct a life; this meant that medicine's modes of communication needed to be equal to the task. For Sacks, to rehabilitate the case history as a form of writing inevitably means that the patient's story becomes the tale of an embattled protagonist striving to preserve a coherent identity in adverse circumstances.[5] Sacks often reminded his audience of the historical drift since the nineteenth century that occurred in science writing – and in medicine in particular – towards greater classification at the expense of detailed descriptions of the patient's idiosyncratic experience. His attention to the idiosyncratic details, and the care he took in presenting them, doubtless accounts for his ongoing appeal as a writer and his success as a physician. But are there any tensions between the dramatic impulse of the case history, thus conceived, and the physician's fidelity to the facticity of the case? If the case history is to become germane to medical methodology once more, how are we to think about its production of "truth" (whether for the patient, the doctor and/or the reader)? And most curiously, for me at least, in what ways does the storyteller reveal *himself* in the act of telling *another's* story?

I first engaged with Sacks' work as an undergraduate student of sociology: we were learning to think about the relation between identity, memory, and trauma, both from the personal or autobiographical perspective, and in relation to questions of collective identity in the context of twentieth-century cultural history. In *The Man Who Mistook His Wife for a Hat* (or his *Hat* book, as Sacks called it),[6] we found stories to demonstrate the precariousness of personal identity. Critically, for the student of sociology, Sacks' work offered an unusual lens – what we might call the lens of "neurological self-hood" – for viewing how one's capacity to sustain a stable sense of self can be disrupted.

Some years later, when I returned to Sacks' work, it was with a view to thinking about the affinities between his research questions and those of psychoanalysis. In 2013, I had the opportunity to ask Dr. Sacks to reflect on the place of psychoanalysis, and of Sigmund Freud, in his life and work; it was clear that there were several lines of thought to pursue. Freud, the writer of case histories, provides a clear precedent for Sacks. Then there is the *therapeutic* experience of psychoanalysis to consider, especially its clinical practice of reading the self beyond its most obvious presentations. Indeed, Sacks discussed with me how his long-standing personal analysis may have strengthened his habit and skill as a listener. But perhaps it is the early Freud – the neurologist in gradual pursuit of a scientific psychology – that Sacks was most able to admire.[7] In the course of our interview, Sacks told me about his great love for marine biology, and how at one point in his career – "between the chemical days and the medical days" – he had wanted to spend his life's work on the nervous systems and behaviors of invertebrates. If it is difficult to reconcile such a wish with the deeply *human* commitment to medicine and science for which Sacks is now renowned, we should remember that the impulse to keep these dimensions distinct – to carve up the world according to different *kinds* in order to limit one's engagement with it – runs counter to Sacks' general approach. Sacks told me that one of the things Freud had a very clear feeling about was the importance of *continuity* between all life forms: "in his paper on crayfish ganglia [Freud] brings out that the nerve cells are essentially similar to the nerve cells of mammals or human beings; it's not the nerve cells ... which are different, but their number and organisation." The provocative question that Sacks raises from Freud's commitment to continuity concerns the boundaries of mental life: where does mental life begin and end? For Sacks' Freud, the mental is not confined to human beings.

When I met with Dr. Sacks, he warned me that he had a tendency to "gabble" and that my questions were "liable to release ten minutes of nonsense" from him. Nothing could have been further from the truth, but we did hit upon a felicitous affinity between his areas of research expertise and the particular mode of attention that allows for productive meanderings off topic (or *seemingly* off topic). I had asked about the rituals that attach themselves to his writing habit. Sacks, by and large, has always been a hand writer. His desk was sectioned with different papers, pads, and numerous pens ordered for various purposes, and his shelves were stacked with journals and notebooks going back years; there were three journals (A5 hardback notebooks) that contained notes from a single month in 1987. He mentioned his preference for a particular thick-paged notebook in which one can write on both sides and, critically, that has no lines. "Do you know what delirium means, literally?" asked Sacks. "It means not staying between the lines." A quick consultation with the nearby dictionary confirmed it: delirium from *dēlīrāre:* prefix *de* as in from, and *lira* as in furrow; "so it's to turn, to turn away from the furrow." Likewise, he told me, *Hallucinations* – the title of his most recent book – connotes a wandering in mind, or not sticking to the point.

Many of the wanderings our conversation took have not been captured in the extract below: for example, the importance of recognizing the existence of mental life in non-human species; the distinction between "mind" and "brain"; the possibility of a basic incompatibility between "organic" etiologies and what we might call "psychosocial" ones. Such are the omissions of this particular write-up. What follows focuses on the line of discussion to which we kept returning: namely, what it means to write a case history. By the end of our time together, Sacks had impressed on me the challenge of being "essentially faithful" to the clinical material in question whilst not disavowing the inevitable "gap between experience and art."

***

OS: I'm in a writing spell now [September 2013], but I wasn't a month ago and I had an arid time in the summer.

JW: Can you sit quite comfortably with that?

OS: No! I'm a miserable person then, and I make other people miserable.

JW: Unless you're writing?

OS: When I'm writing I become much happier; the neuroses fall away, I don't bother people, I see the best of people, I elicit the best of people. And, in this way, writing is absolutely essential for my health and well-being.

JW: One of the questions you ask in your work, and it's a problem I'm also very taken by, is the question of what constitutes a *tenable life*. I noticed in *The New York Times* recently,[8] you evoked the Freudian wisdom whereby what makes a life tenable is the capacity to love and work.[9] It's interesting to hear you reflect on the fact that writing, for you, makes your life tenable, so to speak. I think this really does key into your emphasis on the value of narrative, doesn't it?

OS: On the value of work.

JW: Yes, and work.

OS: Yes, in particular *your* work; *one's work*, which is also one's identity, or part of one's identity. Although I don't know that I've ever quite identified myself as a writer. I was asked in an interview some years ago, what are you first, a physician or a writer? I said a physician but they inverted the order and said a writer, which sort of annoyed me. Though I think the real answer is that they tend to go together and perhaps (as if I were a novelist) people around me – my friends as well as my patients – are in danger, so to speak, because they may be turned into material!

Although, with my patients I'm slow to write about them, I feel I have to know them fairly well, and then I will discuss the matter with them and see how they feel. I'm not satisfied with a formal consent; I have to feel they would be comfortable and I will usually send them what I write and ask them to correct or comment. By that time they may say, I've changed my mind, leave me out.

JW: Ah, okay, and will you do that, if they have changed their mind?

OS: If it's a radical change of mind I might. Or there may be minor changes. This was the case with one relatively early piece of mine on a man with Tourette's called *Witty Ticcy Ray* which was later collected in the *Hat* book.[10] [When I wrote the piece] I'd been seeing him at that point for ten years, since '71. And I asked Ray (this was not his real name) if he'd care to read it and he said, "no, that's okay, I trust you." And I said, "well I think you should read it," and he said, "well, okay, why don't you come to dinner on Friday?" As he was reading it, I noticed various tics and I was getting nervous and he said rather explosively, "*you take some liberties!*" I pulled out my red pen and said, "what should I erase, what should I change?" In the end, he shook his head and said, "leave it, it's *essentially true*," he said, "but don't publish here in New York – why don't you publish it in England?" So it was published in *The London Review of Books*. At that point I thought that if I published in London it would, to some extent, protect my patients in New York – although I'd learned with *Awakenings* that this was not always the case. One of my *Awakenings* patients, a very bright woman who got wind of the fact that the book had been published in England, somehow got a copy. And now, if I write a piece, it's "out there."

Which reminds me, I'm bewildered and often horrified about the nature of blogs, which seem to erase some of the distinction between private and public, and I think they're rather dangerous.

JW: But isn't that also a danger that your work inevitably encounters?

OS: Yes.

JW: So, Ray's response, "you take some liberties" is relevant here. First of all, there's the very simple truth that we can never know whether the patient is going to be able to say, "yes, that does me justice," or "yes, that accords with my own understanding of the situation," or "that is essentially true." And this is precisely one of the dangers of clinical writing; the inevitable misrepresentations and moments that expose a disconnect between two different accounts of an experience. It can be quite anxiety inducing! But then again, and I think your work demonstrates this so well, clinical writing is also enjoyable. In my own work, I worry about that enjoyment. Because, well, it's a difficult type of enjoyment – or pleasure – to take, isn't it?

OS: It is. And it's a very central thing for me. My *Migraine* book has only little vignettes and there are really no recognizable characters. But then in 1970, I submitted some letters – medical letters – to the *Lancet* about some of my patients on L-dopa. A few weeks later the sister of one of my patients came up to me holding the *New York Daily News* in her hand and she said, "is this your medical discretion?" Unknown to me, the *Lancet* had released the letter to a wire service, and it had been picked up by a newspaper here. She wasn't upset or offended, she said probably no one but immediate family would have recognized her sister. But this worried me somewhat. I usually make some disguise, alter identifying details, but obviously in that letter I had not disguised enough.

JW: And perhaps even the notion of "disguise" is problematic?

OS: Yes.

JW: Because that's actually about literary creation, isn't it? So, in ethically disguising the identity of the patient, one is also creatively dissembling.

OS: Yes.

JW: And fictionalizing!

OS: Right. Yes, well with Ray it was fairly light: I changed his name and I changed where he lived. But to what extent is dissembling, as you put it, compatible with truth? Big question!

JW: It is the big question!

OS: Something drifted in and out of my mind. I want to say this: It has been brought up in various forms, sometimes rather traumatic forms; a critic called Tom Shakespeare once called me "the man who mistakes his patients for a literary career," which hurt, and which stays in my mind even thirty years later. I feel that first as a physician I have to respect the patient, and to be tactful and delicate. There are some things where curiosity would make me want to push further and I have to say, no, at least not now. I hope my writings, such as they are, are in the mode of delicacy and respect.

I was very pleased when Mrs. P, the woman mistaken for a hat, after her husband's death, went to see the opera by Michael Nyman.[11] I watched her closely at the performance, wondering what [she'd make of the piece], but she came up to us, the script writer and the musician and myself, and she said, "You have done honor to my husband." And that was very nice; we all gave a big gasp of relief.

JW: Yes! So I wonder if your solemn feeling of responsibility impacts on whether or not you wish to collaborate with others in your writing? I mean I've noticed that you include your readers and the correspondence you get with your readers as part of your practice.

OS: I do now.

JW: So in a way I suppose we can think of your use of letters as a collaborative writing practice. But, exempting the artworks, have you ever wanted to actually sit down and write collaboratively with another?

OS: I think the simple answer is no. Peter Brook phoned me some years ago and said he wanted to do a theatre evening called "The Man Who..." drawing on many things. I introduced him to one or two patients, and I then basically said, "it's up to you." And I felt the same with Pinter when he wrote *A Kind of Alaska*.[12] In the movie of *Awakenings*, I was there only as a sort of technical advisor, for medical details.[13] I disliked one scene in the movie when there's a sort of fight in the lobby of the hospital and I walked off the set angrily. When I saw it made no difference, I came back to the set quietly and kept my mouth shut and thought, it's theirs, not mine.

JW: I'm really curious to hear how you understand the relationship between your clinical writing and the writing of your own memoir; your own case history. These two modes of writing have to be in dialogue somehow. And I think my feeling is that all writing is autobiographical.

OS: Yes, Tolstoy said that everything he wrote was part of one giant confession. And then of course Joyce talks about the artist being ubiquitous but invisible. I fear I've let myself become more and more visible!

JW: And why would that be a fear?

OS: Well, in *Awakenings*[14] more than *Migraine* I had become a figure in patients' lives. I got the drug, I watched them, I felt guilty and appalled when they started to get bad effects of one sort or another, and when one of my patients then called L-dopa "Hell-dopa." I lived through the whole experience with them. But in a way, my *Leg* book [*A Leg to Stand On*][15] became a sort of case history of myself, and in *The Mind's Eye*,[16] I've given an explicit account of being a patient. But also, I think in other books I've sort of thrown myself in, as I would throw anyone in, because of a particular phenomenon or symptom. So say in my chapter on *amusia*, in *Musicophilia*,[17] I mention a couple of times when I had *amusia* with a migraine, as part of a migraine aura. And in *The Mind's Eye*, when I'm writing about *alexia*, I again mention a personal example.

JW: So, you become a character in the lives of your patients, and you can also use yourself as a resource when you've been a patient in a particular medical context. But there's another context in which your patient-hood is at stake, and you allow us just a slight glimpse of this in your *Hallucinations* book.

OS: Oh yes, my Chapter Six.

JW: Yes, your chapter on "Altered States." So, you tell us that in the mid-sixties you entered an analysis following your friend's astute observation that your experimentation with mind-altering drugs may in fact be masking some inner conflicts. I'd be very interested to hear about what it was like to be that type of patient, and also to think with you about how the experience of analysis may have mapped on to the development of your ethos and your style as a writer.

OS: Well, in December, New Year's Eve of '65, when I was fizzing and sort of manic with amphetamine, and had lost a great deal of weight, I had a sort of lucid moment when I saw my gaunt – my then gaunt – face in the mirror and I said to myself, "you will not see another New Year's Day unless there's intervention." I had been seeing an analyst a little bit in Los Angeles, it didn't seem to get anywhere, partly I think because I was always stoned when I saw him, or often stoned. This allowed me to produce some associations with vertiginous rapidity but they were somehow, you know, all on the surface of my mind; nothing really got in, or went deep. In Los Angeles when Dr. Bird said to me, "why are you here?" I said, "ask Dr. Bonnard, she referred me!" So, you know, my heart wasn't in it. Whereas in '66, I sought help for myself, knowing I was in danger. The analyst I saw then is still my analyst; I saw him yesterday and we are now in our forty-seventh, forty-eighth year.

JW: My goodness me!

OS: I see him twice a week and if I'm away somewhere I will phone if I can. I've even phoned from a cell phone from the middle of a desert, or something like that. And I dedicated my *Hat* book to him.

I think that the habit and skill of listening carefully, not interrupting too much, and trying to divine what may be going on behind the words is a sort of – I think this has to be the case with all doctors and maybe with all people – has been strengthened by seeing him.

I think one no longer speaks of analysts as "Freudian" or whatever, but although my own analyst has the *Collected Works* [of Freud], doubtless, he is very sensitive to biological factors as well. I think I mentioned this actually in *Hallucinations* in the chapter on delirium: I'd started having some very peculiar dreams when I was in Brazil, but I'd had diarrhea and a fever and this and that, and I thought they would settle down but they didn't. I had these extraordinary Jane Austen-like dreams which were very atypical and I would wake and have a cup of tea and go back and I would be in the same dream except it would have moved on a chapter, or two months later. I had the feeling it was a narrative saying itself, whether I was awake or asleep. After about a couple of weeks, my analyst said, "you've produced more dreams in the last two weeks than in the previous twenty years, are you on something?" And I said, "no," and then I said, "well, actually I am, I was started on Lariam to prevent malaria." Lariam used to be given to all the armed forces here, and may have played a part in their breakdowns and violence when some of them came back. But it is now a drug handled very carefully and it really shouldn't have been given to me, it's only of use for the sort of malaria one has in South East Asia. But Lariam is now well known for producing bizarre dreams, hallucinations, and psychoses. Anyhow this was an example of [my analyst] saying, something else may be going on here.

I should say that he himself [has] written several books and he displays far more reserve and reticence than I do when he talks of his patients. With some difficulty, I detected a possible reference to myself, maybe conflated with others, in one of his books. I was actually rather sorry it wasn't more of a reference.

Notes

1 Breuer, J. and Freud, S. (1955 [1895]), "*Studies on Hysteria*" in *The Standard Edition of the Complete Psychological Works of Sigmund Freud*, Volume II (1893–1895). (Trans. & ed.) James Strachey. London: The Hogarth Press, p. 60.
2 Sacks, O. (1986), "Clinical Tales" in *Literature and Medicine* 5: 16–23.
3 Sacks, O. (1970), *Migraine*. London: Faber and Faber Limited.
4 Sacks, O. (2012), *Hallucinations*. London: Picador.

5 The phrase 'striving to preserve its identity in adverse circumstances' is one that Sacks borrows from Ivy McKenzie whose work on Encephalitis he greatly admires (see for example Sacks 1986, or his Warwick DLS lecture).

6 Sacks, O. (1985), *The Man Who Mistook His Wife for a Hat*. London: Picador.

7 See Sacks' "The Other Road: Freud the Neurologist" (1988).

8 Sacks, O. (2013), "The Joy of Old Age. (No Kidding.)" in *The New York Times* (July 6), accessed online 10 July 2013, www.nytimes.com/2013/07/07/opinion/sunday/the-joy-of-old-age-no-kidding.html?_r=0.

9 Whilst arguably in keeping with the Freudian *Weltanschauung* (or worldview), this phrase *-the capacity to love and work-* is not in fact found in Freud's writing (see www.freud.org.uk/about/faq/).

10 "Witty Ticcy Ray" was first published in the *London Review of Books* (1981) and then collected in *The Man Who Mistook His Wife for a Hat* (1985).

11 *The Man Who Mistook His Wife for a Hat* inspired a Michael Nyman opera in 1986.

12 Harold Pinter acknowledged the influence of *Awakenings* on his 1982 play *A Kind of Alaska*.

13 In 1990 Penny Marshall directed a film adaptation of *Awakenings*.

14 Sacks, O. (1973), *Awakenings*. London: Duckworth.

15 Sacks, O. (1984), *A Leg to Stand On*. New York: Touchstone Books.

16 Sacks, O. (2010), *The Mind's Eye*. New York: Alfred A. Knopf.

17 Sacks, O. (2007), *Musicophilia*. London: Picador.

13 Shame and Plagiarism

Charles Turner

One could try to begin wittily, by asking whether there was anything new to say about plagiarism, but Hillel Schwartz did that in 1996 in *The Culture of the Copy*. I read Schwartz's book when it came out but had long since forgotten the remark about plagiarism when last year I read (for the first time) Christopher Ricks' 1998 British Academy lecture on the subject. If Ricks felt that Schwartz had deprived him of a *bon mot*, his reference to something so recent may also have been an assertion of his own up-to-dateness; Schwartz got there before me, but not by very much. That is not very convincing: Schwartz is surely only one of a long line of people to whom the same gag has occurred. Paul Valery once wrote in his diary, "last night I dreamt of Freud: what does that mean?" As he did so not long after the *Traumdeutung* was published, we might grant him a measure of paternity, but he can't have been the only one to dream it up, the later ones not so much thieves or usurpers as reasonably alert readers kicking at the same open door. I once "invented" the joke that American men prefer to wear T-shirts because they believe in the right to bare arms, but I can't have been the first. Maybe, then, I should have just begun by asking whether there was anything new to say about plagiarism, on the (firm) grounds that the old jokes are the best.

If there is nothing new to say about plagiarism, is there something more to say? That there must be is the premise of all inquiry in the human sciences. Fortunately, while some university teachers tell their students, in stone-faced admonishment, that plagiarism is the worst thing they can do, those same students, young and inventive, continue to chip away at an apparently inexhaustible seam, devising new forms of the same transgression and entertaining us with their ingenious/ingenuous excuses. The teachers themselves are not immune from a spot of digging either:

> Stanford University said today it had learned that its teaching assistant's handbook section on plagiarism had been plagiarised by the University of Oregon. Stanford issued a release saying Oregon officials conceded that the plagiarism section and other parts of its

handbook were identical with the Stanford guidebook. Oregon offi-
cials apologised and said they would revise their guidebook.

(New York Times, June 6, 1980)

Note that word: they apologized, no more. We can think of plagiarism
as the eighth deadly sin if we like, but we spoil something for ourselves
if we do, restricting the range of ways in which we can talk about it, and
missing the fact that the responses to it range from punishment and loss
of office to humiliation and ridicule. Doubtless it is an offense, but of
what sort? One way of getting a handle on it is to say that punishment
and ridicule follow from two senses of what the offense consists in and
may be mapped onto two psychological conditions, guilt and shame.
Plagiarism, both the psychology and the sociology of it, occupies an uncertain and shifting ground between the two.

In *Shame and Necessity*, Bernard Williams says:

> What arouses guilt in an agent is an act or omission of a sort that
> typically elicits from other people anger, resentment, or indignation.
> What the agent may offer in order to turn this away is reparation; he
> may also fear punishment or may inflict it on himself. What arouses
> shame, on the other hand, is something that typically elicits from
> others contempt or derision or avoidance. This may equally be an
> act or omission, but it need not be: it may be some failing or defect.
> It will lower the agent's self-respect and diminish him in his own
> eyes. His reaction, as we just saw, is a wish to hide or disappear,
> and this is one thing that links shame as, minimally, embarrassment
> with shame as social or personal reduction. More positively, shame
> may be expressed in attempts to reconstruct or improve oneself.[1]

Williams thinks that the problem of shame opens onto a larger moral
landscape than guilt, that it is both more obscure and psychologically
more interesting. Guilt, he says, can be more readily isolated from the
flow of our experience, it is a discreet feeling, whereas shame entails a
continuity of selfhood. I dare say many would dispute this to the point
of putting matters the other way around, with shame as something tem-
porary that can be shrugged off, and guilt as a dominant cultural motif
able to stabilize the personality.

Rather than enter what is a very old problem, here I follow Williams
when he says at one point that the difference between shame and guilt as
psychological states may be discerned in the internalized figures peculiar
to them: shame involves the internalized figure of the watcher or witness;
guilt involves the internalized figures of the victim and the enforcer.

One initial difficulty is that the act of writing is generally witnessed
only by the writer, the shame that attends it being located more in an
anticipated future act of reading. While the imagined witnesses will of

course include the writer, it is easy to see why PhDs and undergraduate essays are such fertile ground for plagiarism: only two or three people will read them. On the other hand, those two or three people will have read many other things, or rather, many things within the same narrow range the student is being asked to occupy. As we will see, that raises the question of what the determined plagiarist should copy. As for the idea that the psychology of guilt requires the internalized figure of the victim, it is hard to imagine that the student who copies out a few pages of Durkheim and hands it in (how I wish they would!) has any internalized sense that they are traducing Durkheim or exploiting him.

One reason why we might link plagiarism more readily to shame than to guilt is that the emotion of shame not only allows us to come to terms with our errors and omissions but is also, Williams suggests, part of the business of rebuilding a self. University plagiarism committee meetings with the student present have something of this about them: they are more therapeutic shaming ceremonies than tribunals, their chief purpose being to confront the student with what they have done and give them a chance to tell of whatever it was in their life that led them to do it, the point of the exercise being to bring them back into line. In most cases it is clear from the start what the punishment should be. That there is a distinction between the ascertaining of guilt and the performance of shame was made clear to me a few years ago when a colleague and I failed a master's dissertation on the grounds that the first few pages had been copied from a single source on the web. On receiving their mark, the student complained to the university authorities: although we had made a decision on the basis of irrefutable evidence of guilt – which she later openly admitted – the complaint was upheld on the grounds that we had failed to follow proper procedures, that is, to afford her the chance to tell her story. We had not allowed the mechanism of shame to do its work, had withheld from her some of the tools with which she might rebuild herself.

Students are afforded this opportunity because they have a career ahead of them, because the process of building and rebuilding their self is far from complete. Not so government ministers, particularly in Germany, where the proportion of PhDs among members of parliament is especially high, and where in recent years determined online campaigners have been outing those thought to have cut corners in their doctorates to hasten their journey up the greasy pole. Recently this brought to the fore a standard strategy for avoiding the feeling of being watched we associate with shame: present oneself as one of the witnesses, the classic example being the person who, having murdered their own child, joins in the appeals for help at a police press conference. In 2011, German MP Annette Schavan joined in the condemnation of defense minister Karl Theodor von und zu Guttenberg following revelations about his plagiarized PhD. Interviewed by the *Süddeutsche Zeitung* she observed: "As someone who was herself awarded a doctorate 31 years ago and who has supervised several doctoral candidates, I am ashamed...and not just behind closed doors."[2] Two years later, on 9 February 2013, she was forced to resign her own ministerial post after her thesis was found to be plagiarized and was withdrawn by the university that awarded it. Its title was "Person and Conscience." You couldn't make it up. Though that of course is what you are supposed to do.

Before we go any further we could do with a definition. Plagiarism, wrote Samuel Johnson, occurs when

> there is a concurrence of more resemblances than can be imagined to have happened by chance, as where the same ideas are conjoined without any natural series or necessary coherence, or where not only the thought but the words are copied.[3]

According to the OED, plagiarism is "the wrongful appropriation, or purloining, and publication as one's own, of the ideas, or the expression of the ideas (literary, artistic, musical, mechanical) of another." Note here – and this is further grounds to doubt the relevance of the category of guilt to the problem of plagiarism – there is little sense of plagiarism being a legal matter. As the improbably named Laurie Stearns put it, "Plagiarism is not a legal term, and though an instance of plagiarism might seem to be the quintessential act of wrongful copying, it does not necessarily constitute a violation of copyright law."[4] Plagiarism rather is "intentionally taking the literary property of another and passing it off as one's own, having failed to add anything of value to the copied material and having reaped from its use an unearned benefit."[5] Nor do copyright infringement and plagiarism overlap: you can infringe copyright by inadvertent copying, and you can justly be accused of plagiarism for lifting words of phrases that are not under copyright. So plagiarism is not so much a crime without a name as a name without a crime: few have been prosecuted for it, it is not theft, for the literary or ideational property that has been taken cannot be said to be no longer in the hands of the one who created it: an idea is no less mine for the fact that someone else has used it or passed it off as their own. A spectacular example of literary plagiarism was Jakob Epstein's 1978 novel *Wild Oats*, much of which was ripped off from Martin Amis's 1973 novel, *The Rachel Papers*. Ricks says: "Martin Amis did not wrongfully lose credit for his novel; Jacob Epstein wrongfully gained credit for his."[6] That is right, but then Ricks says something that I think is wrong. He says that while plagiarism is by no means obviously a legal matter, it is a straightforwardly moral problem, and moreover one that is not particularly modern; it has, he says, been regarded as a moral offense at least since the time of the Roman poet Martial (AD 40–102), who likened the person who makes use of the words of others to the *plagiarius*, the one who steals other people's children or slaves. Here though, while agreeing with Ricks that awareness of plagiarism as a moral offence may be very old, we may observe that the range of practices at which the charge may be directed, and the frequency with which it is leveled, does vary historically: the proportion of written publications that are expected to be a display of authorial individuality is not constant. As George Kennedy put it, classical writing and oratory were

> to a considerable extent a pastiche, or piecing together of commonplaces, long or short... The student memorized passages as he would letters and made up a speech out of these elements as he would words out of letters... In the Middle Ages handbooks of letter-writing often contained formulae, such as openings and closes, which the student could insert into a letter, and a whole series of formulary rhetorics existed in the Renaissance.[7]

We may go further. There have been otherwise discernibly modern cultures where this accommodating attitude to unoriginality was quite at home. In *Everything was Forever until it was no more*, Alexei Yurchak documented the dilemmas faced by members of the Komsomol, the communist youth league for 14–28 year-olds, which most school leavers joined, in the latter days of the Soviet Union. Integration into the Komsomol took place through a series of assignments: lectures, meetings, speeches, farm work, parades, looking after war veterans, all forms of tertiary socialization. The speeches and how they were constructed are of especial interest: they featured the use of a technique that, by the 1980s, had become an established tradition among party cadres, one of "block writing," in which blocks of text, sometimes whole paragraphs, were used repeatedly, with the result that speeches could be read almost backwards without changing their meaning. Komsomol members, anxious about how to make their first speech, would be routinely advised by a senior figure to copy one he or she had made the year before, with a few words changed here and there, on the grounds that the one from last year would itself have been the product of years of editing, and so well written as to be worthy of imitation. If one wanted to add a new phrase of one's own one could insert some phrases from a recent *Pravda* editorial. The difference between this copying and plagiarism, Yurchak suggests, was that it was not clear that there was an objective fact of the matter that would provide the content of what was copied – what was copied was effectively the form alone. At the same time, Komsomol members were not like the early Wittgenstein: their perpetual editing was not perpetual refinement, the distillation of something unwieldy into a set of tight propositions. It was what we might call manifest intertextuality within a limited range. Richard Rorty once made a distinction between metaphysical and ironic intellectual cultures, the one involving different authors striving to get at a single truth, the other in which they "feed each other lines."[8] In the Soviet Union, different writers fed each other the same lines again and again, so that this culture of copying was as much metaphysical as ironic, even if by the 1980s few people had a sense of what the metaphysical truth was that copying was supposed to serve.

The young people of the Komsomol, then, may have been copying, but they were no more plagiarists than were Church of England priests in the sixteenth century who preferred standardized liturgical formulae to the Puritans' spontaneous sermonizing, and who saw the latter as a threat to the church's identity. They had no less of a need for tradition than have members of any other established institution, and block writing was one way of maintaining its continuous character.

The point here is that, while all cultures have some need for continuity, for the familiar stories without which new ones would be incomprehensible, the Soviet case readily evokes that of the child who, yet to begin his own explorations of the world, insists on having his favorite stories endlessly repeated. Tell me a story he says, only not one I don't already know. Where tradition is repetition, plagiarism is impossible. It only becomes possible when tradition is something more, be it variation, "an historically extended argument... about the goods which constitute that tradition," or the wreckage of history.[9]

I mention this in order to say that plagiarism is an interesting moral question as long as we are not too moralistic about it. That does not mean that there are no limits to the excuses and explanations that we should be ready to countenance. At an exam board a few years ago, a student was heading for a 2:2 degree on the basis of marks that included two fails. An external examiner asked for clarification and I explained that this student had been up before our plagiarism committee and been docked marks for "bad academic practice" (how different would the academic landscape be were a charge with this title leveled more often!). The examiner then noticed that the student had gained a first in Islamic Law, and asked whether he/she was a Muslim and so perhaps had a different understanding of plagiarism from the rest of us.

At the time, I thought the examiner deserved her share of the derision attendant on shameful utterances in public, but I should have known better, because it turns out that there is a theory to this effect. It was put forward by Keith Miller. Not the original Keith Miller, of course, the 1950s Australian cricketer and *bon viveur*, but Professor Keith Miller of Arizona State University. Miller developed his theory of "voice merging" in the early 1990s, and it came to prominence during the furor surrounding the revelation that Martin Luther King Jr. (a borrowed name if ever there was one) had lifted entire sections of his 1955 Boston University PhD from a 1952 Boston University PhD, by the splendidly-named Jack Boozer. In his 1993 article "Redefining plagiarism," Miller encouraged his readers "to appreciate the difficulties that some minorities may have in negotiating the boundaries between oral and print traditions," and that "King's plagiarisms must have derived from his inability to separate himself from his homiletic tradition [that is the one of borrowing sermons] and to comprehend the standards of an alien white culture."[10]

So much for cultural sociology, or at least what has become of it. What of psychology?

I will confine myself here to what I call the temporal pressures faced by the plagiarist. I say "the plagiarist" advisedly because we know that plagiarists come in many guises: the student who, asked to produce a 3,000 word essay, hands in a 7,000 word article copied from an academic journal that includes reminiscences about "a lecture I recently gave to students in Lithuania" is clearly doing something that feels more like a cry for help than cheating. Indeed, in the more spectacular cases, the individual may well be wanting precisely to have something seen and publicly witnessed, to be attended to, noticed; a colleague in another department who was sacked a few years ago for plagiarism already had an alternative career as a painter lined up and perhaps saw the revelation of his offense (not his crime or his sin) as helping him make that career-changing decision; whatever shame he felt may have been part of that process of rebuilding a self to which Williams refers. Jakob Epstein's case was one of willful self-destruction; he lifted passages not from someone unknown but from Martin Amis, who being Martin Amis was bound to react. Martin Luther King Jr. was less likely to face recriminations from Jack Boozer.

Notwithstanding the fact that Epstein was immediately exposed while King remained undetected until 20 years after his death, one thing they have in common was that the time between original and copy was noticeably short. One might think that a common strategy of the determined plagiarist would be to pick on something long forgotten and recycle it. The difficulty here though is that the plagiarist is usually, like the rest of us, faced with the shameful prospect of being seen to be outdated or old-fashioned. Doctoral students in particular are expected to be abreast of the latest research and so if they want to copy another's thesis it is going to have to be a fairly recent one. If you are going to meet the deadline by resurrecting some dead lines, the body should not be too long gone. The risk here is exemplified by the case of the Oxford student who, having spent years not writing his thesis on Karl Mannheim, in desperation found one on Mannheim in the Bodleian Library, copied it and submitted it as his own. Sadly he had failed to reckon with the possibility that the external examiner chosen to examine his thesis would be the same one who had examined the original only a few years before, and who, unlike Lord Desai in the case of Muhammar Ghaddafi's son at the LSE, would be capable of smelling a rat.[11] For novelists there seems to be more latitude, though Jakob Epstein in 1979 wouldn't have gotten away with writing in the style of the 1920s because that style, if not the content, would have been recognized for what it was. One way out of this was found by the Indian writer Indrani Aikath-Gyultsen, whose 1994 novel *Cranes Morning*, set in India, was copied from Elizabeth Goudge's 1956 novel *The Rosemary Tree*, set in Devon. This was eventually detected, though not before the novel had received a gushing review from one Paul Kafka (yes) in *The Washington Post*: "at once achingly familiar and breathtakingly new."[12] The book was published in India and the US but not in the UK where Elizabeth Goudge had been a popular writer, though of the sort of books that are quickly forgotten. Theodore Pappas uses this story as contextualization for his own bitter experience when he wrote up the story of Martin Luther King Jr.'s plagiarism and was widely attacked for doing so:

> A second rate novel that was originally panned by the critics as little more than a penny dreadful when it was originally published in the 1950s had become a monumental work of literature 40 years later once plagiarised and set in a third world country.[13]

Yet perhaps Pappas misses something here: for all we know the original novel might have been panned by critics only because they were ignorant of its true qualities, so that it had to wait 40 years for proper recognition, with the plagiarist performing the valuable service of restoring to prominence one who had been unjustifiably forgotten. In some cases, it may be that not only is it doubtful whether the plagiarized writer should be seen as a "victim"; they may end up as beneficiary, with the act of plagiarism being not so much theft as a belated kiss of life.

Something like this actually happened to Ludwik Fleck. Fleck's *Genesis and Development of a Scientific Fact* of 1935 might never have been translated into English (in 1979) and thereby gained wider recognition had it not been for the suggestion in the late sixties that Thomas Kuhn had leaned heavily on it for *The Structure of Scientific Revolutions* of 1962. What we have here is an interesting variation on a process that Erving Goffman wrote about in *Stigma*. A stigma is of course a discrediting mark or trait, one that the individual has to manage interactionally, and one of Goffman's finest observations is that those who manage to cover those marks, say by corrective surgery, may still end up being perceived as "people who have corrected a fault." It is a pity that Goffman never wrote about what one might call the stigma of obscurity, for he might have been able to tell us about the ambivalences at work when the original is rescued from obscurity by the plagiarist. Who is Ludwik Fleck? The Polish microbiologist who wrote an important work in the philosophy of science and then survived Auschwitz, or the author of a book that influenced Thomas Kuhn more than Kuhn cared to say, and who was later rescued from obscurity by those with an axe to grind against Kuhn? Borges said that all authors create their own precursors, but when the author is a plagiarist, he may be disturbing the ground, or dusting off something that had been languishing untouched and forgotten.[14] Max Weber says that the meaning of our work is that it is chained to the course of progress and we have to want it to be surpassed, but how many of us would baulk at the thought of seeing our own ideas live on, even if they were unacknowledged?

Fleck's and Kuhn's books were less than 30 year apart and so it was not difficult for readers to see an affinity between Fleck's "thought collective" and Kuhn's "paradigm." The connection between Elizabeth Goudge and Indrani Aikath-Gyultsen was harder to discern but it was eventually spotted.

This latter case is interesting because, as Pappas suggests, in contrast to cases where the sense of a wrong having been done depended on an identity between the original and the copy, on the same words meaning the same thing at different times, a shift in cultural context may turn something mediocre into something more impressive. Or for that matter, the other way around. Borges offered a logical/illogical variation on this in one of his most celebrated stories, "Pierre Menard, author of the Quixote," in which Pierre Menard sets out, in the 1920s, to write parts of *Don Quixote*, not by transcribing or copying the original, nor by becoming Cervantes and undergoing his experiences – that, Borges says, would be too easy – but precisely by remaining Pierre Menard. When he succeeds we are given the radical historicist punchline: "Cervantes' text and Menard's are verbally identical. But the second is almost infinitely richer."[15] Like many of Borges' stories, "Pierre Menard" appears to achieve its effects by means of a contrast between an impossible world and our own, or by presenting at most an ideal typical scenario. Yet while an ideal type is the one-sided exaggeration of empirical reality, the Pierre Menard example is uncomfortably close to being just that, an example of a phenomenon that academic life, in particular, throws up more often than we might think.

The joke by means of which the historicist point is made runs like this:

> Cervantes writes: "...truth, whose mother is history, rival of time, depository of deeds, witness of the past, exemplar and adviser to the present, and the future's counsellor." Written in the seventeenth century, written by the "lay genius" Cervantes, this enumeration is a mere rhetorical praise of history. Menard on the other hand writes: "truth, whose mother is history, rival of time, depository of deeds, witness of the past, exemplar and adviser to the present, and the future's counsellor." History, the mother of truth: the idea is astounding. Menard, a contemporary of William James, does not define history as an inquiry into reality but its origin. Historical truth, for him, is not what has happened: it is what we judge to have

happened...The contrast in style is also vivid. The archaic style of Menard...suffers from certain affectations. Not so that of his forerunner, who handles with ease the current Spanish of his time.[16]

It is one of Borges' best jokes, but it may fall flat in the face of what I can only call some examples of contemporary Menardism, some of them even more pointed.

In 1989, the Cambridge anthropologist Paul Connerton published a much-praised book, *How Societies Remember*. Shortly after it came out, I discussed its fine style with him, and he told me that as a student he was advised by one of his teachers that if he wanted to write well he should try to write in such a way that someone reading 50 years ago would understand. It was only much later that I realized how much he had taken this advice to heart, for at one point he appears to have set out to write a fragment of Elias Canetti's *Crowds and Power*, published in 1960, by the classically Menardian method of remaining Paul Connerton.

> Rank and power are traditionally connected with certain postures and from the way in which men group themselves we can deduce the amount of authority which each enjoys. We know what it means when one man sits raised up while everyone around him stands; when one man stands and everyone else sits; when everyone in a room gets up as someone comes in; when one man falls on his knees before another; when a new arrival is not asked to sit down.[17]

"We know what it means," Canetti says, as though his autodidactic cod anthropology were a matter of course, of "of course." Canetti, an author who, after the success of his youthful novel *Die Blendung*, has never stopped believing himself destined for the Nobel prize for literature (he probably spent years practicing his acceptance speech in front of the mirror (thank you to Alasdair Gray for that)), writes with the complacent self-confidence of the man of letters who treats his musings on authority and verticality as universal truth, without any reference to particular historical societies. Connerton on the other hand writes:

> Power and rank are commonly expressed through certain postures relative to others; from the way in which they group themselves and the dispositions of their bodies relative to the bodies of others, we can deduce the degree of authority which each is thought to enjoy or to which they lay claim. We know what it means when one person sits in an elevated position when everyone around them stands; when one person stands and everyone else sits; when everyone in a room gets up as someone else comes in; when someone bows, or curtseys, or, in extreme circumstances, falls to their knees before another who remains standing.[18]

Here, in one brilliant sentence at the end of the 1980s, and at the end of a long and heroic mining of the anthropological record, Connerton challenges the cognitivist-symbolic paradigm that had for so long dominated the study of culture, and restores the body, in its very corporeality, to its rightful place, a place that had been usurped by "discourse." His "we know" is no mere appeal to common sense, but points rather to the wisdom of the gesture; it is a vindication of Wittgenstein's remark that there is a way of understanding a rule that is not and never need be an interpretation.

While it is hard to see Canetti being rescued from obscurity by Connerton in the way that Ludwik Fleck was by Kuhn, it is all too easy to see just this happening in the following case, what we might call "one for the price of two" Menardism. In 2004, John Keane, the Australian political theorist and biographer of Tom Paine and Vaclav Havel, adopted the first method that was proposed and rejected by Menard. He set out to be the person whose work he wished to reproduce. In this case, that person was the Australian political theorist and biographer of Tom Paine and Vaclav Havel, John Keane, and he did so even while John Keane was still alive. In his *Reflections on Violence* from 1996, John Keane had written:

> The scale and ferocity of violence produced by such 20th century conflicts have fascinated, shocked and sickened the whole world. Words cannot easily describe their cruelty, and their attempted theorisation seems at first glance to be a self-indulgent act of blandiloquence. Those who do attempt to reflect on such patterns of violence are easily gripped by feelings of shame that they are uninvited witnesses of events littered by corpses sweet with the smell of doom.[19]

Written in the immediate aftermath of the break-up of Yugoslavia and the genocide in Rwanda, these words see the author failing to gain any measure of distance, and substituting emotion, or pseudo-emotion, for sober analysis. "Words cannot easily describe their cruelty." Indeed not, but even if they could, is this the social scientist's task? "Blandiloquence" may have sounded good at the time, but any self-respecting copy editor would have had it removed. And he or she ought to have heard the pornography in "corpses sweet with the smell of doom." In *Violence and Democracy* from 2004, John Keane writes:

> The scale and ferocity of violence produced by uncivil wars have fascinated, shocked and sickened the whole world. Words cannot easily describe their cruelty, and their attempted theorisation seems at first glance to be a self-indulgent act of blandiloquence. Those who attempt to reflect on such patterns of violence are easily gripped by feelings of shame that they are uninvited witnesses of events littered by corpses sweet with the smell of doom.[20]

Here, a full decade after the terrible events of Bosnia and Rwanda, John Keane reminds a readership already in danger of forgetting them what these conflicts were about, that they were "uncivil wars" and not simply "20th century conflicts," and so rescues them from beneath the mountain of "blandiloquent" commentary that has been piled higher than any mound of sweet smelling corpses. Ancient hatreds, system collapse, neo-liberalism, the dark side of democracy, religious fanaticism, none of these theorizations can take away the feelings of shame that attend them, a shame that Keane is honest enough to admit that he himself feels.

In fact, Keane is less than true to the spirit of Menard, because unlike Menard he set out to write not only a chapter or a fragment of *Reflections on Violence* of 1996, but the entire book. We wonder whether for this herculean task he employed an assistant and whether it was he or she who was tempted to amend and edit the text here and there. John Keane writes:

> These points made by Bauman are salutary, and yet his conclusion that modern civility is the ally of barbarism has its costs, one of which is his dogmatic pessimism.[21]

The condescension here is unmistakable, the man from the Antipodes lecturing one from a generation and a continent that knows more than he or his will ever know about the horrors of war. "Dogmatic pessimism" is hyperbole, reflecting a desperation to make a point that might as easily be made without the sneering adjective. John Keane, on the other hand, writes:

> The key point made by Bauman, that civility is prone to barbarism, is salutary. Yet his conclusion that modern civility is the ally of barbarity has its costs, one of which is his dogmatic existentialism.[22]

Civility: prone to barbarism but not an ally of it. A subtle but crucial distinction that needs to be made by anyone who wants to defend the virtues of civility and look barbarism in the face. "Dogmatic existentialism" is a reminder, and again a necessary one, of the fact that even philosophies that, in the name of openness and flexibility, appear to eschew ideological content can take on the appearance of rigidity.

The target of this repeated/varied charge – Keane told readers of his 2003 *Global Civil Society?* that his critique of "dogmatic pessimism" could be found in his 1998 book, *Civil Society: Old Images, New Ideas* (!) – has been accused of something more shameful/shameless than this.[23] It has been suggested that Zygmunt Bauman was no John Keane, engaging in a Borgesian experiment; he was merely a self-plagiarist. His writing career – more than 40 books between retirement in 1990 and his death in 2017 – might in fact have made a good Borges story. According to his accusers, though, he only managed to be so productive by repeating the same thing – the same words – again and again. If Bauman's response to the allegations appears not to have satisfied everyone, it reminds us once again of the grey zone in which plagiarism seems most at home, one where the goalposts are easily moved: from self-plagiarism to recycling to bad academic practice, and finally to perhaps most serious of all in the eyes of academics struggling with obscurity: meeting the publishers' need for prompt copy by copying, and making lots of money in the process. Compared to working for the security police in postwar Poland and having innocent people arrested, it might be considered small beer of course, but then again, after so many years, the internalized figures of guilt, victim and enforcer, may have faded, while those of shame, the watchers and witnesses, the readers, glow ever brighter.

The last word on the new Bauman affair may not be said for some time. Who should have the last word here, on this topic where the problem is, in a sense, that of who had the first word? One is tempted to give it to poor old Jack Boozer, the non-victim of Martin Luther King Jr. Instead, I will give it to another. Christopher Hitchens liked Theodore Pappas' work on the King affair so much that he copied passages from it for an article he wrote on plagiarism in *Vanity Fair*. Confronted with this, he remarked: "I'm in favour of plagiarism and always have been. Wouldn't be able to write without it."[24]

Notes

1 Bernard Williams, *Shame and Necessity* (Berkeley: University of California Press, 1993), 89–90.
2 Nicholas Kullish and Chris Cottrell, "German Fascination with Degrees Claims Latest Victim: Education Minister," *New York Times*, February 9, 2013, www.nytimes.com/2013/02/10/world/europe/german-education-chief-quits-in-scandal-reflecting-fascination-with-titles.html [accessed 20 March 2017].
3 Samuel Johnson, *The Works of Samuel Johnson*, Vol. II (London: George Cowie, 1825), 106.
4 Laurie Stearns, "Copy Wrong: Plagiarism, Process, Property and the Law," in *Perspectives on Plagiarism and Intellectual Property in a Postmodern World*, ed. Lise Buranen and Alice M. Roy (New York: State University of New York Press, 1999), 6.
5 Stearns, "Copy Wrong," 7.
6 Christopher Ricks, *Allusion to the Poets* (Oxford: Oxford University Press, 2002), 240.
7 George Kennedy, *Classical Rhetoric and Its Christian and Secular Tradition from Ancient to Modern Times* (Chapel Hill: University of North Carolina, 1980), 28–29.
8 Richard Rorty, *Contingency, Irony, and Solidarity* (Cambridge: Cambridge University Press, 1989), 39.
9 Alasdair MacIntyre, *After Virtue: A Study in Moral Theory* (Norfolk: Duckworth, 1980), 222.
10 Theodore Pappas, *Plagiarism and the Culture War: The Writings of Martin Luther King, Jr. and Other Prominent Americans* (Tampa: Halberg Publishing Corp, 1993), 77.

11 Saif Gaddafi had been awarded a PhD at the London School of Economics in 2008. When the crisis in Libya began in 2011, concerns were raised both about the LSE's having accepted a £1.5million donation from the Gaddafi regime, and about the originality of the thesis. Lord Desai had been one of the examiners.

12 Molly Moore, "A Mysterious Passage in India," *Washington Post*, April 27, 1994, www.washingtonpost.com/archive/lifestyle/1994/04/27/a-mysterious-passage-in-india/3679104c-75b9-48ec-b90d-9761b2c45b58/?utm_term=.495f584c1eaf [accessed 20 March 2017].

13 Pappas, *Plagiarism*, 33.

14 Jorge Luis Borges, *The Total Library: Non-Fiction 1922–86* (London: Penguin, 1999), 365.

15 Jorge Luis Borges, *Labyrinths* (Harmondsworth: Penguin, 1970), 69.

16 Borges, *Labyrinths*, 69.

17 Elias Canetti, *Crowds and Power* (Harmondsworth: Penguin, 1960), 449.

18 Paul Connerton, *How Societies Remember* (Cambridge: Cambridge University Press, 1989), 74.

19 John Keane, *Reflections on Violence* (London: Verso, 1996), 131.

20 John Keane, *Violence and Democracy* (Cambridge: Cambridge University Press, 2004), 110.

21 Keane, *Reflections*, 37.

22 Keane, *Violence and Democracy*, 68.

23 John Keane, *Global Civil Society?* (Cambridge: Cambridge University Press, 2003), 200.

24 Theodore Pappas, "Christopher Hitchens and Vanity Fair," *Chronicles: A Magazine of American Culture*, June 1, 1996, www.chroniclesmagazine. org/1996/July/20/7/magazine/article/10838257/ [accessed 20 March 2017].

14 "Dance Like Nobody's Watching"

The Mediated Shame of Academic Publishing

Martin Paul Eve

In 1987, Susanna Clark and Richard Leigh composed a set of lyrics for their country song, "Come from the Heart," that have subsequently found a mass-audience afterlife in several internet memes: "You've got to sing like you don't need the money / Love like you'll never get hurt / You've got to dance like nobody's watchin' / It's gotta come from the heart if you want it to work." For academic scholarly communications, however, the well-known humorous Twitter persona of @NeinQuarterly (Eric Jarosinski) perhaps reformulated this best when he cynically wrote: "Tweet like nobody's reading. / Because: / They're not."[1]

Indeed, in recent years the open-access movement has sought to broaden the potential audiences for scientific and scholarly publications by removing price and permission barriers for readers.[2] This has often been rationalized through critiques of the limited readership of paywalled journal articles and expensive scholarly monographs that are disseminated only to academic libraries.[3] In many ways, the goals of the open-access movement are noble in their quest to ensure that as many citizens of the world as possible can access and read high quality research and scholarship.

Yet, as Clark and Leigh knew just as well as Foucault, the belief that one might be being watched can trigger a shame reaction that inhibits practices, from dancing through to publishing writing, even though both are acts that intrinsically call for attention. In this chapter, I examine a set of theoretical questions surrounding observation, readership, and openness for niche, esoteric research practices across a range of disciplines. These include: What behavioral changes might we expect to see in a world of mass readership? How does a new set of publics sit alongside emergent managerial practices at institutions focusing on public "impact?" And might there be a certain "shame" that cuts both ways here: a shame at exposing our work to an imagined plurality of gazes that may misunderstand, misconstrue, or simply interpret the work differently to our authorial intentions, even while feeling ashamed at hiding our writings on the understanding that all our potential audiences may remain disinterested?

As a launch pad for the work in this chapter, I take the autoethnographic, self-writing approach of Elspeth Probyn in her well-known piece, "Writing Shame."[4] Of particular interest to me here is the opening portion of Probyn's work, in which she writes of the shame of writing within an academic framework alongside the physical, embodied shame response that she has in considering her own inability to convey interest to others. This is split in Probyn's piece across structural academic anxieties, nervousness about the relationship of writing to reality, bodily responses, shame and glory, the importance of proximity and distance, and the specific case of the writing of Primo Levi.[5] While Probyn's work in this piece – and indeed more broadly in her book on the subject, *Blush: Faces of Shame* – is brave and self-exposing, I also feel critical of how it disregards the *media* through which academics communicate, within a piece that is fundamentally about a shameful inadequacy of communication.

For if there is any truth in the assertion that the medium is still the message, then it is important that we consider, within a variety of contexts of "shame," how the structural elements of scholarly communications condition different types of shame. As Juliet Jacquet has framed it, "[e]ach time communication was transformed, shaming was as well."[6] The niche modes that have historically developed to facilitate the communication of academic ideas have done so in a way conditioned by economic and material systems that drastically limit the audience for academic writing. If shame in writing is, as Probyn contends, "sheer disappointment in the self" amplified "to a painful level," then it is much easier to be content with one's self-performance if the audience for the work is limited to those predisposed to receive it well: fellow academics.[7] Of course, there can still be shame in writing for peer review and academic colleagues, especially if one makes an oversight or gets something wrong. However, as I will go on to discuss, the fears around a broader, unknown public audience, particularly for some of the humanities disciplines, carries a far greater potential for the amplification of shame.

Observation, Discipline, and Societies of Control

Before it is possible to venture any remarks upon shame in academic publishing and readership, it is first necessary to give some definition of shame that could work within the scholarly communications context and to explain how it would be linked to observation and visibility, the subjects focused upon by the open-access movement. This is at least in part because, in recent years, shame has been tightly coupled to being *seen* within social contexts. Jacquet has explicitly defined shame as a fear of reputational damage through exposure to the specific, but historically mutable, social conditions within which an individual exists.[8] Yet, for Jacquet, this socialized experience of shame is contrasted with guilt as a personal and unsociable experience, which she claims is a more prominent affective experience within a highly individualized society (drawing on the earlier anthropological work of Ruth Benedict and Margaret Mead).[9]

If we acknowledge, then, that Jacquet's definition of shame as opposed to guilt is incomplete, but functionally well-suited to her project's goal of using shaming as a social justice tool, we can still agree that observation has a role to play in the emotion of shame.[10] Indeed, Deleuze's account of shame in T.E. Lawrence, for example, uses the Spinozean concept of autonomous corporeal responses as being linked to shame. For Deleuze's Lawrence, "the body never ceases to act and react *before the mind moves it*" and these involuntary weaknesses make the mind – which is nonetheless perceived as inseparable from the body – ashamed *for* the body.[11] Most tellingly, though, these reflexive bodily actions that the mind cannot condition (in this case an erection) make Lawrence wish to "crawl away and hide until the shame was passed," implying that the observation is here key.[12] Yet the way in which Probyn extends Deleuze's observed bodily shame is also to frame shame as a productive force that can be seen through intersubjective *interest*.[13] It may not quite be that "in shame we are reduced to being an object only for the other's jurisdiction," as framed by Jennifer Biddle, but it does nonetheless seem true that, as Probyn puts it, unless you *care* about the observing or observed object, there can be no shame: "only something or someone that has interested you can produce a flush of shame."[14]

Alongside many other commentators, however, Gilles Deleuze rightly recognizes that "Foucault located the *disciplinary societies*" of regulatory observation, "in the eighteenth and nineteenth centuries" and that they "reach their height at the outset of the twentieth."[15] The system of individualization and discipline by enclosure, in other words, is a historically localized, not contemporary, phenomenon. Foucault himself saw this, stating that "[p]ower is not discipline; discipline is a possible procedure of power" and that "[c]onsequently these analyses can in no way, to my mind, be equated with a general analytics of every power relation."[16] While this implied injunction against using discipline as a catch-all description of contemporary power relations has not been thoroughly heeded, Deleuze himself proposes a successor: the societies of control.

Societies of control, for Deleuze, are not like disciplinary societies. Where disciplinary societies must individualize by segregation, Deleuze claimed in 1990 that we are "now in a generalized crisis in relation to all the environments of enclosure."[17] The replacement of factories (as spaces of disciplinary enclosure) in the contemporary West by "gas"-like corporations that permeate the entirety of society instigates, for Deleuze, a mode of control. In other words, the society may be open not enclosed, apparently free not imprisoned, but thanks to your smart phone, your boss's emails can reach you wherever you are. Schooling is replaced, in Deleuze's societies of control, by a "permanent training" of corporations, a continuing professional development, in which the young are "motivated" to request such training.[18] From a prescient viewpoint of 1990, Deleuze successfully described the dominant power mechanisms of the early twenty-first century, at least in abstract terms. It is the *open prison* that matters, less the total surveillance mode.

Shame then may be an "experience of the self by the self," as Silvan Tomkins put it in the 1950s, but it still is about that self "increas[ing] its visibility" in order to generate "the torment of self-consciousness."[19] For Tomkins, this is located within a contemporary "taboo on looking" that acts as an amplifier of shame-humiliation affects.[20] This focus on a shame affect engendered by surveillance and systems of watching also links to one of the core things that "theory knows today," in the (ironic) words of Eve Kosofsky Sedgwick and Adam Frank, namely that "[t]he bipolar, transitive relations of subject to object, self to other, and active to passive, and the physical sense (sight) understood to correspond most closely to these relations, are dominant organizing tropes" for theory "to the extent that their dismantling as such is framed as both an urgent and interminable task."[21] In other words, if we sit within societies of control with disciplinary cores, we should expect the taboo on looking to create a heightened web of shame, a network of internalized humiliation based on internalized societal norms.

Yet, before moving back to publishing, it does seem that the society of control is *less effective* than the disciplinary society. This can be seen by the fact that, when individuals do not succumb to the control society's mechanisms of media for self-surveillance, a disciplinary regime is reinstigated. We still have supermax prisons that isolate "deviant" individuals under intense surveillance by a relatively scarce number of guards in order to bring prisoners into line. Put otherwise: although the broader societies of control have replaced a mass disciplinary movement, the panoptic, isolating, and individualizing mechanisms of Foucault's disciplinary societies – supposed, we are told, to have vanished into the past – exist as a subform of the contemporary. What we actually seem to have are societies of control that house societies of discipline.

Academic Publishing

We can see some of these subsocieties of discipline at work in contemporary institutions. Hospitals have disciplinary teams, prisons have disciplinary regimes, and universities have disciplines. While the shackles of disciplinarity have been under threat from demands for interdisciplinary approaches for many years, these have not fully been shrugged.[22] Indeed, as Alexander R. Galloway recently put it, interdisciplinarity has a skewed benefit away from a home discipline that usually takes another discipline and merely uses it, creating an asymmetric relationship of benefit:

> [u]ltimately it comes down to this: if you count words in Moby-Dick, are you going to learn more about the white whale? I think you probably can – and we have to acknowledge that. But you won't learn anything new about counting.[23]

Medical humanists might argue differently, claiming that the hermeneutic approaches of the humanities could bring benefit to both medics and humanists (in the reading and interpretation of radiograms for instance), but many instances of interdisciplinarity are more of the type sketched by Galloway. The disciplines – which bring professionalization and specialization through isolation – are alive and well in the academy.

These disciplinary subsocieties also have strictly codified and, from the outside at least, bizarre sets of disciplinary practices to which the inside denizens must adhere. These curious practices range from the wearing of traditional robes and gowns to arcane graduation ceremonies, but they find, I think, an important locus in the systems of dissemination of research material produced by the academy.

Academic publishing is a space where intellectual freedom must be key and this accounts for some of the eccentricities of the academic remuneration system when compared to other endeavors. For universities are among the last contemporary places where researchers are paid to produce work to which they own the copyright and that they are free to give away to whichever publisher they wish. Peter Suber believes that a system like this may emerge in any advanced research ecosystem, since it gives a form of *academic freedom* to those who work beneath it.[24] This freedom is specifically a freedom of researchers from certain types of market practice. Researchers are not dependent upon a market of *selling research* to make their living (although in many higher education environments, they are dependent upon a market of so-called student recruitment through teaching). This freedom from the market is good for research, though, because it allows the investigation of niche and esoteric areas that would not find a large-scale market audience but that are important for the sake of knowledge.[25] Long before the discourses of marketization entered widespread circulation, the university designed structures for the production of speculative knowledge, even if such structures were bound within other elitist educational models of liberal humanism.

Such freedom is also important because the markets that might form in academic publishing are strange and not necessarily like other markets. First, although the potential audience is small, at maybe 200–250 copies for a humanities monograph, the audience is somewhat captive. Because universities demand field mastery from academics, they must have read all relevant material. This means that the relatively small audience has a relatively high incentive to purchase material. Second, as novelty is usually a criterion of academic publishing, there can be little genuine competition between items. If an academic needs to read a specific research article or book, then no substitute good will achieve that purpose. One cannot suggest reading a different article or book since the research work within the originally sought piece holds a "micro-monopoly" (Peter Suber's term) on that knowledge. Both of these measures – the small but motivated audience and the micro-monopolistic situation – conspire to frustrate any price-setting mechanism of a market based on downwards price pressure. At the same time, these measures make it difficult or impossible, in many disciplines, for an academic to make a living purely by selling research work.

Yet, the problem here is that while researchers are free to investigate niche topics through their university salaries, even when soft power mechanisms may be used to drive researchers towards "impactful" topics, publishers are not in the same position. Publishers must usually work within this unusual market, selling the work of academics to which they have contributed. For there are many different forms of publisher labor that stretch from commissioning, typesetting, copyediting, proofreading, (digital) preservation, printing, distribution, marketing, finance, legal, among others that must be remunerated. While academics may be freer from some specific market pressures to make a living, then, publishers are not. This is part of the reason why some have suggested that open access – in which researchers *and* publishers disseminate material online in a way that is free to read and reuse – should be paid for by universities; it would offer, then, the same type of freedom to publishers.

As a result of this strange market, the academic publishing environment is also somewhat twisted. The market, estimated to be worth about £10 billion per year, is dominated by a relatively small number of players (Elsevier, Wiley, Sage, Taylor & Francis, Oxford University Press, Cambridge University Press, Nature), the most commercially aggressive of which makes approximately 36 percent profit per year, with the longtail of the market dwindling to a set of smaller mission-driven publishers who sit perhaps only one lawsuit away from bankruptcy.[26] This dysfunctional market, with a few very large players and a captive audience, whose monopolistic elements derive from the micro-monopolies inherent in the novelty that academia requires, sits at the heart of university-level research.

The Shame of Limited Circulation

As mentioned above, there are a number of reasons why academic material has limited circulation. The first is that research material is niche and esoteric, usually highly segregated into disciplinary silos, and therefore often of interest to a limited number of parties. This is not to say that there will not be other interested audiences who should have access, it is to point out that the main readers of research articles and books are academics and students. The challenge, though, is that we do not have good evidence that this would be the case were there no paywalls to access research worldwide.

That said, in the Latin American context, where a great deal more research is born both digital and open, Juan Pablo Alperin has shown that 9 percent of access to the SciELO platform (the major publishing platform there) is by those outside the academy; the general public.[27] Furthermore, in that demographic survey, 50 percent of users of SciELO were students, of which 20 percent were most likely still in high school.[28] Indeed, more broadly, the "Who Needs Access?" site has made its mission to chart the demographics and stories of people who do not have access to the research from publicly funded research but would benefit from it. Among the categories of people they list are: translators, research organizations, small businesses, people working with the developing world, doctors and dentists, nurses, teachers, politicians, consumer organizations, patients, patient groups, amateur palaeontologists, astronomers and ornithologists, Wikipedia contributors, bloggers, unaffiliated scholars working into their retirement, professional researchers, independent researchers, publishers, and artists.[29] In fact, even if only 1 percent of the general public wanted access to research material (a low estimate, as above), rounding a 2013 approximation of a world population down to seven billion, this would have been 70,000,000 people. Taking this figure at 10 percent and this 70 million becomes 700 million people.

That said, anecdotal conversations with researchers (particularly in the humanities) lead to denials of this claim. I have been told by peers and peer reviewers that the biggest shame comes from indifference and the fact that many researchers know that they are producing work that few will read. I refuse to believe that this is entirely the case, though. Indeed, on the open-access journal platform that I founded and run, the Open Library of Humanities, the 909 articles that we published in our first twelve months were viewed 118,686 times (counting unique views). That is an average of 131 views per article, although clearly the spread is not even and what a "view" really means (we mean: they stayed on the page for more than 20 seconds) could be divided from the idea of a "reader."[30] There is an emergent ambiguity here in the face of the assertion that nobody *wants* to read such work: namely, why are we so certain?

Indeed, to deny access to between the aforementioned 70 million and 700 million people for research that we have allowed researchers to give away (in some limited senses) seems to be a shame. Sites such as "Who Needs Access?" are meant to foster a self-aware shame in academics and publishers through an amplification in visibility. As well as providing narrative evidence, it is clear that the site is meant to shame academics for squandering their claimed freedom. Yet the move to make research material openly available meets with continued resistance and skepticism for a variety of reasons. David Wojick, previously a consultant with the Office of Scientific and Technical Information at the U.S. Department of Energy in the area of information and communication science, noted in early 2016 on the conservative scholarly communications blog *The Scholarly Kitchen* that "I personally doubt that there are large numbers of people who (1) have the expert knowledge required to read and benefit from the scholarly literature but who (2) cannot find a way to access what they need."[31] To the first of these points, approximately 40 percent –50 percent of the populations of Canada, the U.K., the U.S., Norway, Australia, France, and Sweden have attended university and therefore almost half of the national populations have the expert knowledge required to read and benefit from the scholarly literature.[32] The second point is harder to query but centers around ideas of discoverability in scholarly communications that merits one further detour here.

With many types of goods, it is possible to know whether or not they are wanted before purchase. If I dislike a foodstuff, for example, then I am unlikely to buy it. I must, at some point in my life, though, have eaten the foodstuff to know this, although there are also irrational foodstuff fears that may be attributional to shame.[33] This usually means that on one occasion I will have bought mushrooms, but probably on one occasion only. With research material, this is, again, not possible. Every single article or book is different and unique. I cannot usually have enough foreknowledge of an article's content and use to me to merit the $30 single article price or a yearly subscription in advance. There are, of course, other goods that are a little like this. Music sold on compact discs, for example. Except that usually record stores will allow potential customers to listen to the CD in advance or to stream the entire album online. The same does not go for the micro-monopolistic world of research material where often it is only an abstract or micro-portion of a work that is available beforehand. This inhibits discoverability through pricing.

The specific form of shame that is shaped within the context of limited circulation of research material here is of a political and negative historico-charitable nature. To understand this, we must properly conceive of education (and higher education research) in the Western tradition, at least, within a backdrop of a liberal humanist theory of education. Such a stance would see education as necessary for the creation of an enlightened population, capable of participating coherently within a democratic system. We see this continued to this day in several aspects. The first is the continued defense of the humanities system against marketization using this very logic. Indeed, as Michael Bérubé charts it, recounting a letter from his Dean, "[a] traditional liberal arts education has theoretically affirmed the belief in the existence of a certain kind of knowledge or wisdom – as opposed to information, or content – that is timeless and universally valuable to the human spirit."[34] Bérubé does not himself hold this view, but there is something enduring about the liberal-humanist myth, even while humanists cannot claim this viewpoint explicitly "in good conscience," since the anti-historicism and universality of the claim is opposed to most contemporary humanistic discourse.[35]

More broadly, though, in the early twenty-first century, the collapse of the (nonetheless false) liberal humanist myth is at least partially linked to a history of charity law and its undoing through privatization initiatives. In most jurisdictions with charity laws, the advancement of education has been set aside as a legitimate charitable purpose. Indeed, in the U.S., section 501(c)(3) of the Internal Revenue Code specifies the "advancement of education or science" as a valid claim for federal tax relief, and in the U.K., the Charity Commission has a similar clause.[36] These laws are rooted in a history of "public benefit" that also finds an etymological and theological locus in the term *caritus*. Most importantly for the way in which education is framed, however, there is supposed to be a relationship of superiority of the giver over the receiver in a charitable transaction. Indeed, charity is often framed as giving to the unfortunate and there is meant to be an element of humility, or even shame, in accepting charity; at least under present discourse. Yet, religious organizations and universities, alongside private schools, are often charitable organizations that can accept donations or state funding. These educational organizations, claiming a public benefit, are now all but private in many parts of the world, though. The well-known descent of publicly funded higher education substituted for fees and income-contingent repayment loans can lead us to question what the public benefit of the university might actually be.[37]

There is a good argument that the continued public benefit of universities lies within their research function, even as teaching is commodified into an income generating service. However, when that research is behind expensive paywalls and largely inaccessible to the general public, this charitable history is compromised. Thus, while profiting from tax relief for public benefit, institutions of higher education can become shameful recipients of charity that are also unable to make good on any publicly available benefit. This is a shame of unrepaid debt. Researchers, of course, can change this through making their work open access. However, as I will now discuss, the combination of a symbolic economy and a shame linked to visibility often makes this less likely.[38]

Shamed in the Public Gaze

Let us assume, though, that researchers do begin to make their works publicly available. What are the risks here with respect to shame and visibility? What behavioral changes might we expect as works are made more broadly accessible? And what do tabloid media norms about certain disciplinary practices do to shape a space of shaming?

The first point to note is that open access has met with vociferous resistance from some academic researchers in respect to public access. Robin Osborne, for example, states that it is the case that (and should be the case that) "the primary beneficiary of research-funding is the re-searcher" and that "[a]cademic research is a process – a process which universities teach (at a fee)." For Osborne, a Cambridge-based classi-cist writing about the humanities, the risks are that making the end-publication available neither captures the act of performing the research itself nor exposes the research to an informed audience since "academic research publication is a form of teaching that assumes some prior knowledge."[39] This line of attack misses the fact that there is a public appetite for research publications and a large number of university-level educated readers who cannot afford access. It also, though, strikes me as betraying a shame, centered around notions of observed norm viola-tion. In fact, Osborne closes his piece with the adage that "[m]uch more will be downloaded; much less will be understood," which I will argue fits well with many of the observational related shame paradigms that I outlined earlier in this piece.[40] For there is certainly an intra-academic norm for reception here, which Osborne frames as "understanding". The violation of that norm leads to a fear that research – especially from the humanities disciplines – will be misused and recontextualized within a culture where it does not make the same sense. If that norm is more broadly held and the piece is seen as nonsensical by a broader popula-tion, it is likely to trigger a shaming reaction.

Indeed, there have been a number of occasions where various right wing tabloid newspapers have picked up on research stories – often on the advice of so-called think tanks – in order to attempt to ridicule and shame the research and researchers. Examples include the U.K.'s *Daily Mail* attacking research into human-chicken interactions and *The Times* and *The Telegraph* both running stories attacking research into "why cookies crumble" and "why don't woodpeckers get headaches."[41] Of course, within a university context, such questions can easily be re-framed: "how are the musculoskeletal systems of woodpeckers able to withstand intense, repetitive shock without the onset of cephalalgia?" or the surely useful to the biscuit industry: "what causes particular disin-tegration of some baked goods over others?" These research questions, which have valid contexts, are here taken by the press, decontextualized and ridiculed. By insinuating a new norm for the soundness of research, through ridicule and humiliation, in order to serve the paper's (or think tank's) political goals of cutting public funding of higher education, such news publications are attempting to use shame as a mechanism to dele-gitimate the academy.

These examples of the popular press decontextualizing serious aca-demic research are often in the sciences or social sciences. However, the humanities are also at risk in an open-access world. Should the tabloids get their hands on various poststructuralist readings of literary texts – as one example – they would easily be able to cause a storm of ridicule and shame for the institutions and researchers that they targeted. Sometimes, though, this shaming comes from within the academy itself. The philosopher Denis Dutton's "Bad Writing Contest" famously pointed to the prose of William V. Spanos and Judith Butler as models of obscurantism.[42] It is possible, though, that such intra-academic shaming (also seen in areas of quality control, such as that in the Sokal affair/hoax) is more prevalent in a culture of closed publication, since there must be the added element of revelation or "full exposure" for the humiliation to work. Dutton's contest held general public appeal because there was no way for the general public, usually, to read academic writing and judge the levels of opacity that such prose can reach, and, further, account for the arguments a writer such as Butler might make defending opaque prose as more expressive and truthful than a populist writing style. Popular shaming of opacity through revelation and exposure does seem to be a risk of open access.

In turn, this potential for public shame may prompt behavioral changes among researchers and universities. Indeed, institutions now employ press managers and public relations consultants to attempt to manage the way in which work is displayed in popular venues. As such institutions become ever more dependent upon donations from wealthy alumni, it is certainly the case that such management is financially prudent. However, researchers have become accustomed to working within a symbolic economy that is somewhat altered by an open-access world. What I mean by this is that the system of patronage that constitutes academic remuneration (where researchers, remember, are not tied directly to the need to sell their work to live) is one that is founded on a system of prestige. Traditionally, this is accrued by researchers who can pass the toughest peer-review procedures and produce the most high-quality work, thereby affiliating themselves with the "brand" name of respected presses and journals. As with all of Pierre Bourdieu's symbolic economies, however, those who can fare well in the medium of prestige can translate that back into a salary in cold, hard cash through job appointments, promotions, and more.

General public exposure of these venues (presses and journals) changes the norms by which academics are usually evaluated. When the situation is one of talking to one's peers within known contexts, the arguments can be nonetheless intensely fierce. When such work is recontextualized to a broader public for evaluation, the standards and background contexts that are brought to bear on the work are different. This is why phenomena such as the impact agenda in the United Kingdom – implemented for the Research Excellence Framework in 2014 – have come under fire from various parties. "Impact" is here defined (loosely by the Higher Education Funding Council for England) as a desirable causal effect outside academia that can be attributed to the reach and significance of research outputs.[43] While the panels that evaluated such "impact" are composed of academics, the evidence base that must be marshalled in order to score highly in this exercise must include members of the public who will not necessarily share the academic contexts within which the original research was conducted. In some disciplines, such as translational bio-medicine, this is not so problematic. Developing drugs that can change people's lives is fairly easy to demonstrate, even if the original work was hard to do. On the other hand, the educational benefits of humanities research are often harder to slot into such a paradigm. In any case, the kickback against this was again one of academic freedom. If it is neces-sary to satisfy a broader cross section of the public in terms of impact then there are implicit restrictions placed upon the research topics that researchers may wish to prudently investigate.

The same can be said for open publication. It is not known what effects we might see from widespread access to academic research and a new set of norms forming around its evaluation. That said, there may be no harm whatsoever in insisting that the university speak beyond its own walls, in an effort to integrate an otherwise sealed academy back into society. In terms of the observational paradigms under which this might fall, I would suggest that the academy currently remains a disciplinary struc-ture sitting within a broader society of control. Open publication prac-tice denormalizes the disciplinary procedures via which research work is usually read and understood, extending evaluation throughout a societal totality. Of course, it is well known that if you want to change behavior, the easiest thing to do is to measure the aspect that you wish to alter. In a society of control and open publication, academic unease can often be expressed as a fear of shaming. For in order to know how to behave, one must know how one is to be evaluated. In a society-wide system of evalu-ation, it is far harder to predict how such norms will coalesce.

Publish Like Nobody's Reading?

In this chapter, I have examined two opposed sets of shameful practice in the academy, both centered around access. For the first part, I have set out the reasons why the current limited circulation of academic material can be considered shameful, rooted in a history of charitable education meeting a set of new technologies that reconfigure the labor practices of publication. The fact that the means exist to disseminate material glob-ally at nearly unlimited levels, but go unused, despite the patronage-like structures within the academy that permit academic ownership, triggers a type of shame that is akin to being seen to be hiding. The shame of being found to be trying to be invisible when one is nonetheless sought. On the other hand, widespread circulation of academic material recon-textualizes the norms of reception for a previously insular conversation.

In the tabloid press, for instance, this can lead to challenging personal and institutional situations that do not understand the purpose of work. On the other hand, the broad spectrum of individuals among the general population who possess academic degrees and *can* understand research work is frequently underestimated. Indeed, the potential for shaming can be undone by researchers working for a better understanding of their own fields among wider publics. For it strikes me that as the shame of hiding is intensified and visibility is sought, the risks of public shaming will only increase. Academics must, therefore, work to foster norms throughout society that are accepting of good research practices and to ensure that we can publish like nobody is watching, even when the whole world actually is.

Notes

1 @NeinQuarterly, "Tweet like Nobody's Reading. Because: They're Not", *Twitter*, 2013 https://twitter.com/neinquarterly/status/630538393219407872 [accessed 18 January 2014].
2 Peter Suber, *Open Access*, Essential Knowledge Series (Cambridge, MA: MIT Press, 2012) http://bit.ly/oa-book; Martin Paul Eve, *Open Access and the Humanities: Contexts, Controversies and the Future* (Cambridge: Cambridge University Press, 2014) http://dx.doi.org/10.1017/CBO9781316161012.
3 Philip M. Davis, "Open Access, Readership, Citations: A Randomized Controlled Trial of Scientific Journal Publishing", *FASEB Journal: Official Publication of the Federation of American Societies for Experimental Biology*, 25.7 (2011), 2129–34 http://dx.doi.org/10.1096/fj.11-183988.
4 Elspeth Probyn, "Writing Shame", in *The Affect Theory Reader*, ed. by Melissa Gregg and Gregory J. Seigworth (Durham, NC: Duke University Press, 2010), pp. 71–90.
5 Probyn, "Writing Shame", pp. 71–76.
6 Jennifer Jacquet, *Is Shame Necessary?: New Uses for an Old Tool* (London: Penguin Random House, 2016), p. 18; Ruth Benedict, *The Chrysanthemum and the Sword: Patterns of Japanese Culture*, Reprint [der Ausg.] Cleveland, Meridian Books, 1967 (Boston: Houghton Mifflin Co, 1989).
7 Probyn, "Writing Shame", p. 73.
8 Jacquet, p. 9.
9 Jacquet, pp. 11, 36.
10 I also have extreme reservations about the positive spin that Jacquet puts on shaming as a tool for transforming corporate practices since the practice seems to me to more often be used to prey upon specific, often gendered, groups in the online space.
11 Gilles Deleuze, "The Shame and the Glory: T.E. Lawrence", in *Essays Critical and Clinical*, trans. by Daniel W. Smith and Michael A. Greco (Minneapolis: University of Minnesota Press, 1997), pp. 115–25 (p. 123).
12 T.E. Lawrence, *The Seven Pillars of Wisdom: A Triumph* (Garden City, NY: Doubleday, Doran, 1935), III, p. 188.
13 Elspeth Probyn, *Blush: Faces of Shame* (Minneapolis: University of Minnesota Press, 2005).
14 Jennifer Biddle, "Shame", *Australian Feminist Studies*, 12.26 (1997), 227–39 (p. 227) doi:10.1080/08164649.1997.9994862; Probyn, *Blush*, pp. ix–x.
15 Gilles Deleuze, "Postscript on the Societies of Control", *October*, 59 (1992), 3–7 (p. 3).

16 Michel Foucault, "Politics and Ethics: An Interview", in *The Foucault Reader*, ed. by Paul Rabinow, trans. by Catherine Porter (London: Penguin, 1991), pp. 373–80 (p. 380); See also, Stuart Elden, *Foucault's Last Decade* (Malden, MA: Polity, 2016), p. 208.

17 Deleuze, "Postscript on the Societies of Control", pp. 3–4.

18 Deleuze, "Postscript on the Societies of Control", p. 7.

19 Tomkins, p. 136.

20 Tomkins, pp. 145–48.

21 Eve Kosofsky Sedgwick and Adam Frank, "Reading Silvan Tomkins", in *Shame and Its Sisters: A Silvan Tomkins Reader*, ed. by Eve Kosofsky Sedgwick and Adam Frank (Durham, NC: Duke University Press, 1995), pp. 1–28 (p. 1).

22 And the debate has raged for some time. See, for instance, Stanley Fish, "Being Interdisciplinary Is so Very Hard to Do", *Profession*, 1989, 15–22. doi:10.2307/25595433.

23 Melissa Dinsman and Alexander R. Galloway, "The Digital in the Humanities: An Interview with Alexander Galloway", *Los Angeles Review of Books* https://lareviewofbooks.org/article/the-digital-in-the-humanities-an-interview-with-alexander-galloway/ [accessed 19 April 2016].

24 Suber, p. 10.

25 It is also important to add that various government and funding agendas can also have a type of market-like soft power effect on the choice of research topic. For instance, the U.K.'s 'impact agenda' rewards institutions with funding when they can demonstrate that the research work that is undertaken has resulted in behavioral change outside of the academy. This, to some extent, then incentivizes both a choice of popular research topic and late-stage translational work. Both of these aspects leads to a type of populism that is similar to a market-based system. However, the point that I seek to make here is that there remains, at least in theory, a system of remuneration for producing research in the university that is different to other spaces.

26 For more see Stuart Lawson, Jonathan Gray and Michele Mauri, "Opening the Black Box of Scholarly Communication Funding: A Public Data Infrastructure for Financial Flows in Academic Publishing", *Open Library of Humanities*, 2.1 (2016). doi:10.16995/olh.72; Eve.

27 Juan Pablo Alperin, "The Public Impact of Latin America's Approach to Open Access", (unpublished PhD, Stanford, 2015), p. 49 https://purl.stanford.edu/jr256tk1194 [accessed 21 April 2016].

28 80 percent of respondents who claimed only to having completed a high school education also claimed they were undergraduate students, leaving 20 percent who were students but not undergraduates claiming the lowest tier: high school. Alperin, p. 50.

29 "Who Needs Access? You Need Access!", *Who Needs Access? You Need Access!* https://whoneedsaccess.org/ [accessed 21 April 2016].

30 "The Open Library of Humanities: Year One", *Open Library of Humanities*, 2016 https://about.openlibhums.org/2016/09/12/the-open-library-of-humanities-year-one/ [accessed 10 October 2016].

31 David Wojick, "Comment on Sci-Hub and the Four Horsemen of the Internet", *The Scholarly Kitchen*, 2016 https://scholarlykitchen.sspnet.org/2016/03/02/sci-hub-and-the-four-horsemen-of-the-internet/#comment-158522 [accessed 21 April 2016].

32 See, for instance OECD, *Education at a Glance 2011: OECD Indicators*, 2011, pt. Indicator A1: To What Extent have People Studied? Table A1.3a. Population with Tertiary Education (2009) www.oecd.org.

33 Of course, a range of other sociocultural factors may also influence supposed 'market' choices in this respect, such as class, upbringing, unconscious associations and more.

34 Michael Bérubé, "Value and Values", in *The Humanities, Higher Education, and Academic Freedom: Three Necessary Arguments*, ed. by Michael Bérubé and Jennifer Ruth (New York: Palgrave Macmillan, 2015), pp. 27–56 (p. 29).

35 Again, see Bérubé, p. 29.

36 I apologise for the Anglocentric bias in this survey of charity laws. I have gone with the areas with which I am most familiar. Internal Revenue Service, "Exempt Purposes – Internal Revenue Code Section 501(c)(3)", 2015 www.irs.gov/Charities-&-Non-Profits/Charitable-Organizations/Exempt-Purposes-Internal-Revenue-Code-Section-501(c)(3) [accessed 5 May 2016]; The Charity Commission, UK, 'Charitable Purposes', 2013 www.gov.uk/government/publications/charitable-purposes [accessed 5 May 2016].

37 For more on this, see Andrew McGettigan, *The Great University Gamble Money, Markets and the Future of Higher Education* (London: Pluto Press, 2013).

38 See Eve, chapter 2.

39 Robin Osborne, "Why Open Access Makes No Sense", in *Debating Open Access*, ed. by Nigel Vincent and Chris Wickham (London: British Academy, 2013), pp. 96–105 (p. 104).

40 Osborne, p. 105.

41 Luke Salkeld, "A Birdbrained Idea? Outrage as Academics Are Handed £2m to Study How Humans Interact with CHICKENS", *Mail Online*, 2013 www.dailymail.co.uk/sciencetech/article-2425213/Outrage-academics-handed-2m-study-humans-interact-CHICKENS.html [accessed 6 May 2016]; Greg Hurst, "Prove Research Is Useful or Lose Funds, Universities Are Told", *The Times (London)* (London, 16 December 2015), section Education www.thetimes.co.uk/tto/education/article4642025.ece [accessed 6 May 2016]; Javier Espinoza, "Universities Wasting Public Money on 'Pointless' Research, Says Think Tank", *The Telegraph* (London, 22 July 2015) www.telegraph.co.uk/education/educationnews/11756727/Universities-wasting-public-money-on-pointless-research-says-think-tank.html [accessed 6 May 2016].

42 Denis Dutton, "Language Crimes: A Lesson in How Not to Write, Courtesy of the Professoriate", *The Wall Street Journal* (New York, 5 February 1999).

43 Higher Education Funding Council for England, "Assessment Criteria and Level Definitions : REF 2014", 2014 www.ref.ac.uk/panels/assessmentcriteriaandleveldefinitions/ [accessed 11 May 2016].

15 Cultural Capital and the Shameful University

Thomas Docherty

In 1989, at the end of a decade of great political turbulence, Kazuo Ishiguro published his novel, *The Remains of the Day*. The novel's Prologue is dated 1956, a year of crises, including Khrushchev's "secret speech" at the Twentieth Congress of the Communist Party attacking Stalinism, the Suez Crisis, and the Hungarian Uprising. 1956 is a pivotal year, exactly halfway between the year of the novel's publication and the period in which the narrative is largely set, the 1930s, another period of huge political turbulence. What have these two periods in common, and why might the historical culture of the 1930s be available and important to a novelist at the end of the 1980s?

The 1930s saw the rise of Fascism and Nazism across Europe; the 1980s saw the ostensible fall of Communism in the face of an emergent neoliberal economic consensus, culminating in the fall of the Berlin Wall. For those with an historical eye, the later 1980s were dominated by a series of high-profile prosecutions of elderly Nazis from the 1930s, including John Demjanjuk and Klaus Barbie. These men, like Rudolph Hess who committed suicide on 17 August 1987, straddle this historical period. The specter of Nazism – and the fear that it had persisted and secretly triumphed – also haunted a major international institution: it was alleged in 1985 that Kurt Waldheim, UN Secretary General 1972–1981, might have been deeply implicated in Nazi atrocities.

The Waldheim affair provides the political unconscious that shapes *Remains*. In his "Ein letztses Wort," a "final word" written at the remains of Waldheim's days, Waldheim alluded to those allegations, acknowledging that "Ja, ich habe auch Fehler gemacht" – "Yes, I have also made mistakes."[1] It is this idea of Nazism as a "mistake" that forges the specific cultural link here. In *Remains*, the central character, Stevens, served Lord Darlington of Darlington Hall as butler in the 1930s. Darlington had been a Nazi sympathizer who, at one point, requires the dismissal – by a compliant Stevens – of any Jewish staff. Even when the extent of his Nazism has become clear, Stevens exculpates him, reducing Darlington's Nazi allegiance to "mistakes." "Lord Darlington," he says, "wasn't a bad man. He wasn't a bad man at all. And at least he had the privilege of being able to say at the end of his life that he had made his own mistakes."[2]

"Mistakes" constitute the core of the narrative. Stevens is on his 1956 tour, revisiting Miss Kenton, because he needs a rest, as he had been "responsible for a series of small errors in carrying out my duties."[3] These errors cause him embarrassment, or shame; and it is the link between such shame and the political "error" of Nazism – or political "errors" of totalitarian and authoritarian governance as a whole, errors that, like those of Stalinism, are grounded in the cult of personalities – that will ground my argument here.

Towards the end of *Remains*, Stevens and Dr. Carlisle, the doctor in the village of Moscombe, discuss politics, especially the politics of Harry Smith, the local working-class man who is extremely concerned to engage "ordinary" people with the political process. This sequence, like the entire narrative, is driven by social class. Smith has stressed the "dignity" of the ordinary working individual, identifying dignity with democracy itself: "Dignity's not just something for gentlemen."[4] Stevens regards this view, emanating as it does from the working-class Smith, as not worthy of "serious consideration."[5] Suddenly, Carlisle asks Stevens very directly, "What do *you* think dignity's all about?" Dignity obsesses Stevens, as it does Smith; but Stevens equates dignity with value or worthiness generally, and he identifies such value with class and social standing. Surprised by the directness of the question, he replies, with equally uncharacteristic directness, that "I suspect it comes down to not removing one's clothes in public."[6]

This particular basic statement relates value or capital in the form of "dignity" to broader questions of the relations between the private and the public. Further, it relates these issues to corporeal matters of the materiality of the body, of flesh, even of sex. It hints at the frailty of the physical body. It reveals that, for Stevens, the opposite of dignity – and what therefore gives it its full meaning – is shame; and such shame relates to the fact that, as physical human beings, we are subject to the frailty whose realization is death itself. Shame becomes characterized in terms of a relation between *la vita nuda*, Agamben's "bare life," and its public manifestation in politics: it is, as it were, conditioned by a logic of privatization as such.[7]

I will here explore shame as a condition – even as a determining precondition – of value as such, even to capital; and will find how it relates to moral capital and to cultural capital. Intrinsic to this is an argument about our contemporary institutions of value, and above all the institution that prides itself on the advancing of cultural capital, the "public" university, an institution menaced by the logic of privatization.

I will structure the argument through some exemplary texts. Ishiguro's *Remains* examines moral capital; *The Noise of Time* by Julian Barnes extends the argument into the conditions of institutional capital where criticism itself is colored by the shame of cowardice; and J.M. Coetzee's *Disgrace* explores the relations of cultural capital (and the university as

its privileged site) to a new feudalism, where real estate and the ownership of private land become the determinants of all forms of value.

Two texts are earlier precursors. Tolstoy, in "Shame" (1896), inserts
ethics into politics, thus individualizing a political situation, thereby
raising issues of individual and liberal value (humaneness) against systemic constructions of value (or bureaucracy); and, closer to our own
predicaments, Kafka's *Zur Frage der Gesetze* puts the issue of shame at
the heart of politics itself.

Tolstoy: A Politics of Shame

"Shame" is a short narrative and an allegorical tract. Its subject is what
Tolstoy saw as a "legalized crime," the constitutional standing of corporal punishment, specifically punishment by flogging or the imposition of
political law directly onto the *vita nuda*. For Tolstoy, this issue is clearly
marked by politics, class, and education. In 1890s Russia, even in the
military, corporal punishment has been seen as regressive, repugnant,
and barbaric and has therefore long been abandoned. In civic life, it
persists as something that is visited upon individuals from the peasant
classes. However, it is not applied to all the peasants, "but only those
who have not finished a course in a popular school." Flogging becomes
emblematic of a crime that is, in effect, structured around class, admin-
istered by the upper classes to the less-educated members of the peasant
or working classes. Education and class combine to determine the legalization of this barbaric crime. The logical structure here implies that
education is itself an insurance against domination by class.

This – education as protection against an intrinsic class domination
based on prejudice and unauthorized, illegitimate ideas of innate superiority of one class of people over others – is nowadays a cliché. It relates
to the idea that knowledge is power, that education offers social mobility
(upwards) between classes, and that while an education may not yield
money, it nonetheless offers the rewards of "soft power" in cultural or
intellectual capital. The rarely noted downside of this is that to be less
well educated – and, even worse, to be under-educated working or peasant class (like Ishiguro's Harry Smith) – is itself somehow intrinsically
shameful. The tacit ideology supporting "social mobility" is that it is a
shaming moral failing for a working-class person not to want to escape
her or his class position and condition. The class prejudice thus revealed
at the core of "cultural capital" is something that is morally or ethically
dubious (even repellent), based as it is on unwarranted claims to innate
class superiority – disparagement of the working class – as a structural
principle for the organization of society.[8]

The very existence of corporal punishment is, for Tolstoy, intrinsically
shaming. Consequently, he argues, "such things must be arraigned, because these things, when the aspect of legality is given to them, only

disgrace all of us who live in the state where such acts are committed."[9] "Shame" is one such shaming arraignment of the practice: a shaming story intended to deploy shame itself as a means of changing conduct.

This structures the text's internal logic: shame can be a positive factor in changing shameful activities. The narrative concerns a thieving, frequently drunk soldier, caught repeatedly in various disreputable or nefarious acts. He expects the habitual physical punishment; but his commanding officer simply admonishes him and asks him to change his ways. The effect is powerful: "the soldier was so surprised at this new way of being treated that he changed completely and became a model soldier."

There is an economic structure here; and the commanding officer's action calls a prior economy into question and institutes a new one. Crime is no longer "matched" or economically "paid for" by punishment, but is instead met by grace or graciousness. Grace rejects an intrinsically shaming economy based on the exercising of corporal punishment for perceived wrongdoing. Tolstoy mocks the idea that there can be a "calm discussion" of economics, of "how many rods" are germane and applicable to a specific instance, as if wrongdoing has a rationalized tariff. Any such tariff must be essentially arbitrary; and it therefore lacks the very rationality that it claims as the ground for its legality, making flogging irrational, illegal, and therefore shameful.

The logic here should be followed through: if corporal punishment brings shame upon us, we might equally say, inversely, that shame as such is the condition of our being ruled by the arbitrariness of a law that is based upon the crude power of class (especially if that is legitimized by our ideologies of education-as-social-mobility) instead of reason. Only if we become ashamed at this shame will we do what is required to avoid the legalization of the crime involved in class-based corporal punishment.

Tolstoy establishes a profound link between the claims of an ostensibly positive cultural capital on one hand, and the shameful prejudices of arbitrary class-based social order on the other. He is clear on the fundamental illegitimacy and moral worthlessness of the resulting arbitrary law. "If we have to speak at all of this monstrousness," he writes,

> we can only say that there can be no such law, signatures, or command of the czar that can make a law of a crime, and that, on the contrary, the vesting of such a crime with the form of law proves better than anything else that, where such an imaginary legalization of a crime is possible, no laws exist, but only savage arbitrariness of rude power.

This "rude power" is essentially unearned authority: an authority that may be legal constitutionally but which lacks any proper legitimacy within modern democratic arrangements because it has been imposed autocratically or in a quasi-feudal manner. It is power without authority: tyranny. The point is that some forms of "soft power" in cultural capital will reveal themselves, in fact, to be themselves a form of "rude power."

The only way beyond such barbarity, argues Tolstoy, comes not when any individual peasant escapes flogging "but only when the ruling classes will recognize their sin and meekly confess to it." Change can only happen when the ruling classes, like the converted soldier in the text, see themselves publicly shamed. The text becomes itself an articulation of the position of the commanding officer, an admonishment of the ruling class; and, like that officer, it acknowledges that change requires patience.[10]

Kafka revisits the motif, in *Zur Frage der Gesetze*, or "On the Question of our Laws," published in 1931 (though probably written as early as 1920, in the immediate aftermath of the Russian Revolution). Kafka writes: "Our laws are unfortunately not widely known, they are the closely guarded secret of the small group of nobles who govern us."[11] From the beginning, according to this account, law divides society, but also establishes class bonds – in this case, the nobility bound together in complicit possession, literal possession, of the laws, laws that are essentially made for the personal interests of the nobility. Further, being in possession of the law, the nobility themselves stand "outside the law, and that is why the laws seem to have been given exclusively into their hands."

Some dispute the actual existence of these laws, writes Kafka; and those of this disposition "try to show us that, if any law exists, it can only be this: the Law is whatever the nobles do." The only way around the paradoxes here would be a revolutionary act through which to effect the overthrow of the nobility – like the Russian Revolution that just preceded this text. Yet, even though that would be popular, "no one dares to reject the nobility." Kafka concludes his short piece with the observation that "the only visible unquestionable law that has been imposed on us is the nobility, and who are we to rob ourselves of the only law we have?"[12]

This, too, is a shameful condition. Kafka's text laments this cravenness before the nobility, and hankers for a time when the people will own the laws and the nobility will vanish. This isn't because of hatred of the nobility. Instead, "We are more inclined to hate ourselves, because we have not yet shown ourselves worthy of being entrusted with the laws."

Between Tolstoy and Kafka lies the fundamental question at issue here: how do shame, worthiness, and dignity regulate themselves as values? More succinctly, how do we construct value itself – cultural value or cultural capital – from the interplay of shame and dignity? Ishiguro explores precisely this terrain.

Ishiguro and the Failure of Moral Capital

The Remains of the Day offers a means of establishing value through its explicit opposition between shame and dignity. The key shaming episode relates to Miss Kenton, the housekeeper at Darlington Hall, working alongside Stevens; and the shame in question is not just moral but also political. Lord Darlington's Nazi sympathies lead him to dismiss two Jewish maids, Ruth and Sarah, under the influence of a shadowy Mrs. Carolyn Burnet. Miss Kenton is horrified, and threatens to resign if Stevens goes ahead and fires the two young women. She sees the immorality, and is also aware of its politics, in a way that Stevens – deliberately and willfully blind at this point to what he will later call the "errors" of his lord – does not. However, after the two are fired, she stays on after all, despite her earnest threats. The threat to resign is founded in ideas of dignity and integrity: Miss Kenton does not subscribe to the view that the Jewishness of the maids indicates a lesser worth, as workers or as human beings. Yet she is unable to sustain her dignified position, and to maintain her integrity.

At the close of the novel Miss Kenton explains that this was because of her own moral cowardice: "Had I been anyone worthy of any respect at all, I dare say I would have left Darlington Hall long ago." So why didn't she? "It was cowardice, Mr. Stevens. Simple cowardice... There," she concludes, "that's all my high principles amount to. I feel so ashamed of myself."[13]

The resignation threat is recognizably consistent with a fundamental principle of all criticism, perhaps especially of criticism that has serious material high stakes risks at its core. The dignity of her stance resides in her will to be in solidarity with those who are wronged, especially those wronged through the exercise of arbitrary and unjustified power by the nobility. Criticism, especially in our contemporary institutionalized formulation of it, often depends precisely upon the willingness to take similar risks, especially risks that jeopardize the survival or livelihood of the speaker or critic herself. In this respect, "free" speech can be a costly business.[14]

In establishing solidarity with the underdog, the critic puts herself willingly in that precarious position, speaking back to the arbitrariness of barbaric "rude power" the better to expose its lack of legitimacy. The moral standing of such a speaker rises: she or he has foregone advancement or financial reward, say, for an increase in *moral capital*. In criticism, moral value can be accompanied by the logic of self-sacrifice. Conventional economics would monetize this, based perhaps on a calculation of loss of earnings. Yet the point is that this critical stance fundamentally rejects conventional monetized economics: its governing principles are not determined by financial considerations.

Miss Kenton, however, fails to sustain her dignified position: she is aware of the price that her stance might cost; and, afraid that she will be unemployed if she leaves, with no means of survival, she avoids risk, fails to bear witness critically to Darlington's anti-Semitic Nazi politics. Her avowed "cowardice" is conditioned by the economic demand for self-preservation.[15] When the maids are sacked, there is no recourse to law to mitigate the "error" of Darlington. As Stevens acknowledges, it was simply a matter of carrying out their lordship's wishes in a professional manner, for it was "a task...that demanded to be carried out with dignity."[16] As it remains legally permissible for Darlington to sack the maids because they are Jewish, Miss Kenton's only recourse is to morality: "if you dismiss my girls tomorrow, it will be wrong, a sin as any sin ever was one."[17]

This is as close as anyone comes to acknowledging how seriously wrong is Darlington's anti-Semitism. When, one year later, Darlington whimsically changes his tune, he too acknowledges that "It was wrong what happened and one would like to recompense them [Ruth and Sarah] somehow."[18] Darlington seems also to accept the view that a wrong can be "recompensed," in terms of the economic logic of the "tariff" that Tolstoy had exposed as intrinsically irrational and shameful. Money is still key here, for all parties. Miss Kenton loses moral stature because she can't resign, needing the financial security of her job; Darlington thinks that handing over money can right or erase a moral wrong. For the latter, financial capital can eradicate moral shame: you can buy your way into "justice" like buying indulgences in medieval, feudal societies.

Darlington distances himself from responsibility for the action: "it was wrong what happened," as if "what happened" did not derive from him. This is precisely the same position as that of Stevens himself, who acts as he does because he regards it as "dignified" professionally simply to carry out unquestioningly the will of the lord. In the prevailing feudal structure here, responsibility for actions is evaded by being effectively "outsourced." Mrs. Burnet outsources her anti-Semitism to Darlington, who outsources the responsibility for leaving Ruth and Sarah potentially destitute to Stevens. Behind all this lies the arbitrary "rude power" of feudal pre-capitalist servility.

Theoretically, then, "dignity" depends upon a distancing of the self from the material realities of ethical action. Dignity is a matter of establishing and maintaining a "private self," withdrawn from the struggles of the world, above the bodily materiality of class struggle or even just rational argument. This is the meaning of restraint and propriety for Stevens. It is important that one does not remove one's clothes in public: it is important that there be a distance between the self and the world. Dignity needs the mediation of a distancing protocol, even if that means the refusal to risk changing one's status by entering into a reasoned debate.[19] "Propriety" becomes intimate with its near cognate, "property"; and, in this bizarre logic, dignity is the privatization of such property.

The point of class distinctions is to allow those who claim to be inherently superior to distance themselves from their social and ethical responsibilities to other people. The fundamental issue here is the "shame of privilege." Fredric Jameson wrote about something similar in 1997.

In "Culture and Finance Capital," he argued that, in contemporary politics, "we sense that the problems of ideological analysis are enormously simplified, and the ideologies themselves far more transparent." Privilege is becoming shamelessly brazen in parading itself, and in establishing greater distances between the privileged class or 1 percent (Kafka's contemporary "nobility") and the rest. Jameson goes on:

> Now that, following master thinkers like Hayek, it has become customary to identify political freedom with market freedom, the motivations behind ideology no longer seem to need an elaborate machinery of decoding and hermeneutic reinterpretation; and the guiding thread of all contemporary politics seems much easier to grasp, that the rich want their taxes lowered.[20]

In the face of this, criticism that relies on moral capital will always fail, because in material terms, finance capital trumps moral capital. But what about a more particular form of cultural capital: musical aesthetics? This is the subject of Julian Barnes' 2016 novella, *The Noise of Time*.

Barnes: The Critic as Coward

In *The Noise of Time*, Barnes depicts Shostakovich, accurately enough, as a composer whose life was often in jeopardy because of his music. What endangered him is the relation between his musical cultural capital and political power, a power that governed society through the primacy of fear. For Shostakovich here, "Fear normally drives out all other emotions as well; but not shame. Fear and shame swilled happily together in his stomach."[21]

As with Ishiguro's Miss Kenton, shame marks a specific value, allowing us to consider the relation of criticism to cowardice. First, though, it yields a direct link back to Tolstoy. Barnes describes Shostakovich punishing his child, Maxim, for some naughtiness; and we find that "the boy's shame was often such that it felt as if the punishment were being visited back upon the father."[22] Corporal punishment, here conditional upon nothing more "rational" than the supposed superiority of age and experience is, as in Tolstoy, a recipe for shame, the shame that we should feel at the very existence of irrational and unjustified privilege which, in the final instance, rests on the threat of violence.

The Noise of Time is structured around Shostakovich's "conversations with power." These conversations are shadowed by the threat of a violence that might be perpetrated upon Shostakovich at any time. In this instance, power is not class-based but is *institutional*. Stalin has established legal and cultural institutions that operate as vehicles for the maintenance of his own power. Those who make the institutions operable are his apparatchiks, bureaucrats who function as the instruments of power. It is the simple knowledge of how this system works – a con-science, as it were – that, as in *Hamlet*, makes cowards of everyone, both inside and outside the vectors of the institutions themselves.[23]

This yields the dark inversion of moral capital. Barnes exposes how rude power hijacks the soft power of moral capital – the very core component of what makes cultural criticism valuable in the first place – and converts it to a principle of fear. The bureaucratic institution makes cowards of all of the citizens who have to live through it. A criticism that wants to produce action and material change becomes almost impossible, and certainly stymied. As in the Stalinist state, criticism is mute under compliant conformity.[24]

Shostakovich imagined that he would resist the demands of rude power, figuring himself an ethical critic, able to retain legitimate authority in the face of unearned brutal power. He is mistaken. At a crucial moment, he is given the Russian text of a speech that he must make in America. As he starts to read it out, he realizes that it is an attack on his most favored composer, Stravinsky. By this stage, he has realized that it would be a folly, threatening his own life, if he were to denounce the speech. In despair, he simply stops reading; but his translator continues to deliver the speech, despite Shostakovich's silence. His shame is enormous at this point, worsened when he does denounce Stravinsky in the questions-and-answer session, in direct response to a provocation from Nicolas Nabokov.

The denunciation is inevitable yet shaming. Shostakovich ponders the difference between himself and a composer like Prokofiev. Prokofiev thought it possible to make an accommodation with power – to compromise diplomatically, as it were. That, however, is precisely the problem: in believing this, Prokofiev "completely failed to see the tragic dimension of what was happening."[25] Far from ethical criticism reaching an accommodation with rude power, the opposite is occurring: even oppositional criticism becomes encompassed by power, such that it is completely neutered, rendered complicit with barbarity.

Thus, Shostakovich sees the limits of a criticism based in the cultural capital contained in his music: it is neutered in the face of another form of capital. In this instance – and this is the next stage after Ishiguro's Miss Kenton – it is not financial capital that it loses out to, but *institutional capital*. "Those words of his," – words of defiance – he realizes, "had been at best a foolish boast, at worst a mere figure of speech. And Power had no interest in figures of speech." There are, in fact, only two types of composers in the face of the forms of Power that are grounded in institutional capital such as that of Stalin's bureaucracy: "those who were alive and frightened; and those who were dead."[26]

Shostakovich puts this explicitly in terms of different types of capital. He survives; and he had been good at managing to survive and yet to keep faith with his art. He had been good at doing what was needed, rendering to Caesar that which was Caesar's, but

> Yes, he had been naïve about Caesar. Or rather, he had been work-ing from an outdated model. In the old days, Caesar had demanded tribute money, a sum to acknowledge his power, a certain percent-age of your calculated worth. But things had moved on, and the new Caesars of the Kremlin had upgraded the system: nowadays your tribute money was calculated at the full 100% of your worth. Or, if possible, more.[27]

This is the coercion that makes a virtue of complicity with institutional rude power, our contemporary version of the "nobility." It is based upon fear; and it is yet more "efficient" in preserving privilege because, in such systems, the apparatchik will always over-comply, doing more than is re-quired by tyrannical power (more than the "full 100% of your worth").

Yet the institutional apparatchik has also internalized fear; and she or he deals with that fear by becoming themselves someone to be feared. They can shame those who would criticize the institution by informing on them; and while the effect of such shame may not be life-threatening, it can certainly be livelihood-threatening. The apparatchik knows that capital is gained by encouraging fear, by a general economics of "growth," an increase in the "circulation" not of money but of fear, and its corollary shame, swilling together in the stomach. In the face of this, the critic's only possible mode of self-preservation is through the acceptance of cowardice as a mode of survival. That cowardice entails, in turn, the production of more fear. Yet, as Shostakovich has said, at least those who are fearful are still alive, still in employment. When Khrushchev succeeds Stalin, things seem less threatening: disagreement becomes possible. But Shostakovich senses the real difference: "Before, they had tested the extent of his courage; now, they tested the extent of his cowardice...".[28]

Institutional capital achieves its goal by co-opting the idea of criticism as morally uplifting. *Pravda* articulates Stalin's hint, giving the ethical judgment that *Lady Macbeth of Mtensk* is "muddle instead of music." It fails to edify the public, fails to offer the kind of uplift that good art should give. In making this judgment – the judgment that blights Shostakovich's career and life – Stalin's institutional power has quite simply fully co-opted the idea of the critic as heroic individual standing up for the ordinary underdog. It is a political tactic common to many totalitarian social structures and to many authoritarian institutional structures.

Can there be a way out of this predicament? Perhaps we can turn to the very central institution of cultural capital, the university, to find out.

Coetzee: Knowledge and Capitalized Land

"Shame makes human beings of us," says the character of Wunderlich to Coetzee's alter-ago, Elizabeth Costello, in *The Lives of Animals*[29]. It is in Coetzee that we see shame operating most forcefully as a driver of economic relations. Interestingly, the relation between shame and economics, between morality and capital, focuses on land ownership. It takes us back not just to financial capital (money) outweighing cultural capital (the institutions of knowledge, criticism) and moral capital (ethics); worse than this, it takes us back to an essentially feudal structure in which capital and values are tied intimately and incontrovertibly to the ownership of land.

Most criticism of Coetzee's much-lauded and controversial 1999 novel, *Disgrace*, focuses on issues of personal shame. Almost without exception, the focus is on the shame that accrues around the issues of rape (especially inter-racial rape) and sexual harassment (in the context of the university institution).

Derek Attridge, for example, writes about the vexing shame in which David Lurie, the academic, abuses his position to take sexual advantage of a student, Melanie Isaacs. This shame derives from a man being caught with pants down: it is the opposite of Stevens' dignity. It is a "public shame," writes Attridge, that "can only be canceled by... public esteem, disgrace redeemed by honor." Coetzee, therefore, is not offering "a practical commitment to improving the world, but a profound need to preserve the ethical integrity of the self,"[30] Attridge concludes.

Myrtle Hooper takes Attridge to task for failing to address "the rights and responsibilities that we would expect to be met in the real world" as against Attridge's claim of the "higher ethical stance" associated with his ethical prioritization of the self or of selfhood. Nonetheless, Hooper also sees Coetzee as valorizing privacy, over against an embarrassment that involves the making public of the private: "David elects disgrace, in dramatic, histrionic, hysterical ways. But he eschews embarrassment – and Coetzee does not enable it – even disables it – on his behalf."[31]

Katherine Hallemeier notes that these readings, among others, "suggest that, in Coetzee's work, the shame of privilege is concomitant to the shame of writing and that, in either case, shame holds the ethical promise of extending an equality that yet respects an absolute alterity."[32] This focuses attention on the act of writing itself; and we can extend this to questions of the institutionalized value of writing.

All of these critics, however, share one ideological predilection. They all take shame really as a matter of character: they are incipiently moral-psychoanalytic. Yet what if we take shame – the shame of privilege and especially the privilege of the writing that constitutes Lurie's employment (and Coetzee's profession) – in terms of capital, or as an issue of value as such, put into an economy with grace or with dignity or honor? This changes our understanding of shame, and it shifts the "disgrace" issue on to a general idea of value associated with "property" and ownership.

The central question concerns the ownership of land. The story of Lurie taking advantage of Melanie is paralleled with the story of the burglary attack on Lurie and his daughter Lucy, who is also gang-raped. Lurie is troubled by the fact that Lucy will not go public with the story of her rape; and he sees this as the basic demonstration of the rude power of the rapists. The attackers will read the reports of their actions in the newspapers, but they will see that the rape is not referred to there, because, for Lucy, what happened to her "is a private matter." "It will dawn on them that over the body of the woman silence is being drawn like a blanket. *Too ashamed*, they will say to each other, *too ashamed to tell*, and they will chuckle luxuriously."[33]

Lurie contemplates why the crime happened at all, and thinks it

> A risk to own anything... Not enough to go around, not enough cars, shoes, cigarettes... What there is must go into circulation, so that everyone can have a chance to be happy for a day. That is the theory....Not human evil, just a vast circulatory system, to whose workings pity and terror are irrelevant.[34]

The circulation of finance has no relation to cultural form such as tragedy, and simply ignores it: money and property are absolute. But, above all, what Lucy owns – and what is desired by others, especially Petrus, her worker who will eventually acquire it – is land. As she puts it, "They see me as owing something. They see themselves as debt collectors, tax collectors. Why should I be allowed to live here without paying?"[35]

With Lucy pregnant from the rape, running her smallholding becomes almost impossible, physically and spiritually. Petrus assumes increasing importance in running things; and, eventually, she becomes willing to sign the land over and become a tenant on what is now Petrus's land. She and Lurie both agree that this reversal of fortunes is "humiliating," but, for Lucy, "perhaps that is a good point to start from again... With nothing. Not with nothing but. With nothing. No cards, no weapons, no property, no rights, no dignity... Like a dog."[36]

That phrase, "like a dog," does two things. First, it refers us back to Kafka, whose novel *The Trial* ends with precisely this phrase. *The Trial* is an extended version of *Zur Frage des Gesetze*. Secondly, the phrase refers us to Coetzee's own interest in animal rights. Within *Disgrace*, the dignity of animals is considered insistently. When Lurie first arrives at Lucy's farm, he and Lucy take her dogs for a walk. One of the dogs defecates: "The bitch continues to strain, hanging her tongue out, glancing around shiftily as if ashamed to be watched."[37] But the shame of the dog will, in the course of the novel, be transferred to the shame of the owners.

Just as in Tolstoy, where floggings reflect badly on those in the position of master, so also, here – but with a major political component and inflection. Here, when Petrus takes over the land, we are invited to consider the situation as one in which the revolutions of Tolstoy and of Kafka take place: a revolutionary but feudal reversal of roles between lord/landowner and servant/serf. Coetzee's focus on the dog – recalling the cynic Diogenes – will yield a substantial argumentative advance.

While living with Lucy, Lurie starts to work occasionally at the "Animal Welfare House" run by Bev Shaw, her friend. Bev takes care of abandoned dogs. In many cases, they must be slaughtered. On Lucy's farm, Petrus took care of her dogs, and he was called a "dog-man," inviting the direct allusion to Diogenes, the cynic. Diogenes, apocryphally, knew no shame; and, by knowing no shame himself, he was able to shame his society. This is how cynical reason works: it is shame converted to cultural and political capital. Not much is known of the historical figure of Diogenes himself; but he was probably involved in economic business, somewhat like banking, as was his father, and he rejected money for the search after knowledge and wisdom, ostensibly therefore prioritizing cultural capital over financial capital.

After Petrus takes possession of Lucy's land, Lurie starts visiting Bev Shaw regularly; and he, now, becomes referred to as the dog-man. His task in the Animal Welfare House is chastening. The dogs are victims of their own productivity and copulation: they are "too menny." Bev runs the Animal House in terms that explicitly invite comparison with the Nazi death-camps; and Lurie's task is to be with the dogs when they are killed and then to dispose of the corpses. By this point, shame is fully associated with the simple fact of death itself, as if the necessity of dying – for humans as for animals – is a reminder of the shamefully simple physicality of life. As with Stevens in Ishiguro, or men who "shat in their pants" in Barnes, embodiment itself becomes a condition of shame.

In debasing pretension, death makes shame the human condition: death cannot be outsourced, and is the ultimate bond between the self and the materiality of history. The upper classes find it an impropriety. Stevens, in *Remains*, ignores his own dying father while serving his lord. Lurie in *Disgrace* senses that the dogs instinctively turn against him as they go to be killed:

> If, more often than not, the dog fails to be charmed, it is because of his presence: he gives off the wrong smell... the smell of shame... They flatten their ears, they droop their tails, as if they too feel the disgrace of dying.[38]

Finally, this – the cynicism of the death camp – is the condition of our shame. It makes us realize that there is a profound limitation in anything that tries to redeem capital by relocating it to culture and knowledge, both of which serve to fracture the solidarity of class by promising social mobility. We must remember Lurie's profession: he is an academic, and one who has become somewhat cynical about the condition of the camp – the campus – or institution of knowledge, the University. This is tantamount to saying that he has come to realize the false pretense – the pretensions – of human knowing: there is no form of cultural capital that can outweigh the shame of our dying. Death, as Baudrillard once told us, is the end of any form of exchange, especially that of capital.[39]

That is so in a capitalist society; but it is not so in a feudal one.

This is our predicament: in a state of affairs where value is inscribed in culture, we drive a wedge between conscience and history, between theory and the world. We hanker after the belief that while financial capital is transitory, knowledge can transcend its moment or occasion of production, giving us a soft power that outweighs the realities of money. Yet what contemporary society also knows is that money itself is increasingly "soft" too. It has lost its link to labor, for example; and has even lost its link to value as such.[40] Now, capital turns to what it once knew as the sure foundation and cornerstone of superiority and power: the ownership of land, the reality of "real" estate. We are witnessing a return to feudalism. It is the extreme form of privatization.

Lurie tells his daughter: "These are puritanical times. Private life is public business. Prurience is respectable, prurience and sentiment. They wanted a spectacle: breast-beating, remorse, tears if possible. A TV show, in fact. I wouldn't oblige."[41] This – the "puritanism" that makes private life public – is simply one side of a coin that is minted in privatization. In making a fetish of the private, it also valorizes "culture" as the marketization of shame.

The University and the Politics of Shame

Amartya Sen frequently rehearses J.S. Mill's definition of democracy as "governance by discussion." The idea – as in Habermas – is that rational societies seek, through non-coercive discussion, the better argument. We thereby propose and jointly agree on the best solution to predicaments or issues. This ideal is moot, for, in all real-life argument, there is an attempt at persuasion by all parties, and such persuasion can itself be characterized as the desire to make the other party agree. In short, all argument involves the attempt to prove one position to be superior to another.

It is here that democracy itself can become contaminated and destabilized by shame. The texts I have discussed here, in which shame is the instrument by which we can change shameful activity, are all politically motivated by a desire for greater democracy and by a challenge to unearned and class-based authority. They appeal to the "better argument"; and, in the end, the better argument is always characterized by an argument based in sound rational thinking. The place where we usually encourage such thought is, in its highest formulation, the University institution. We come now to a concluding observation about the now shameful University.

The point of any argument is to prove that "my" case is better than "yours"; and, ideally, this is a substantial positive force in bringing a society together. However, it is now actually conditioned by shame, and becomes a negative force. How? Reason becomes conditioned by shame when the winner of an argument shames the loser by demonstrating a superior intellectual grasp of issues in a specific debate. But under what conditions might I feel such shame at losing? Shame and humiliation occur if and only if I feel myself to be *personally* implicated, *privately* beaten in argument, such that it is not the argument that is lost, but "I" that am lost. Shame occurs when the private individual and not her or his argument is interpellated.

Shame, we can therefore say, occurs as a condition of the identification of the individual with an argumentative case: in short, shame is a condition of a reason that has been essentially "privatized." In this, reason itself becomes characterized as elitist, demeaning the loser personally and privately through argument.[42] "The personal is political" is a slogan that is complicit with this privatization of the political as such.

The contemporary University is an institution that is increasingly driven precisely by that privatization of reason, and of all economic, social, moral and political interests. It is also, as a result, a quasi-feudal institution. Its lordly VC/President undemocratically identifies himself as "the" University, like a medieval earl of Warwick, York, Sussex and so on. He demands fealty, crushing academic freedom in the desire for brand conformity. Criticism brings him into disrepute, and he will therefore jeopardize the livelihood of those who voice it. He demands feu duty in the form of grant capture; and, when he gets it, he claims a salary increase based on the productivity of staff and performance of students. Above all, he presides over an institution that is shaped by the privatization of all interests, and not just the commodification of knowledge. The contemporary institution depends, thus, on an economic structure akin to corporal punishment in Tolstoy. We need, as Kafka knew, a revolution to overthrow this new nobility; we need to change the shameful University.

Notes

1 See http://derstandard.at/2920415/Im-Wortlaut-Das-Waldheim-Vermaechtnis, [accessed 20 March 2017].
2 Kazuo Ishiguro, *The Remains of the Day* (London: Faber & Faber, 1989; repr. 1990), 243.
3 Ishiguro, *Remains*, 5.
4 Ishiguro, *Remains*, 185–186.

5 Ishiguro, *Remains*, 194.
6 Ishiguro, *Remains*, 210.
7 See Giorgio Agamben, *Homo Sacer* (Torino: Einaudi, 1995), *passim*. In his characterization of "la vita nuda," Agamben owes much to Hannah Arendt's work, but see, especially, her *The Human Condition* (Chicago, IL: University of Chicago Press, 1998).
8 For the contemporary exploration of this, see Owen Jones, *Chavs* (London: Verso, 2011); and see also, Lynsey Hanley, *Estates* (London: Granta, 2007), and *Respectable* (London: Penguin, 2016). See also Robert Hewison, *Cultural Capital* (London: Verso, 2014), on the perversions of cultural capital into cultural capitalism.
9 Leo Tolstoy, "Shame!," www.nonresistance.org/docs_htm/Tolstoy/Shame. html for the full text of "Shame" in English. All subsequent quotations are from this web version, [accessed 20 March 2017].
10 It is worth noting dates. Tolstoy writes in the early years of the reign of Tsar Nicholas II, who retained the idea of autocratic rule. Just two years after the publication of "Shame" (and, despite Lenin's 1895 exile, and in the face of decrees banning the formation of political parties), the Russian Social Democratic Workers' Party was formed, endorsing fundamentally Marxist principles. "Shame" sits at the center of a period when the class system itself is coming under extreme pressure from within the class system itself; and "Shame" plays its part in shaming and thus undermining the claims to authority of a ruling class.
11 Franz Kafka, "On the Question of our Laws," trans. Michael Hofmann, *London Review of Books*, 37: 14, July 16, 2015, 23. All subsequent references are from this source.
12 We have a word for our own contemporary "nobility": the 1%.
13 Ishiguro, *Remains*, 152–153.
14 It is interesting to consider "free" speech in such economic terms, for it brings into question a play of "values" other than freedom-as-such. See, for interesting discussions, Anthony Lester, *Five Ideas Worth Fighting For* (Place: Oneworld, 2016), ch. 3, and Timothy Garton Ash, *Free Speech* (London: Alantic Books, 2016).
15 This is also the position of individuals such as Kurt Waldheim. Hannah Arendt pointed out that some Nazis exculpate themselves by suggesting that, in doing as they did, they "saved" others from having to do terrible deeds.
16 Ishiguro, *Remains*, 148.
17 Ishiguro, *Remains*, 149.
18 Ishiguro, *Remains*, 151.
19 This is the logic of the "Aristocracy of Culture," in Pierre Bourdieu, *Distinction*, trans. Richard Nice (London: Routledge, 1972), 3–9.
20 Fredric Jameson, "Culture and Finance Capital," *Critical Inquiry*, 24:1 (1997), 247.
21 Julian Barnes, *The Noise of Time* (London: Jonathan Cape, 2016), 61.
22 Barnes, *Noise*, 73.
23 The reference here is to Hamlet's most famous soliloquy, in which Shakespeare pits a critical conscience against action; and the consequence is the critic as cowardly procrastinator of action. It is a lesson we are still learning.
24 Many academics will recognize the contemporary university behind this: an institution that demands social conformity and political compliance.
25 Barnes, *Noise*, 104.
26 Barnes, *Noise*, 48
27 Barnes, *Noise*, 55.

28 Barnes, *Noise*, 131.
29 J.M. Coetzee, *Lives of Animals* (Princeton, NJ: Princeton University Press, 1999), 40.
30 Derek Attridge, *J.M. Coetzee and the Ethics of Reading* (Chicago, IL: University of Chicago Press, 2004), 178, 187.
31 Myrtle Hooper, "'Scenes from a Dry Imagination': *Disgrace* and Embarrassment," in *J.M. Coetzee's Austerities*, eds. Graham Bradshaw and Michael Neill (Farnham: Ashgate, 2010), 143.
32 Katherine Hallemeier, *J.M. Coetzee and the Limits of Cosmopolitanism* (Basingstoke: Palgrave Macmillan, 2013), 113.
33 J.M. Coetzee, *Disgrace* (London: Vintage, 2000), 112, 110.
34 Coetzee, *Disgrace*, 98.
35 Coetzee, *Disgrace*, 158.
36 Coetzee, *Disgrace*, 205.
37 Coetzee, *Disgrace*, 68.
38 Coetzee, *Disgrace*, 142–143.
39 See Jean Baudrillard, *L'échange symbolique et la mort* (Paris: Gallimard, Paris, 1976).
40 See André Gorz, *L'Immatériel* (Paris: Galilée, Paris, 2003) for a good discussion of this.
41 Coetzee, *Disgrace*, 66.
42 In relation to this, witness UK Justice Secretary and former Education Secretary, Michael Gove, explicitly decrying education during the 2016 Brexit debates: "the people of this country have had enough of experts." See www.ft.com/cms/s/0/3be49734-29cb-11e6-83e4-abc22d5d108c.html#ax-zz4Cry2n3QQ, [accessed 20 March 2017].

Index